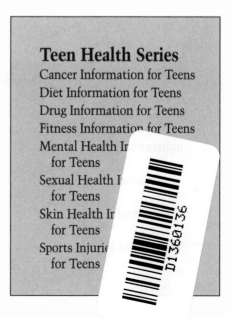

Back and Neck
SOURCEBOOK

Second Edition

Health Reference Series

Second Edition

Back and Neck
SOURCEBOOK

*Basic Consumer Health Information about Spinal
Pain, Spinal Cord Injuries, and Related Disorders,
Such as Degenerative Disk Disease, Osteoarthritis,
Scoliosis, Sciatica, Spina Bifida, and Spinal Stenosis,
and Featuring Facts about Maintaining Spinal
Health, Self-Care, Pain Management, Rehabilitative
Care, Chiropractic Care, Spinal Surgeries, and
Complementary Therapies*

*Along with Suggestions for Preventing Back and
Neck Pain, a Glossary of Related Terms, and a
Directory of Resources*

Edited by
Amy L. Sutton

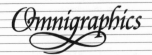

Omnigraphics

615 Griswold Street • Detroit, MI 48226

Bibliographic Note

Because this page cannot legibly accommodate all the copyright notices, the Bibliographic Note portion of the Preface constitutes an extension of the copyright notice.

Edited by Amy L. Sutton

Health Reference Series

Karen Bellenir, *Managing Editor*
David A. Cooke, M.D., *Medical Consultant*
Elizabeth Barbour, *Permissions Associate*
Dawn Matthews, *Verification Assistant*
Laura Pleva Nielsen, *Index Editor*
EdIndex, Services for Publishers, *Indexers*

* * *

Omnigraphics, Inc.

Matthew P. Barbour, *Senior Vice President*
Kay Gill, *Vice President—Directories*
Kevin Hayes, *Operations Manager*
Leif Gruenberg, *Development Manager*
David P. Bianco, *Marketing Director*

* * *

Peter E. Ruffner, *Publisher*

Frederick G. Ruffner, Jr., *Chairman*

Copyright © 2004 Omnigraphics, Inc.

ISBN 0-7808-0738-3

Library of Congress Cataloging-in-Publication Data

Back and neck sourcebook : basic consumer health information about spinal pain, spinal cord injuries, and related disorders, such as degenerative disk disease, osteoarthritis, scoliosis, sciatica, spina bifida, and spinal stenosis, and featuring facts about maintaining spinal health, self-care, pain management, rehabilitative care, chiropractic care, spinal surgeries, and complementary therapies; along with suggestions for preventing back and neck pain, a glossary of related terms, and a directory of resources / edited by Amy L. Sutton.-- 2nd ed.
    p. cm. -- (Health reference series)
  Includes bibliographical references and index.
  ISBN 0-7808-0738-3 (hardcover : alk. paper)
  1. Backache--Treatment--Popular works. 2. Neck pain--Treatment--Popular works. 3. Back--Care and hygiene--Popular works. 4. Neck--Care and hygiene--Popular works. I. Sutton, Amy L. II. Health reference series (Unnumbered)
  RD771.B217B2935 2004
  617.5'64--dc22

                                                                    2004018091

Table of Contents

Visit www.healthreferenceseries.com to view *A Contents Guide to the Health Reference Series*, a listing of more than 10,000 topics and the volumes in which they are covered.

Part II: Maintaining Spinal Health

Part V: Chronic Disorders Associated with Back and Neck Pain

Part VI: Medications and Rehabilitative Therapies for Spinal Problems

Part VII: Information about Spinal Surgeries

Part VIII: Additional Help and Information

Preface

About This Book

According to the American Academy of Orthopaedic Surgeons, four out of five adults will experience low back pain at some time during their lives. All told, low back pain, the second most common neurological ailment in the United States after headache, costs Americans $50 billion each year. The upper spine is also a frequent source of pain, and the Centers for Disease Control and Prevention (CDC) reports that 14% of Americans experience pain in the neck area. In addition, every year more than 10,000 people in the U.S. suffer traumatic spinal cord injuries as a result of automobile accidents, acts of violence, falls, sports injuries, and other causes. Although back and neck disorders are responsible for significant suffering, new treatments, medications, exercise programs, and surgical advances are bringing hope to many patients with spinal concerns.

This *Sourcebook* provides information about diseases, disorders, and injuries that affect the spinal column, including degenerative disk disease, osteoarthritis, scoliosis, sciatica, spina bifida, spinal stenosis, ankylosing spondylitis, and sprains, strains, and fractures. It also describes proper spine function and includes suggestions for maintaining spinal health. For patients with spinal problems, it offers helpful information about medications and rehabilitative and complementary therapies, along with facts about surgical techniques and the use of chiropractic care to prevent and treat spinal injuries and pain. A glossary, directory of resources for further help and information, and suggestions for additional reading are also provided.

How to Use This Book

This book is divided into parts and chapters. Parts focus on broad areas of interest. Chapters are devoted to single topics within a part.

Part I: Understanding Back and Neck Problems identifies causes, prevalence, symptoms, and risk factors for spinal disorders. It provides information about the anatomy and function of the spine, describes the risk of back and neck disorders among different age groups, and explains how aging affects the spine. Tips on preparing for a medical consultation with a spine specialist are also included.

Part II: Maintaining Spinal Health describes methods for preventing pain and disability with good body mechanics and proper posture. It includes exercises for preventing back and neck pain, including yoga and Pilates, and discusses the incidence and prevention of spinal pain at school, home, and work. It also offers tips for easing spinal pain during pregnancy.

Part III: Chiropractic Care provides an explanation of chiropractic adjustment and subluxation and addresses concerns and questions consumers often have when seeking chiropractic care. It offers tips on choosing a chiropractor, describes what to expect during the first visit, and answers questions parents may have about chiropractic care for children and adolescents.

Part IV: Acute Injuries to the Back and Neck outlines first-aid treatment for spinal injuries. It also identifies acutely painful back and neck injuries, including stingers, whiplash, and cervical, thoracic, and lumbar spinal fractures. In addition, it offers guidance on understanding and adapting to spinal cord injuries that cause permanent disability.

Part V: Chronic Disorders Associated with Back and Neck Pain includes chapters on spinal conditions such as ankylosing spondylitis, cauda equina syndrome, degenerative disk disease, scoliosis, osteoarthritis, sacroiliac joint syndrome, spina bifida, spinal stenosis, and spinal tumors and cysts.

Part VI: Medications and Rehabilitative Therapies for Spinal Problems identifies common medications used to reduce the pain associated with spinal disorders such as nonsteroidal anti-inflammatory medications and spinal injections. Other nonsurgical pain relief treatments, including physical therapy, back and neck braces, ice massage, heat therapy, and hydrotherapy exercise programs, are also described.

Part VII: Information about Spinal Surgeries details traditional surgical treatments for spinal disorders, including spinal fusion surgery, bone grafts, minimally invasive spinal surgery, as well as cutting-edge treatments, such as artificial disk replacement, intradiscal electrothermal annuloplasty (IDET), and percutaneous vertebral augmentation.

Part VIII: Additional Help and Information offers a glossary of important terms and directory of government agencies and private organizations that provide help and information to patients with spinal disorders. Also included is a suggested list of books, magazines, and journal articles for further reading.

Bibliographic Note

This volume contains documents and excerpts from publications issued by the following U.S. government agencies: Agency for Healthcare Research and Quality (AHRQ); National Center for Complementary and Alternative Medicine (NCCAM); National Institute of Arthritis and Musculoskeletal and Skin Diseases (NIAMS); National Institute of Neurological Disorders and Stroke (NINDS); National Institutes of Health (NIH); and the U.S. Food and Drug Administration (FDA).

In addition, this volume contains copyrighted documents from the following organizations and individuals: Acupuncture Today; A.D.A.M., Inc.; AgSafe; American Academy of Orthopaedic Surgeons (AAOS); American Academy of Physical Medicine and Rehabilitation; American Association of Neurological Surgeons (AANS); American Chiropractic Association; American Physical Therapy Association (APTA); Howard S. An, M.D. and Kristen Karl Juarez, R.N., M.S.N.; Baylor College of Medicine Office of Health Promotion; Cleveland Clinic Foundation; DePuy Spine, Inc.; Dynamic Chiropractic; Dystonia Medical Research Foundation; Dave Edell; Federation of Chiropractic Licensing Boards; Healthcommunities.com, Inc.; International Chiropractors Association; the McGraw Hill Companies (*Physician and Sportsmedicine*); Nemours Center for Children's Health Media;

North American Spine Society; George D. Picetti, M.D.; John Regan, M.D.; Spina Bifida Association of America; Spine-health.com; Spondylitis Association of America; University of Alabama at Birmingham Board of Trustees; and the University of Pittsburgh Medical Center.

Full citation information is provided on the first page of each chapter. Every effort has been made to secure all necessary rights to reprint the copyrighted material. If any omissions have been made, please contact Omnigraphics to make corrections for future editions.

Acknowledgements

Thanks go to the many organizations, agencies, and individuals who have contributed materials for this *Sourcebook* and to medical consultant Dr. David Cooke, verification assistant Dawn Matthews, and document engineer Bruce Bellenir. Special thanks go to managing editor Karen Bellenir and permissions specialist Liz Barbour for their help and support.

About the Health Reference Series

The *Health Reference Series* is designed to provide basic medical information for patients, families, caregivers, and the general public. Each volume takes a particular topic and provides comprehensive coverage. This is especially important for people who may be dealing with a newly diagnosed disease or a chronic disorder in themselves or in a family member. People looking for preventive guidance, information about disease warning signs, medical statistics, and risk factors for health problems will also find answers to their questions in the *Health Reference Series*. The *Series*, however, is not intended to serve as a tool for diagnosing illness, in prescribing treatments, or as a substitute for the physician/patient relationship. All people concerned about medical symptoms or the possibility of disease are encouraged to seek professional care from an appropriate health care provider.

Locating Information within the Health Reference Series

The *Health Reference Series* contains a wealth of information about a wide variety of medical topics. Ensuring easy access to all the fact sheets, research reports, in-depth discussions, and other material contained within the individual books of the series remains one of our highest priorities. As the *Series* continues to grow in size and scope, however, locating the precise information needed by a reader may become more challenging.

A Contents Guide to the Health Reference Series was developed to direct readers to the specific volumes that address their concerns. It presents an extensive list of diseases, treatments, and other topics of general interest compiled from the Tables of Contents and major index headings. To access *A Contents Guide to the Health Reference Series*, visit www.healthreferenceseries.com.

Medical Consultant

Medical consultation services are provided to the *Health Reference Series* editors by David A. Cooke, M.D. Dr. Cooke is a graduate of Brandeis University, and he received his M.D. degree from the University of Michigan. He completed residency training at the University of Wisconsin Hospital and Clinics. He is board-certified in Internal Medicine. Dr. Cooke currently works as part of the University of Michigan Health System and practices in Brighton, MI. In his free time, he enjoys writing, science fiction, and spending time with his family.

Our Advisory Board

We would like to thank the following board members for providing guidance to the development of this *Series*:

Dr. Lynda Baker, Associate Professor of Library and Information Science, Wayne State University, Detroit, MI

Nancy Bulgarelli, William Beaumont Hospital Library, Royal Oak, MI

Karen Imarisio, Bloomfield Township Public Library, Bloomfield Township, MI

Karen Morgan, Mardigian Library, University of Michigan-Dearborn, Dearborn, MI

Rosemary Orlando, St. Clair Shores Public Library, St. Clair Shores, MI

Health Reference Series *Update Policy*

The inaugural book in the *Health Reference Series* was the first edition of *Cancer Sourcebook* published in 1989. Since then, the *Series* has been enthusiastically received by librarians and in the medical community. In order to maintain the standard of providing high-quality health information for the layperson the editorial staff at Omnigraphics felt it was necessary to implement a policy of updating volumes when warranted.

Medical researchers have been making tremendous strides, and it is the purpose of the *Health Reference Series* to stay current with the most recent advances. Each decision to update a volume will be made on an individual basis. Some of the considerations will include how much new information is available and the feedback we receive from people who use the books. If there is a topic you would like to see added to the update list, or an area of medical concern you feel has not been adequately addressed, please write to:

Editor
Health Reference Series
Omnigraphics, Inc.
615 Griswold Street
Detroit, MI 48226
E-mail: editorial@omnigraphics.com

Part One

Understanding
Back and Neck Problems

Chapter 1

Anatomy and Function of the Spine

Introduction

Your spine is one of the most important parts of your body. It gives your body structure and support. Without it you could not stand up or keep yourself upright. It allows you to move about freely and to bend with flexibility. The spine is also designed to protect your spinal cord. The spinal cord is a column of nerves that connects your brain to the rest of your body, allowing you to control your movements. Without a spinal cord you could not move any part of your body, and your organs could not function. Keeping your spine healthy is vital if you want to live an active life. Learn about the spine including:

- how the spine functions
- what differentiates the cervical, thoracic, and lumbar spinal segments
- what important structures make up the spine

Anatomy

What exactly is the spine?

The spine is made up of 24 bones, called vertebrae. Ligaments and muscles connect these bones together to form the spinal column. The spinal column gives the body form and function. The spinal column holds and protects the spinal cord, which is a bundle of nerves that sends signals to other parts of the body. The many muscles that connect to the spine help support the upright posture of the spine and move the spine.

The spinal column has three main sections—the cervical spine, the thoracic spine, and the lumbar spine. The first seven vertebrae form the cervical spine. The mid back, called the thoracic spine, consists of 12 vertebrae. The lower portion of the spine, called the lumbar spine, is usually made up of five vertebrae. However some people have a sixth lumbar vertebra.

The normal spine has an S-like curve when looking at it from the side. This allows for an even distribution of weight. The S curve helps a healthy spine withstand all kinds of stress. The cervical spine curves slightly inward, the thoracic slightly outward, and the lumbar slightly inward. Even though the lower portion of your spine holds most of the body's weight, each segment relies upon the strength of the others to function properly.

Cervical Spine (Neck)

The cervical spine is made up of the first seven vertebrae in the spine. It starts just below the skull and ends just above the thoracic spine. The cervical spine has a lordotic curve, a backward C-shape— just like the lumbar spine. The cervical spine is much more mobile than both of the other spinal regions. Think about all the directions and angles you can turn your neck.

Unlike the rest of the spine, there are special openings in each vertebra in the cervical spine for arteries (blood vessels that carry blood away from the heart). The arteries that run through these openings bring blood to the brain.

Two vertebrae in the cervical spine, the atlas and the axis, differ from the other vertebrae because they are designed specifically for rotation. These two vertebrae are the reason your neck can move in so many directions.

The atlas is the first cervical vertebra—the one that sits between the skull and the rest of the spine. The atlas does not have a vertebral body, but it does have a thick forward (anterior) arch and a thin back (posterior) arch with two prominent sideways masses.

The atlas sits on top of the second cervical vertebra, the axis. The axis has a bony knob called the odontoid process, which sticks up

4

through the hole in the atlas. Special ligaments between the atlas and the axis allow for a great deal of rotation. It is this special arrangement that allows the head to turn from side to side as far as it can.

The cervical spine is very flexible, but it is also very much at risk for injury from strong, sudden movements, such as whiplash-type injuries. This high risk of harm is due to the limited muscle support that exists in the cervical area, and the fact that this part of the spine has to support the weight of the head—an average of 15 pounds. This is a lot of weight for a small, thin set of bones and soft tissues to bear. Sudden, strong head movements can cause damage.

Thoracic Spine (Mid Back)

The thoracic spine is made up of the middle 12 vertebrae. These vertebrae connect to your ribs and form part of the back wall of the thorax (the ribcage area between the neck and the diaphragm). The thoracic spine's curve is kyphotic, a C-shaped curve with the opening of the C in the front. This part of the spine has very narrow, thin intervertebral disks. Rib connections and smaller disks in the thoracic spine limit the amount of spinal movement in the mid back compared to the lumbar or cervical parts of the spine. There is also less space inside the spinal canal.

Lumbar Spine (Low Back)

The lowest part of the spine is called the lumbar spine. This area usually has five vertebrae. However, sometimes people are born with a sixth vertebra in the lumbar region. The base of your spine (called the sacrum) is a group of specialized vertebrae that connects the spine to the pelvis. When one of the bones forms as a vertebra rather than part of the sacrum, it is called a transitional (or sixth) vertebra. This occurrence is not dangerous and does not appear to have any serious side effects.

The lumbar spine's shape has a lordotic curve-shaped like a backward C. If you think of the spine as having an S-like shape, the lumbar region would be the bottom of the S. The vertebrae in the lumbar spine area are the largest of the entire spine. The lumbar spinal canal is also larger than in the cervical or thoracic parts of the spine. The size of the lumbar spine allows for more space for nerves to move about.

Low back pain is a very common complaint for a simple reason. Since the lumbar spine is connected to your pelvis, this is where most of your weight bearing and body movement takes place. Typically this is where people tend to place too much pressure, such as when lifting up a heavy box, twisting to move a heavy load, or carrying a heavy object. These activities can cause repetitive injuries that can lead to damage to the parts of the lumbar spine.

Important Structures of the Spine

Vertebrae

Your spine is made up of 24 small bones, called vertebrae. The vertebrae protect and support the spinal cord. They also bear the majority of the weight put upon your spine. Vertebrae, like all bones, have an outer shell, called cortical bone, which is hard and strong. The inside is made of a soft, spongy type of bone, called cancellous bone.

The vertebral body is the large, round portion of bone. Each vertebra is attached to a bony ring. When the vertebrae are stacked one on top of the other, the rings create a hollow tube for the spinal cord to pass through. Each vertebra is held to the others by groups of ligaments. Ligaments connect bones to bones; tendons connect muscles to bones. There are also tendons that fasten muscles to the vertebrae.

The bony ring attached to the vertebral body consists of several parts. The laminae extend from the body to cover the spinal canal, which is the hole in the center of the vertebra. The spinous process is the bony portion opposite the body of the vertebra. You feel this part if you run your hand down a person's back. There are two transverse processes (little bony bumps), where the back muscles attach to the vertebrae. The pedicle is a bony projection that connects the laminae to the vertebral body.

Intervertebral Disk

Between each vertebra is a soft, gel-like cushion, called an intervertebral disk. These flat, round cushions act like shock absorbers by helping absorb pressure. The disks prevent the bones from rubbing against each other.

Each disk has a strong outer ring of fibers called the annulus, and a soft, jelly-like center called the nucleus pulposus. The annulus is the strongest area of the disk. It helps keep the disk's center intact. The annulus is actually a strong ligament that connects each vertebra together.

6

The mushy nucleus of the disk serves as the main shock absorber. The nucleus is made up of tissue that is very moist because it has high water content. The water content is what helps the disk act like a shock absorber—somewhat like a waterbed mattress.

Facet Joints

The spinal column has real joints (just like the knee, elbow, etc.) called facet joints. The facet joints link the vertebrae together and give them the flexibility to move against each other. The facets are the bony knobs that meet between each vertebra. There are two facet joints between each pair of vertebrae, one on each side. They extend and overlap each other to form a joint between the neighboring vertebra facet joint. The facet joints give the spine its flexibility.

The facet joints are synovial joints, structures that allow movement between two bones. The ends of the bones that make up a synovial joint are covered with articular cartilage, a slick spongy material that allows the bones to glide against one another without much friction. Synovial fluid inside the joint keeps the joint surfaces lubricated, like oil lubricates the parts of a machine. This fluid is contained inside the joint by the joint capsule, a watertight sac of soft tissue and ligaments that fully surrounds and encloses the joint.

Neural Foramen

The spinal cord branches off into 31 pairs of nerve roots, which exit the spine through small openings on each side of the vertebra called neural foramen. The two nerve roots in each pair go in opposite directions when traveling through the foramina. One goes out the left foramina; the other goes out through the right foramina. The nerve root allows nerve signals to travel to and from your brain to the rest of your body.

Spinal Cord

The spinal cord is a column of millions of nerve fibers that carries messages from your brain to the rest of your body. It extends from the brain to the area between the end of your first lumbar vertebra and top of your second lumbar vertebra. Each vertebra has a hole in the center, so when they stack on top of each other they form a hollow tube (spinal canal) that holds and protects the entire spinal cord and its nerve roots.

The spinal cord only goes down to the second lumbar vertebra. Below this level, the spinal canal contains a group of nerve fibers, called the cauda equina. This group of nerves goes to the pelvis and lower limbs.

A protective membrane called the dura mater covers the spinal cord. The dura mater forms a watertight sac around the spinal cord and the spinal nerves. Inside this sac, the spinal cord is surrounded by spinal fluid.

Nerve Roots

The nerve fibers in your spinal cord branch off to form pairs of nerve roots that travel through the small openings between your vertebrae. The nerves in each area of the spinal cord connect to specific parts of your body. This is why damage to the spinal cord can cause paralysis in certain areas and not others. It depends on which spinal nerves are affected. The nerves of the cervical spine go to the upper chest and arms. The nerves of the thoracic spine go to the chest and abdomen. The nerves of the lumbar spine reach to the legs, pelvis, bowel, and bladder. These nerves coordinate and control all the body's organs and parts, and allow you to control your muscles.

The nerves carry electrical signals back to the brain that allow you to feel sensations. If your body is being hurt in some way, your nerves signal the brain. Damage to the nerves themselves can cause pain, tingling, or numbness in the area where the nerve travels. Without nerve signals, your body would not be able to function.

Paraspinal Muscles

The muscles next to the spine are called the paraspinal muscles. They support the spine and provide the motor for movement of the spine. Joints allow flexibility, and muscles allow mobility. There are many small muscles in the back. Each controls some part of the total movement between the vertebrae and the rest of the skeleton. These muscles can be directly injured, such as when you have a pulled muscle or muscle strain. They can also cause problems indirectly, such as when they are in spasm after injury to other parts of the spine.

A muscle spasm is experienced when your muscle tightens up and will not relax. Spasms usually occur as a reflex (meaning that you cannot control the contraction). When any part of the spine is injured—including a disk, ligament, bone, or muscle—the muscles automatically go into spasm to reduce the motion around the area. This mechanism is designed to protect the injured area.

8

Muscles that are in spasm produce too much lactic acid, a waste product from the chemical reaction inside muscle cells. When muscles contract, the small blood vessels traveling through the muscles are pinched off (like a tube pinched between your thumb and finger), which causes a buildup of lactic acid. If the muscle cells cannot relax and too much lactic acid builds up, it causes a painful burning sensation. The muscle relaxes as the blood vessels open up, and the lactic acid is eventually washed away by fresh blood flowing into the muscle.

Spinal Segments

Doctors sometimes look at a spinal segment to understand and explain how the whole spine works. A spinal segment is made up of two vertebrae attached together by ligaments, with a soft disk separating them. The facet joints fit between the two vertebrae, allowing for movement, and the neural foramina between the vertebrae allow space for the nerve roots to travel freely from the spinal cord to the body. The spinal segment allows physicians to examine the repeating parts of the spinal column to understand what can go wrong with the various parts of the spine.

Chapter 2

Understanding Pain

Introduction: The Universal Disorder

You know it at once. It may be the fiery sensation of a burn moments after your finger touches the stove. Or it's a dull ache above your brow after a day of stress and tension. Or you may recognize it as a sharp pierce in your back after you lift something heavy.

It is pain. In its most benign form, it warns us that something isn't quite right, that we should take medicine or see a doctor. At its worst, however, pain robs us of our productivity, our well being, and, for many of us suffering from extended illness, our very lives. Pain is a complex perception that differs enormously among individual patients, even those who appear to have identical injuries or illnesses.

In 1931, the French medical missionary Dr. Albert Schweitzer wrote, "Pain is a more terrible lord of mankind than even death itself." Today, pain has become the universal disorder, a serious and costly public health issue, and a challenge for family, friends, and health care providers who must give support to the individual suffering from the physical as well as the emotional consequences of pain.

"Pain—Hope Through Research" is published by the National Institute of Neurological Disorders and Stroke (NINDS), November 7, 2001. Available online at http://www.ninds.nih.gov; accessed April 2004.

11

The Two Faces of Pain: Acute and Chronic

What is pain? The International Association for the Study of Pain defines it as: An unpleasant sensory and emotional experience associated with actual or potential tissue damage or described in terms of such damage.

It is useful to distinguish between two basic types of pain, acute and chronic, and they differ greatly.

- **Acute pain,** for the most part, results from disease, inflammation, or injury to tissues. This type of pain generally comes on suddenly, for example, after trauma or surgery, and may be accompanied by anxiety or emotional distress. The cause of acute pain can usually be diagnosed and treated, and the pain is self-limiting, that is, it is confined to a given period of time and severity. In some rare instances, it can become chronic.

- **Chronic pain** is widely believed to represent disease itself. It can be made much worse by environmental and psychological factors. Chronic pain persists over a longer period of time than acute pain and is resistant to most medical treatments. It can—and often does—cause severe problems for patients.

Types of Pain That Affect the Back and Neck

Hundreds of pain syndromes or disorders make up the spectrum of pain. There are the most benign, fleeting sensations of pain, such as a pin prick. There is the pain of childbirth, the pain of a heart attack, and the pain that sometimes follows amputation of a limb. There is also pain accompanying cancer and the pain that follows severe trauma, such as that associated with head and spinal cord injuries. A sampling of common pain syndromes follows, listed alphabetically.

Back pain has become the high price paid by our modern lifestyle and is a startlingly common cause of disability for many Americans, including both active and inactive people. Back pain that spreads to the leg is called sciatica and is a very common condition. Another common type of back pain is associated with the disks of the spine, the soft, spongy padding between the vertebrae (bones) that form the spine. Disks protect the spine by absorbing shock, but they tend to degenerate over time and may sometimes rupture. Spondylolisthesis is a back condition that occurs when one vertebra extends over another, causing pressure on nerves and therefore pain. Also, damage to nerve roots is a serious condition, called radiculopathy, that can be extremely painful. Treatment for a damaged disk includes drugs such as painkillers, muscle relaxants, and steroids; exercise or rest, depending on the patient's condition; adequate support, such as a brace or better mattress and physical therapy. In some cases, surgery may be required to remove the damaged portion of the disk and return it to its previous condition, especially when it is pressing a nerve root. Surgical procedures include discectomy, laminectomy, or spinal fusion.

Muscle pain can range from an aching muscle, spasm, or strain, to the severe spasticity that accompanies paralysis. Another disabling syndrome is fibromyalgia, a disorder characterized by fatigue, stiffness, joint tenderness, and widespread muscle pain. Polymyositis, dermatomyositis, and inclusion body myositis are painful disorders characterized by muscle inflammation. They may be caused by infection or autoimmune dysfunction and are sometimes associated with connective tissue disorders, such as lupus and rheumatoid arthritis.

Neuropathic pain is a type of pain that can result from injury to nerves, either in the peripheral or central nervous system. Neuropathic pain can occur in any part of the body and is frequently described as a hot, burning sensation, which can be devastating to the affected individual. It can result from diseases that affect nerves (such as diabetes) or from trauma, or, because chemotherapy drugs can affect nerves, it can be a consequence of cancer treatment.

Sciatica is a painful condition caused by pressure on the sciatic nerve, the main nerve that branches off the spinal cord and continues down into the thighs, legs, ankles, and feet. Sciatica is characterized by pain in the buttocks and can be caused by a number of factors. Exertion, obesity, and poor posture can all cause pressure on the sciatic nerve. One common cause of sciatica is a herniated disk.

Sports injuries are common. Sprains, strains, bruises, dislocations, and fractures are all well-known words in the language of sports. Pain is another. In extreme cases, sports injuries can take the form of costly and painful spinal cord and head injuries, which cause severe suffering and disability.

Spinal stenosis refers to a narrowing of the canal surrounding the spinal cord. The condition occurs naturally with aging. Spinal stenosis causes weakness in the legs and leg pain usually felt while the person is standing up and often relieved by sitting down.

Surgical pain may require regional or general anesthesia during the procedure and medications to control discomfort following the operation. Control of pain associated with surgery includes presurgical preparation and careful monitoring of the patient during and after the procedure.

13

Trauma can occur after injuries in the home, at the workplace, during sports activities, or on the road. Any of these injuries can result in severe disability and pain. Some patients who have had an injury to the spinal cord experience intense pain ranging from tingling to burning and, commonly, both. Such patients are sensitive to hot and cold temperatures and touch. For these individuals, a touch can be perceived as intense burning, indicating abnormal signals relayed to and from the brain. This condition is called central pain syndrome or, if the damage is in the thalamus (the brain's center for processing bodily sensations), thalamic pain syndrome. It affects as many as 100,000 Americans with multiple sclerosis, Parkinson's disease, amputated limbs, spinal cord injuries, and stroke. Their pain is severe and is extremely difficult to treat effectively. A variety of medications, including analgesics, antidepressants, anticonvulsants, and electrical stimulation, are options available to central pain patients.

How Is Pain Diagnosed?

There is no way to tell how much pain a person has. No test can measure the intensity of pain, no imaging device can show pain, and no instrument can locate pain precisely. Sometimes, as in the case of headaches, physicians find that the best aid to diagnosis is the patient's own description of the type, duration, and location of pain. Defining pain as sharp or dull, constant or intermittent, burning or aching may give the best clues to the cause of pain. These descriptions are part of what is called the pain history, taken by the physician during the preliminary examination of a patient with pain.

Physicians, however, do have a number of technologies they use to find the cause of pain. Primarily these include:

- Electrodiagnostic procedures include electromyography (EMG), nerve conduction studies, and evoked potential (EP) studies. Information from EMG can help physicians tell precisely which muscles or nerves are affected by weakness or pain. Thin needles are inserted in muscles and a physician can see or listen to electrical signals displayed on an EMG machine. With nerve conduction studies the doctor uses two sets of electrodes (similar to those used during an electrocardiogram) that are placed on the skin over the muscles. The first set gives the patient a mild shock that stimulates the nerve that runs to that muscle. The second set of electrodes is used to make a recording of the nerve's electrical signals, and from this information the doctor can determine if there is nerve damage. EP tests also involve two sets of electrodes—one set for stimulating a nerve (these electrodes are attached to a limb) and another set on the scalp for recording the speed of nerve signal transmission to the brain.

- Imaging, especially magnetic resonance imaging or MRI, provides physicians with pictures of the body's structures and tissues. MRI uses magnetic fields and radio waves to differentiate between healthy and diseased tissue.

- A neurological examination in which the physician tests movement, reflexes, sensation, balance, and coordination.

- X-rays produce pictures of the body's structures, such as bones and joints.

How Is Pain Treated?

The goal of pain management is to improve function, enabling individuals to work, attend school, or participate in other day-to-day activities. Patients and their physicians have a number of options for the treatment of pain; some are more effective than others. Sometimes, relaxation and the use of imagery as a distraction provide relief. These methods can be powerful and effective, according to those who advocate their use. Whatever the treatment regime, it is important to remember that pain is treatable. The following treatments are among the most common.

Acetaminophen is the basic ingredient found in Tylenol® and its many generic equivalents. It is sold over the counter, in a prescription-strength preparation, and in combination with codeine (also by prescription).

Acupuncture dates back 2,500 years and involves the application of needles to precise points on the body. It is part of a general category of healing called traditional Chinese or Oriental medicine. Acupuncture remains controversial but is quite popular and may one day prove to be useful for a variety of conditions as it continues to be explored by practitioners, patients, and investigators.

Analgesic refers to the class of drugs that includes most painkillers, such as aspirin, acetaminophen, and ibuprofen. The word analgesic is derived from ancient Greek and means to reduce or stop pain. Non-prescription or over-the-counter pain relievers are generally used for mild to moderate pain. Prescription pain relievers, sold through a pharmacy under the direction of a physician, are used for more moderate to severe pain.

Anticonvulsants are used for the treatment of seizure disorders but are also sometimes prescribed for the treatment of pain. Carbamazepine in particular is used to treat a number of painful conditions, including trigeminal neuralgia. Another antiepileptic drug, gabapentin, is being studied for its pain-relieving properties, especially as a treatment for neuropathic pain.

Antidepressants are sometimes used for the treatment of pain and, along with neuroleptics and lithium, belong to a category of drugs called psychotropic drugs. In addition, anti-anxiety drugs called benzodiazepines also act as muscle relaxants and are sometimes used as pain relievers. Physicians usually try to treat the condition with analgesics before prescribing these drugs.

Antimigraine drugs include the triptans—sumatriptan (Imitrex®), naratriptan (Amerge®), and zolmitriptan (Zomig®)—and are used specifically for migraine headaches. They can have serious side effects in some people and therefore, as with all prescription medicines, should be used only under a doctor's care.

Aspirin may be the most widely used pain-relief agent and has been sold over the counter since 1905 as a treatment for fever, headache, and muscle soreness.

Biofeedback is used for the treatment of many common pain problems, most notably headache and back pain. Using a special electronic machine, the patient is trained to become aware of, to follow, and to gain control over certain bodily functions, including muscle tension, heart rate, and skin temperature. The individual can then learn to effect a change in his or her responses to pain, for example, by using relaxation techniques. Biofeedback is often used in combination with other treatment methods, generally without side effects. Similarly, the use of relaxation techniques in the treatment of pain can increase the patient's feeling of well-being.

Capsaicin is a chemical found in chili peppers that is also a primary ingredient in pain-relieving creams.

Chemonucleolysis is a treatment in which an enzyme, chymopapain, is injected directly into a herniated lumbar disk in an effort to dissolve material around the disk, thus reducing pressure and pain. The procedure's use is extremely limited, in part because some patients may have a life-threatening allergic reaction to chymopapain.

Chiropractic refers to hand manipulation of the spine, usually for relief of back pain, and is a treatment option that continues to grow in popularity among many people who simply seek relief from back disorders. It has never been without controversy, however. Chiropractic's usefulness as a treatment for back pain is, for the most part, restricted to a select group of individuals with uncomplicated acute low back pain who may derive relief from the massage component of the therapy.

Cognitive-behavioral therapy involves a wide variety of coping skills and relaxation methods to help prepare for and cope with pain. It is used for postoperative pain, cancer pain, and the pain of childbirth.

Counseling can give a patient suffering from pain much needed support, whether it is derived from family, group, or individual counseling. Support groups can provide an important adjunct to drug or surgical treatment. Psychological treatment can also help patients learn about the physiological changes produced by pain.

COX-2 inhibitors (superaspirins) may be particularly effective for individuals with arthritis. For many years scientists have wanted to develop a drug that works as well as morphine but without its negative side effects. Nonsteroidal anti-inflammatory drugs (NSAIDs) work by blocking two enzymes, cyclooxygenase-1 and cyclooxygenase-2, both of which promote production of hormones called prostaglandins, which in turn cause inflammation, fever, and pain. Newer drugs, called COX-2 inhibitors, primarily block cyclooxygenase-2 and are less likely to have the gastrointestinal side effects sometimes produced by NSAIDs. In 1999, the Food and Drug Administration approved two COX-2 inhibitors—rofecoxib (Vioxx®) and celecoxib (Celebrex®). [Editor's Note: In September 2004, Merck & Company, Inc. announced a voluntary withdrawal of Vioxx from the market due to concerns regarding an increased risk of cardiovascular events (including heart attack and stroke). For more information from Merck, visit www.merck.com or www.vioxx.com or call 1-888-368-4699. For more information from the U.S. Food and Drug Administration (FDA), visit www.fda.gov/cder/drug/infopage/vioxx/default.htm or call 1-888-INFO-FDA.]

Electrical stimulation, including transcutaneous electrical stimulation (TENS), implanted electric nerve stimulation, and deep brain or spinal cord stimulation, is the modern-day extension of age-old practices in which the nerves of muscles are subjected to a variety of stimuli, including heat or massage. Electrical stimulation, no matter what form, involves a major surgical procedure and is not for everyone, nor is it 100 percent effective. The following techniques each require specialized equipment and personnel trained in the specific procedure being used:

- **TENS** uses tiny electrical pulses, delivered through the skin to nerve fibers, to cause changes in muscles, such as numbness or contractions. This in turn produces temporary pain relief. There is also evidence that TENS can activate subsets of peripheral nerve fibers that can block pain transmission at the spinal cord level, in much the same way that shaking your hand can reduce pain.

- **Peripheral nerve stimulation** uses electrodes placed surgically on a carefully selected area of the body. The patient is then able to deliver an electrical current as needed to the affected area, using an antenna and transmitter.

- **Spinal cord stimulation** uses electrodes surgically inserted within the epidural space of the spinal cord. The patient is able to deliver a pulse of electricity to the spinal cord using a small box-like receiver and an antenna taped to the skin.

- **Deep brain or intracerebral stimulation** is considered an extreme treatment and involves surgical stimulation of the brain, usually the thalamus. It is used for a limited number of conditions, including severe pain, central pain syndrome, cancer pain, phantom limb pain, and other neuropathic pains.

Exercise has come to be a prescribed part of some doctors' treatment regimes for patients with pain. Because there is a known link between many types of chronic pain and tense, weak muscles, exercise—even light to moderate exercise such as walking or swimming—can contribute to an overall sense of well-being by improving blood and oxygen flow to muscles. Just as we know that stress contributes to pain, we also know that exercise, sleep, and relaxation can all help reduce stress, thereby helping to alleviate pain. Exercise has been proven to help many people with low back pain. It is important, however, that patients carefully follow the routine laid out by their physicians.

Hypnosis, first approved for medical use by the American Medical Association in 1958, continues to grow in popularity, especially as an adjunct to pain medication. In general, hypnosis is used to control physical function or response, that is, the amount of pain an individual can withstand. How hypnosis works is not fully understood. Some believe that hypnosis delivers the patient into a trance-like state, whereas others feel that the individual is simply better able to concentrate and relax or is more responsive to suggestion. Hypnosis may result in relief of pain by acting on chemicals in the nervous system, slowing impulses. Whether and how hypnosis works involves greater insight—and research—into the mechanisms underlying human consciousness.

Ibuprofen is a member of the aspirin family of analgesics, the so-called nonsteroidal anti-inflammatory drugs. It is sold over the counter and also comes in prescription-strength preparations.

Low-power lasers have been used occasionally by some physical therapists as a treatment for pain, but like many other treatments, this method is not without controversy.

Magnets are increasingly popular with athletes who swear by their effectiveness for the control of sports-related pain and other painful conditions. Usually worn as a collar or wristwatch, the use of magnets as a treatment dates back to the ancient Egyptians and Greeks. Although it is often dismissed as quackery and pseudoscience by skeptics, proponents offer the theory that magnets may effect changes in cells or body chemistry, thus producing pain relief.

Nerve blocks employ the use of drugs, chemical agents, or surgical techniques to interrupt the relay of pain messages between specific areas of the body and the brain. There are many different names for the procedure, depending on the technique or agent used. Types of surgical nerve blocks include neurectomy; spinal dorsal, cranial, and trigeminal rhizotomy; and sympathectomy, also called sympathetic blockade.

Nonsteroidal anti-inflammatory drugs (NSAIDs) (including aspirin and ibuprofen) are widely prescribed and sometimes called non-narcotic or non-opioid analgesics. They work by reducing inflammatory responses in tissues. Many of these drugs irritate the stomach and for that reason are usually taken with food. Although acetaminophen may have some anti-inflammatory effects, it is generally distinguished from the traditional NSAIDs.

Opioids are derived from the poppy plant and are among the oldest drugs known to humankind. They include codeine and perhaps the most well-known narcotic of all, morphine. Morphine can be administered in a variety of forms, including a pump for patient self-administration. Opioids have a narcotic effect, that is, they induce sedation as well as pain relief, and some patients may become physically dependent upon them. For these reasons, patients given opioids should be monitored carefully; in some cases stimulants may be prescribed to counteract the sedative side effects. In addition to drowsiness, other common side effects include constipation, nausea, and vomiting.

Physical therapy and rehabilitation date back to the ancient practice of using physical techniques and methods, such as heat, cold, exercise, massage, and manipulation, in the treatment of certain conditions. These may be applied to increase function, control pain, and speed the patient toward full recovery.

Placebos offer some individuals pain relief although whether and how they have an effect is mysterious and somewhat controversial. Placebos are inactive substances, such as sugar pills, or harmless procedures, such as saline injections or sham surgeries, generally used in clinical studies as control factors to help determine the efficacy of active treatments. Although placebos have no direct effect on the underlying causes of pain, evidence from clinical studies suggests that many pain conditions such as migraine headache, back pain, post-surgical pain, rheumatoid arthritis, angina, and depression sometimes respond well to them. This positive response is known as the placebo effect, which is defined as the observable or measurable change that can occur in patients after administration of a placebo. Some experts believe the effect is psychological and that placebos work because the patients believe or expect them to work. Others say placebos relieve pain by stimulating the brain's own analgesics and setting the body's self-healing forces in motion. A third theory suggests that the act of taking placebos relieves stress and anxiety—which are known to aggravate some painful conditions—and, thus, cause the patients to feel better. Still, placebos are considered controversial because by definition they are inactive and have no actual curative value.

R.I.C.E.—Rest, Ice, Compression, and Elevation—are four components prescribed by many orthopedists, coaches, trainers, nurses, and other professionals for temporary muscle or joint conditions, such as sprains or strains. Although many common orthopedic problems can be controlled with these four simple steps, especially when combined with over-the-counter pain relievers, more serious conditions may require surgery or physical therapy, including exercise, joint movement or manipulation, and stimulation of muscles.

Surgery, although not always an option, may be required to relieve pain, especially pain caused by back problems or serious musculoskeletal injuries. Surgery may take the form of a nerve block or it may involve an operation to relieve pain from a ruptured disk. Surgical procedures for back problems include discectomy or, when microsurgical techniques are used, microdiscectomy, in which the entire disk is removed; laminectomy, a procedure in which a surgeon removes only a disk fragment, gaining access by entering through the arched portion of a vertebra; and spinal fusion, a procedure where the entire disk is removed and replaced with a bone graft. In a spinal fusion, the two vertebrae are then fused together. Although the operation can cause the spine to stiffen, resulting in lost flexibility, the procedure serves one critical purpose: protection of the spinal cord. Other operations for pain include rhizotomy, in which a nerve close to the spinal cord is cut, and cordotomy, where bundles of nerves within the spinal cord are severed. Cordotomy is generally used only for the pain of terminal cancer that does not respond to other therapies. Another operation for pain is the dorsal root entry zone operation, or DREZ, in which spinal neurons corresponding to the patient's pain are destroyed surgically. Because surgery can result in scar tissue formation that may cause additional problems, patients are well advised to seek a second opinion before proceeding. Occasionally, surgery is carried out with electrodes that selectively damage neurons in a targeted area of the brain. These procedures rarely result in long-term pain relief, but both physician and patient may decide that the surgical procedure will be effective enough that it justifies the expense and risk. In some cases, the results of an operation are remarkable. For example, many individuals suffering from trigeminal neuralgia who are not responsive to drug treatment have had great success with a procedure called microvascular decompression, in which tiny blood vessels are surgically separated from surrounding nerves.

A Pain Primer: What Do We Know about Pain?

We may experience pain as a prick, tingle, sting, burn, or ache. Receptors on the skin trigger a series of events, beginning with an electrical impulse that travels from the skin to the spinal cord. The spinal cord acts as a sort of relay center where the pain signal can be blocked, enhanced, or otherwise modified before it is relayed to the brain. One area of the spinal cord in particular, called the dorsal horn, is important in the reception of pain signals.

The most common destination in the brain for pain signals is the thalamus and from there to the cortex, the headquarters for complex thoughts. The thalamus also serves as the brain's storage area for images of the body and plays a key role in relaying messages between the brain and various parts of the body. In people who undergo an amputation, the representation of the amputated limb is stored in the thalamus.

Pain is a complicated process that involves an intricate interplay between a number of important chemicals found naturally in the brain and spinal cord. In general, these chemicals, called neurotransmitters, transmit nerve impulses from one cell to another.

There are many different neurotransmitters in the human body; some play a role in human disease and, in the case of pain, act in various combinations to produce painful sensations in the body. Some chemicals govern mild pain sensations; others control intense or severe pain.

The body's chemicals act in the transmission of pain messages by stimulating neurotransmitter receptors found on the surface of cells; each receptor has a corresponding neurotransmitter. Receptors function much like gates or ports and enable pain messages to pass through and on to neighboring cells. One brain chemical of special interest to neuroscientists is glutamate. During experiments, mice with blocked glutamate receptors show a reduction in their responses to pain. Other important receptors in pain transmission are opiate-like receptors. Morphine and other opioid drugs work by locking on to these opioid receptors, switching on pain-inhibiting pathways or circuits, and thereby blocking pain.

Another type of receptor that responds to painful stimuli is called a nociceptor. Nociceptors are thin nerve fibers in the skin, muscle, and other body tissues, that, when stimulated, carry pain signals to the spinal cord and brain. Normally, nociceptors only respond to strong stimuli such as a pinch. However, when tissues become injured or inflamed, as with a sunburn or infection, they release chemicals that

22

make nociceptors much more sensitive and cause them to transmit pain signals in response to even gentle stimuli such as breeze or a caress. This condition is called allodynia—a state in which pain is produced by innocuous stimuli.

The body's natural painkillers may yet prove to be the most promising pain relievers, pointing to one of the most important new avenues in drug development. The brain may signal the release of painkillers found in the spinal cord, including serotonin, norepinephrine, and opioid-like chemicals. Many pharmaceutical companies are working to synthesize these substances in laboratories as future medications.

Endorphins and enkephalins are other natural painkillers. Endorphins may be responsible for the "feel good" effects experienced by many people after rigorous exercise; they are also implicated in the pleasurable effects of smoking.

Similarly, peptides, compounds that make up proteins in the body, play a role in pain responses. Mice bred experimentally to lack a gene for two peptides called tachykinins—neurokinin A and substance P— have a reduced response to severe pain. When exposed to mild pain, these mice react in the same way as mice that carry the missing gene. But when exposed to more severe pain, the mice exhibit a reduced pain response. This suggests that the two peptides are involved in the production of pain sensations, especially moderate-to-severe pain. Continued research on tachykinins may pave the way for drugs tailored to treat different severities of pain.

Scientists are working to develop potent pain-killing drugs that act on receptors for the chemical acetylcholine. For example, a type of frog native to Ecuador has been found to have a chemical in its skin called epibatidine, derived from the frog's scientific name, *Epipedobates tricolor.* Although highly toxic, epibatidine is a potent analgesic and, surprisingly, resembles the chemical nicotine found in cigarettes. Also under development are other less toxic compounds that act on acetylcholine receptors and may prove to be more potent than morphine but without its addictive properties.

The idea of using receptors as gateways for pain drugs is a novel idea, supported by experiments involving substance P. Investigators have been able to isolate a tiny population of neurons, located in the spinal cord, that together form a major portion of the pathway responsible for carrying persistent pain signals to the brain. When animals were given injections of a lethal cocktail containing substance P linked to the chemical saporin, this group of cells, whose sole function is to communicate pain, were killed. Receptors for substance P served as a portal or point of entry for the compound.

Within days of the injections, the targeted neurons, located in the outer layer of the spinal cord along its entire length, absorbed the compound and were neutralized. The animals' behavior was completely normal; they no longer exhibited signs of pain following injury or had an exaggerated pain response. Importantly, the animals still responded to acute, that is, normal, pain. This is a critical finding as it is important to retain the body's ability to detect potentially injurious stimuli. The protective, early warning signal that pain provides is essential for normal functioning. If this work can be translated clinically, humans might be able to benefit from similar compounds introduced, for example, through lumbar (spinal) puncture.

Another promising area of research using the body's natural pain-killing abilities is the transplantation of chromaffin cells into the spinal cords of animals bred experimentally to develop arthritis. Chromaffin cells produce several of the body's pain-killing substances and are part of the adrenal medulla, which sits on top of the kidney. Within a week or so, rats receiving these transplants cease to exhibit telltale signs of pain. Scientists, working with support from the NINDS, believe the transplants help the animals recover from pain-related cellular damage. Extensive animal studies will be required to learn if this technique might be of value to humans with severe pain.

One way to control pain outside of the brain, that is, peripherally, is by inhibiting hormones called prostaglandins. Prostaglandins stimulate nerves at the site of injury and cause inflammation and fever. Certain drugs, including NSAIDs, act against such hormones by blocking the enzyme that is required for their synthesis.

Blood vessel walls stretch or dilate during a migraine attack and it is thought that serotonin plays a complicated role in this process. For example, before a migraine headache, serotonin levels fall. Drugs for migraine include the triptans: sumatriptan (Imitrex®), naratriptan (Amerge®), and zolmitriptan (Zomig®). They are called serotonin agonists because they mimic the action of endogenous (natural) serotonin and bind to specific subtypes of serotonin receptors.

Ongoing pain research continues to reveal at an unprecedented pace fascinating insights into how genetics, the immune system, and the skin contribute to pain responses.

The explosion of knowledge about human genetics is helping scientists who work in the field of drug development. We know, for example, that the pain-killing properties of codeine rely heavily on a liver enzyme, CYP2D6, which helps convert codeine into morphine. A small number of people genetically lack the enzyme CYP2D6; when given codeine, these individuals do not get pain relief. CYP2D6 also helps break down certain other drugs. People who genetically lack CYP2D6 may not be able to cleanse their systems of these drugs and may be vulnerable to drug toxicity. CYP2D6 is currently under investigation for its role in pain.

In his research, the late John C. Liebeskind, a renowned pain expert and a professor of psychology at UCLA, found that pain can kill by delaying healing and causing cancer to spread. In his pioneering research on the immune system and pain, Dr. Liebeskind studied the effects of stress—such as surgery—on the immune system and in particular on cells called natural killer or NK cells. These cells are thought to help protect the body against tumors. In one study conducted with rats, Dr. Liebeskind found that, following experimental surgery, NK cell activity was suppressed, causing the cancer to spread more rapidly. When the animals were treated with morphine, however, they were able to avoid this reaction to stress.

The link between the nervous and immune systems is an important one. Cytokines, a type of protein found in the nervous system, are also part of the body's immune system, the body's shield for fighting off disease. Cytokines can trigger pain by promoting inflammation, even in the absence of injury or damage. Certain types of cytokines have been linked to nervous system injury. After trauma, cytokine levels rise in the brain and spinal cord and at the site in the peripheral nervous system where the injury occurred. Improvements in our understanding of the precise role of cytokines in producing pain, especially pain resulting from injury, may lead to new classes of drugs that can block the action of these substances.

What Is the Future of Pain Research?

In the forefront of pain research are scientists supported by the National Institutes of Health (NIH), including the NINDS. Other institutes at NIH that support pain research include the National Institute of Dental and Craniofacial Research, the National Cancer Institute, the National Institute of Nursing Research, the National Institute on Drug Abuse, and the National Institute of Mental Health. Developing better pain treatments is the primary goal of all pain research being conducted by these institutes.

Some pain medications dull the patient's perception of pain. Morphine is one such drug. It works through the body's natural painkilling machinery, preventing pain messages from reaching the brain. Scientists are working toward the development of a morphine-like drug that will have the pain-deadening qualities of morphine but without the drug's negative side effects, such as sedation and the potential for addiction. Patients receiving morphine also face the problem of morphine tolerance, meaning that over time they require higher doses of the drug to achieve the same pain relief. Studies have identified factors that contribute to the development of tolerance; continued progress in this line of research should eventually allow patients to take lower doses of morphine.

One objective of investigators working to develop the future generation of pain medications is to take full advantage of the body's pain "switching center" by formulating compounds that will prevent pain signals from being amplified or stop them altogether. Blocking or interrupting pain signals, especially when there is no injury or trauma to tissue, is an important goal in the development of pain medications. An increased understanding of the basic mechanisms of pain will have profound implications for the development of future medicines. The following areas of research are bringing us closer to an ideal pain drug.

Systems and Imaging: The idea of mapping cognitive functions to precise areas of the brain dates back to phrenology, the now archaic practice of studying bumps on the head. Positron emission tomography (PET), functional magnetic resonance imaging (fMRI), and other imaging technologies offer a vivid picture of what is happening in the brain as it processes pain. Using imaging, investigators can now see that pain activates at least three or four key areas of the brain's cortex—the layer of tissue that covers the brain. Interestingly, when patients undergo hypnosis so that the unpleasantness of a painful stimulus is not experienced, activity in some, but not all, brain areas is reduced. This emphasizes that the experience of pain involves a strong emotional component as well as the sensory experience, namely the intensity of the stimulus.

Channels: The frontier in the search for new drug targets is represented by channels. Channels are gate-like passages found along the membranes of cells that allow electrically charged chemical particles called ions to pass into the cells. Ion channels are important for transmitting signals through the nerve's membrane. The possibility now exists for developing new classes of drugs, including pain cocktails that would act at the site of channel activity.

Trophic Factors: A class of "rescuer" or "restorer" drugs may emerge from our growing knowledge of trophic factors, natural chemical substances found in the human body that affect the survival and function of cells. Trophic factors also promote cell death, but little is known about how something beneficial can become harmful. Investigators have observed that an over-accumulation of certain trophic factors in the nerve cells of animals results in heightened pain sensitivity, and that some receptors found on cells respond to trophic factors and interact with each other. These receptors may provide targets for new pain therapies.

Molecular Genetics: Certain genetic mutations can change pain sensitivity and behavioral responses to pain. People born genetically insensate to pain—that is, individuals who cannot feel pain—have a mutation in part of a gene that plays a role in cell survival. Using "knockout" animal models—animals genetically engineered to lack a certain gene-scientists are able to visualize how mutations in genes cause animals to become anxious, make noise, rear, freeze, or become hypervigilant. These genetic mutations cause a disruption or alteration in the processing of pain information as it leaves the spinal cord and travels to the brain. Knockout animals can be used to complement efforts aimed at developing new drugs.

Plasticity: Following injury, the nervous system undergoes a tremendous reorganization. This phenomenon is known as plasticity. For example, the spinal cord is "rewired" following trauma as nerve cell axons make new contacts, a phenomenon known as "sprouting." This in turn disrupts the cells' supply of trophic factors. Scientists can now identify and study the changes that occur during the processing of pain. For example, using a technique called polymerase chain reaction, abbreviated PCR, scientists can study the genes that are induced by injury and persistent pain. There is evidence that the proteins that are ultimately synthesized by these genes may be targets for new therapies. The dramatic changes that occur with injury and persistent pain underscore that chronic pain should be considered a disease of the nervous system, not just prolonged acute pain or a symptom of an injury. Thus, scientists hope that therapies directed at preventing the long-term changes that occur in the nervous system will prevent the development of chronic pain conditions.

Neurotransmitters: Just as mutations in genes may affect behavior, they may also affect a number of neurotransmitters involved in the control of pain. Using sophisticated imaging technologies, investigators can now visualize what is happening chemically in the spinal cord. From this work, new therapies may emerge, therapies that can help reduce or obliterate severe or chronic pain.

Hope for the Future

Thousands of years ago, ancient peoples attributed pain to spirits and treated it with mysticism and incantations. Over the centuries, science has provided us with a remarkable ability to understand and control pain with medications, surgery, and other treatments. Today, scientists understand a great deal about the causes and mechanisms of pain, and research has produced dramatic improvements in the diagnosis and treatment of a number of painful disorders. For people who fight every day against the limitations imposed by pain, the work of NINDS-supported scientists holds the promise of an even greater understanding of pain in the coming years. Their research offers a powerful weapon in the battle to prolong and improve the lives of people with pain: hope.

Chapter 3

Overview of the Causes and Risk Factors for Back Pain

Overview

Neck and back pain, especially pain in the lower back, is one of the most common health problems in adults. Fortunately, most back and neck pain is temporary, resulting from short-term stress on the muscles or ligaments that support the spine rather than from a serious injury or medical condition such as nerve damage or kidney disease.

Anatomy

The back is an intricate structure of bones, ligaments, muscles, nerves, and tendons. The backbone, or spine, is made up of 33 bony segments called vertebrae:

- 7 cervical (neck) vertebrae
- 12 thoracic (middle back) vertebrae
- 5 lumbar (lower back) vertebrae
- 5 sacral (lowest area of the back) vertebrae
- 4 coccygeal (coccyx, or tailbone) vertebra (made up of several fused segments)

"Back Pain," reprinted with permission. © Healthcommunities.com, Inc., 2004. All rights reserved.

The vertebrae are arranged in a long vertical column and held together by ligaments, which are attached to muscles by tendons. Between each vertebra lies a gel-like cushion called an intervertebral disk, consisting of semifluid matter (nucleus pulposus) that is surrounded by a capsule of elastic fibers (annulus fibrosus).

The spinal cord is an extension of the brain that runs through a long, hollow canal in the column of vertebrae. The meninges, cerebrospinal fluid, fat, and a network of veins and arteries surround, nourish, and protect the spinal cord.

Thirty-one pairs of nerve roots emerge from the spinal cord through spaces in each vertebra. The spinal cord and peripheral nerves perform essential sensory and motor activities of the body. The peripheral nervous system conveys sensory information from the body to the brain and conveys motor signals from the brain to the body.

Incidence and Prevalence

In the United States, back pain is reported to occur at least once in 85% of adults below the age of 50. Nearly all of them will have at least one recurrence. It is the second most common illness-related reason given for a missed workday and the most common cause of disability. Work-related back injury is the number one occupational hazard.

Risk Factors

Aging produces wear and tear on the spine that may result in conditions (e.g., disk degeneration, spinal stenosis) that produce neck and back pain. Having a **previous back injury** puts one at risk for another injury.

Physically demanding **occupations** that require repetitive bending and lifting have a high incidence of back injury (e.g., construction worker, caregiver). Jobs that require long hours of standing without a break (e.g., hairdresser) or sitting in a chair (e.g., keyboard operator) that does not support the back well put a person at risk for neck and lower back injury.

Being **sedentary** (i.e., not exercising regularly or engaging in physical recreation) and being **overweight**, which increases stress on the lower back, are risk factors.

Poor posture, such as slouching in a chair, driving hunched over, standing incorrectly, and using poor body mechanics when lifting and carrying heavy loads are risk factors. Sleeping on a soft or sagging mattress also can lead to back pain.

Sports that involve twisting the back, like golf, can result in back injury or worsen existing lower back pain.

Joint and/or bone disease (e.g., osteoporosis, arthritis) and **infectious disease** (e.g., spinal meningitis) can lead to degeneration, inflammation, and compression.

Causes

Many conditions can cause back and neck pain, ranging from injury to infection to simply twisting the wrong way. An injury sustained in an automobile or other type of accident can damage muscles, joints, ligaments, and vertebrae.

Overuse or underuse of the back is by far the most common cause of back pain that manifests as tightening or spasm of the muscles that connect to the spine. Inflammation and swelling often occur in the joints and ligaments, especially in the cervical and lumbar regions, as people age.

A **herniated disk** occurs when the inner material of the disk (nuclear pulposus), pushes through a tear in the capsule of elastic fibers that surrounds the disk (annulus fibrosus), causing nerve root compression.

The cervical and lumbar regions of the spine have the most mobility and the disks there are more likely to wear down or be injured. Ninety percent of disk herniations occur in the lower two lumbar vertebrae.

Over time, repeated daily stress coupled with minor injury can contribute to **intervertebral disk degeneration**. The annulus fibrosus, the capsule of elastic fibers that surrounds the disk, may develop small tears and form scar tissue.

As more scar tissue forms, the nucleus pulposus, the semifluid inner portion of the disk, begins to dry up. Over time, the disk collapses and significantly narrows the space between vertebrae, causing spinal stenosis.

Spinal stenosis, narrowing of the spine, can cause spinal cord irritation and injury. Conditions that cause spinal stenosis include infection, tumors, trauma, herniated disk, arthritis, thickening of ligaments, growth of bone spurs, and disk degeneration. Spinal stenosis most commonly occurs in older individuals as a result of vertebral degeneration.

A **pinched nerve**, or radiculopathy, occurs when something rubs or presses against a nerve, creating irritation or inflammation. Radiculopathy can result from a herniated disk, bone spur, tumor growing into the nerves, and vertebral fracture, and many other conditions.

Sciatica is a certain type of radiculopathy that involves inflammation of the sciatic nerve. Pain is experienced along the large sciatic nerve, from the lower back down through the buttocks and along the back of the leg.

A **spinal tumor** that originates in the spine (primary tumor) or spreads to the spine from another part of the body (metastatic tumor) can compress the spine or nerve roots and cause significant pain.

An **infection** that develops in the vertebrae (e.g., vertebral osteomyelitis), the disks, the meninges (e.g., spinal meningitis), or the cerebrospinal fluid can compress the spinal cord and result in serious neurological deterioration, if it is not diagnosed and treated immediately.

Facet joints allow movement of the spine. These consist of two knobs, or facets, that meet between each vertebra to form a joint. As facet joints degenerate, they may not align correctly, and the cartilage and fluid that lubricates the joints may deteriorate. Bone then rubs against bone, which can be very painful.

Bone and joint diseases (e.g., osteoporosis, ankylosing spondylitis, osteoarthritis) can cause degeneration, inflammation, and spinal nerve compression.

Pain can radiate to the back from other areas of the body (i.e., referred pain) affected by disease or injury, such as bleeding from the aorta, the large artery that carries blood out of the heart; pancreatic disease; pneumonia; kidney diseases; bladder disorders; and uterine abnormalities.

Signs and Symptoms

Pain can be constant or intermittent. Intensity can vary from a dull ache to searing agony. The onset may be sudden, with or without apparent reason, or gradual.

Most back pain resolves in a few days or weeks with or without treatment. However, some people have chronic pain that lasts months or years. Severe pain lasting more than a few days without improvement may require medical attention. Anyone having difficulty passing urine; numbness in the back or genital area; numbness, pins and needles, or weakness in the legs; shooting pain down the leg; or unsteadiness when standing should see a physician immediately.

Localized pain is often described as aching, tight, stiff, sore, burning, throbbing, or pulling. The pain may worsen while bending, sitting, walking, or standing too long in one position. It may also be more prevalent at different times of the day, such as when a person wakes up in the morning.

Pinched nerves produce numbness or tingling, warm or cold sensations, and burning or stabbing pain that begins in the back and radiates down the leg (e.g., sciatica) or arm. Activities such as coughing, sneezing, or walking may increase pressure on the pinched nerve and aggravate the pain.

Compressed nerves cause numbness and weakness in the muscle associated with the nerve. The muscle may atrophy if the compression is not relieved.

An infection affecting the spinal cord or nerves may produce fever and lethargy as well as symptoms of compression.

Diagnosis

Diagnosing the underlying cause of neck and back pain can be difficult. A medical history is taken and a complete physical examination, which may include a neurological examination, is performed.

Laboratory Tests

X-rays show the alignment of the cervical, thoracic, and lumbar spine; and may reveal degenerative joint disease, fracture, or tumor.

Magnetic resonance imaging (MRI) provides clear images of disk deterioration, pathologies of the spinal cord, spinal stenosis, herniated disks, spinal tumors, and abnormalities in nerves and ligaments. Contrast dye may be injected to highlight problematic areas.

Computerized tomography (CT scan) is an x-ray that utilizes computer technology and can be enhanced with contrast dye. It is used to show abnormalities in bones and soft tissue. CT scan can be used for patients who are unable to tolerate MRI.

Myelography is used to examine the spinal canal and cord. Contrast dye is injected into the cerebrospinal fluid to outline the spinal cord and nerve roots, thus allowing abnormal disk conditions or bone spurs to be visualized with x-ray or CT scan.

Electromyogram (EMG) uses tiny electrodes inserted into muscle tissue to test for abnormal electrical signals, which may indicate that a nerve root is pinched or irritated at the spine.

Spinal tap involves drawing a sample of cerebrospinal fluid and analyzing it for elevated pressure, infection, bleeding, or tumor.

Bone scan locates problems (e.g., fracture, osteoporosis) in the vertebrae. A radioactive tracer is injected into the patient and after several hours, x-ray will reveal bone undergoing rapid changes where large amounts of tracer accumulate.

Chapter 4

How Aging Affects the Spine

Time, old injuries, and bad habits take their toll on the spine as you age. But new treatments and better diagnostic tests can help keep back pain at bay throughout an entire lifetime. There are several diseases that can lead to low back pain in the aging spine including disk degeneration (deterioration), lumbar spinal stenosis, and spondylolisthesis (displacement of a vertebra by the one above it).

"The spine goes through the aging process just like any other part of the body," Stan Pelofsky, M.D., *Neurosurgery Today* Editorial Board Chair and a neurosurgeon in Oklahoma City said. "Many of these conditions reduce the quality of life and patients tend to just accept them as a consequence of getting older. But, it doesn't have to be that way and these patients need to see a neurosurgeon early in the disease stage in order to develop a long-range treatment plan."

For patients with a history of back pain and who are currently experiencing symptoms that are interfering with activities, the first step is proper diagnostic testing to determine the cause of the symptoms and the severity of the problem. A series of imaging tests over a period of time can help the neurosurgeon monitor the disease progression and determine the correct course of treatment.

Studies have shown that age is not a major factor in determining whether someone will benefit from surgery, although some conditions associated with age, such as high blood pressure or diabetes, can influence their surgical risks. "A patient is never 'too old' to undergo surgery," Dr. Pelofsky said. "Spine surgery provides great relief to patients well into their 80s."

Disk Degeneration

One of the most common disorders in the lower spine is disk degeneration, or osteoarthritis in the spine. The spine is made up of bones, or vertebra, and softer, gel-like disks. As the body ages, the disks in the spine dehydrate, or dry out, and lose their ability to act as shock absorbers. The bones and ligaments that make up the spine also become less pliable and thicken. Degeneration in the disks is normal and is not in itself a problem. The problem happens when these disks began to pinch and put pressure on the nearby nerve roots or spinal cord.

Treatment plans for patients with disk degeneration in the spine are often long and conservative with the focus on relieving the pressure on the nerve. Neurosurgeons will often prescribe an array of treatments including physical therapy, anti-inflammatory medications, steroid injections, and a consult by a physiatrist, a physician who specializes in rehabilitative medicine.

Lumbar Spinal Stenosis

Another result of degeneration of the spine is lumbar spinal stenosis (LSS). This disease involves a narrowing of the canal that houses the spinal cord and nerve roots. Because the spinal canal is narrowing, the entire spinal cord is often being compressed, not just a single nerve.

Patients who suffer from LSS often experience weakness and pain in the legs, a dull pain in the lower back when they walk or stand, numbness or pins and needles in their legs or buttocks when they walk or stand, and often get relief when sitting or bending forward when they walk or leaning on a shopping cart. Symptoms of LSS usually occur in patients over the age of 50.

Once a diagnosis has been confirmed and the severity of the stenosis has been assessed, the physician will explore the most appropriate avenue of treatment, including medications, physical therapy, and surgery. Many patients respond well to conservative treatment—which includes anti-inflammatory medications, physical therapy, cortisone injections—for quite a few years. Should surgery become an option, your neurosurgeon will carefully review your history and conduct a physical exam and imaging studies to determine the most appropriate procedure for you. The surgical remedy focuses on opening up the spinal canal and relieving the pressure from any nerves that are being irritated.

"Degeneration and lumbar spinal stenosis are often a package deal and therefore the surgery can be fairly comprehensive," Russell L. Travis, M.D., a frequent lecturer on spine care and a neurosurgeon in Kentucky said. "However, over 80 percent of LSS patients have dramatic increases in their quality of life after spine surgery and can return to their active lifestyles."

Degeneration in the spine also can lead to spondylolisthesis, a condition characterized by the slippage of a vertebra in the spine. In this disease process, a vertebra is displaced out of line with the other adjacent vertebra. Like all other spine disorders, conservative treatment often provides relief and pain doesn't become severe unless a nerve root is irritated.

"The most important thing to remember with back pain is that surgery is one of many possible solutions the neurosurgeon has available," Dr. Travis said. "The important thing is to diagnose what is wrong and to develop a treatment plan that works for you."

Chapter 5

Facts about Low Back Pain

If you have lower back pain, you are not alone. Nearly everyone at some point has back pain that interferes with work, routine daily activities, or recreation. Americans spend at least $50 billion each year on low back pain, the most common cause of job-related disability and a leading contributor to missed work. Back pain is the second most common neurological ailment in the United States—only headache is more common. Fortunately, most occurrences of low back pain go away within a few days. Others take much longer to resolve or lead to more serious conditions.

Acute or short-term low back pain generally lasts from a few days to a few weeks. Most acute back pain is mechanical in nature— the result of trauma to the lower back or a disorder such as arthritis. Pain from trauma may be caused by a sports injury, work around the house or in the garden, or a sudden jolt such as a car accident or other stress on spinal bones and tissues. Symptoms may range from muscle ache to shooting or stabbing pain, limited flexibility and/or range of motion, or an inability to stand straight. Occasionally, pain felt in one part of the body may radiate from a disorder or injury elsewhere in the body. Some acute pain syndromes can become more serious if left untreated.

"Low Back Pain Fact Sheet" from the National Institute of Neurological Disorders and Stroke (NINDS), July 26, 2003. Available online at http://www.ninds.nih.gov; accessed April 2004.

Chronic back pain is measured by duration—pain that persists for more than 3 months is considered chronic. It is often progressive and the cause can be difficult to determine.

What Structures Make up the Back?

The back is an intricate structure of bones, muscles, and other tissues that form the posterior part of the body's trunk, from the neck to the pelvis. The centerpiece is the spinal column, which not only supports the upper body's weight but houses and protects the spinal cord—the delicate nervous system structure that carries signals that control the body's movements and convey its sensations. Stacked on top of one another are more than 30 bones—the vertebrae—that form the spinal column, also known as the spine. Each of these bones contains a roundish hole that, when stacked in register with all the others, creates a channel that surrounds the spinal cord. The spinal cord descends from the base of the brain and extends in the adult to just below the rib cage. Small nerves (roots) enter and emerge from the spinal cord through spaces between the vertebrae. Because the bones of the spinal column continue growing long after the spinal cord reaches its full length in early childhood, the nerve roots to the lower back and legs extend many inches down the spinal column before exiting. This large bundle of nerve roots was dubbed by early anatomists as the cauda equina, or horse's tail. The spaces between the vertebrae are maintained by round, spongy pads of cartilage called intervertebral disks that allow for flexibility in the lower back and act much like shock absorbers throughout the spinal column to cushion the bones as the body moves. Bands of tissue known as ligaments and tendons hold the vertebrae in place and attach the muscles to the spinal column.

Starting at the top, the spine has four regions:

- the seven cervical or neck vertebrae (labeled C1–C7)
- the 12 thoracic or upper back vertebrae (labeled T1–T12)
- the five lumbar vertebrae (labeled L1–L5), which we know as the lower back
- the sacrum and coccyx, a group of bones fused together at the base of the spine

The lumbar region of the back, where most back pain is felt, supports the weight of the upper body.

What Causes Lower Back Pain?

As people age, bone strength and muscle elasticity and tone tend to decrease. The disks begin to lose fluid and flexibility, which decreases their ability to cushion the vertebrae.

Pain can occur when, for example, someone lifts something too heavy or overstretches, causing a sprain, strain, or spasm in one of the muscles or ligaments in the back. If the spine becomes overly strained or compressed, a disk may rupture or bulge outward. This rupture may put pressure on one of the more than 50 nerves rooted to the spinal cord that control body movements and transmit signals from the body to the brain. When these nerve roots become compressed or irritated, back pain results.

Low back pain may reflect nerve or muscle irritation or bone lesions. Most low back pain follows injury or trauma to the back, but pain may also be caused by degenerative conditions such as arthritis or disk disease, osteoporosis or other bone diseases, viral infections, irritation to joints and disks, or congenital abnormalities in the spine. Obesity, smoking, weight gain during pregnancy, stress, poor physical condition, posture inappropriate for the activity being performed, and poor sleeping position also may contribute to low back pain. Additionally, scar tissue created when the injured back heals itself does not have the strength or flexibility of normal tissue. Buildup of scar tissue from repeated injuries eventually weakens the back and can lead to more serious injury.

Occasionally, low back pain may indicate a more serious medical problem. Pain accompanied by fever or loss of bowel or bladder control, pain when coughing, and progressive weakness in the legs may indicate a pinched nerve or other serious condition. People with diabetes may have severe back pain or pain radiating down the leg related to neuropathy. People with these symptoms should contact a doctor immediately to help prevent permanent damage.

Who Is Most Likely to Develop Low Back Pain?

Nearly everyone has low back pain some time. Men and women are equally affected. It occurs most often between ages 30 and 50, due in part to the aging process but also as a result of sedentary lifestyles with too little (sometimes punctuated by too much) exercise. The risk of experiencing low back pain from disk disease or spinal degeneration increases with age.

Low back pain unrelated to injury or other known cause is unusual in preteen children. However, a backpack overloaded with schoolbooks and supplies can quickly strain the back and cause muscle fatigue. The U.S. Consumer Product Safety Commission estimates that more than 13,260 injuries related to backpacks were treated at doctors' offices, clinics, and emergency rooms in the year 2000. To avoid back strain, children carrying backpacks should bend both knees when lifting heavy packs, visit their locker or desk between classes to lighten loads or replace books, or purchase a backpack or airline tote on wheels.

What Conditions Are Associated with Low Back Pain?

Conditions that may cause low back pain and require treatment by a physician or other health specialist include:

- Bulging disk (also called protruding, herniated, or ruptured disk). The intervertebral disks are under constant pressure. As disks degenerate and weaken, cartilage can bulge or be pushed into the space containing the spinal cord or a nerve root, causing pain. Studies have shown that most herniated disks occur in the lower, lumbar portion of the spinal column.

- A much more serious complication of a ruptured disk is cauda equina syndrome, which occurs when disk material is pushed into the spinal canal and compresses the bundle of lumbar and sacral nerve roots. Permanent neurological damage may result if this syndrome is left untreated.

- Sciatica is a condition in which a herniated or ruptured disk presses on the sciatic nerve, the large nerve that extends down the spinal column to its exit point in the pelvis and carries nerve fibers to the leg. This compression causes shock-like or burning low back pain combined with pain through the buttocks and down one leg to below the knee, occasionally reaching the foot. In the most extreme cases, when the nerve is pinched between the disk and an adjacent bone, the symptoms involve not pain but numbness and some loss of motor control over the leg due to interruption of nerve signaling. The condition may also be caused by a tumor, cyst, metastatic disease, or degeneration of the sciatic nerve root.

- Spinal degeneration from disk wear and tear can lead to a narrowing of the spinal canal. A person with spinal degeneration may experience stiffness in the back upon awakening or may feel pain after walking or standing for a long time.

- Spinal stenosis related to congenital narrowing of the bony canal predisposes some people to pain related to disk disease.

- Osteoporosis is a metabolic bone disease marked by progressive decrease in bone density and strength. Fracture of brittle, porous bones in the spine and hips results when the body fails to produce new bone and/or absorbs too much existing bone. Women are four times more likely than men to develop osteoporosis. Caucasian women of northern European heritage are at the highest risk of developing the condition.

- Skeletal irregularities produce strain on the vertebrae and supporting muscles, tendons, ligaments, and tissues supported by spinal column. These irregularities include scoliosis, a curving of the spine to the side; kyphosis, in which the normal curve of the upper back is severely rounded; lordosis, an abnormally accentuated arch in the lower back; back extension, a bending backward of the spine; and back flexion, in which the spine bends forward.

- Fibromyalgia is a chronic disorder characterized by widespread musculoskeletal pain, fatigue, and multiple tender points, particularly in the neck, spine, shoulders, and hips. Additional symptoms may include sleep disturbances, morning stiffness, and anxiety.

- Spondylitis refers to chronic back pain and stiffness caused by a severe infection to or inflammation of the spinal joints. Other painful inflammations in the lower back include osteomyelitis (infection in the bones of the spine) and sacroiliitis (inflammation in the sacroiliac joints).

How Is Low Back Pain Diagnosed?

A thorough medical history and physical exam can usually identify any dangerous conditions or family history that may be associated with the pain. The patient describes the onset, site, and severity of the pain; duration of symptoms and any limitations in movement; and history of previous episodes or any health conditions that might be related to the pain. The physician will examine the back and conduct neurologic tests to determine the cause of pain and appropriate treatment. Blood tests may also be ordered. Imaging tests may be necessary to diagnose tumors or other possible sources of the pain.

A variety of diagnostic methods are available to confirm the cause of low back pain:

- X-ray imaging includes conventional and enhanced methods that can help diagnose the cause and site of back pain. A conventional x-ray, often the first imaging technique used, looks for broken bones or an injured vertebra. A technician passes a concentrated beam of low-dose ionized radiation through the back and takes pictures that, within minutes, clearly show the bony structure and any vertebral misalignment or fractures. Tissue masses such as injured muscles and ligaments or painful conditions such as a bulging disk are not visible on conventional x-rays. This fast, noninvasive, painless procedure is usually performed in a doctor's office or at a clinic.

- Discography involves the injection of a special contrast dye into a spinal disk thought to be causing low back pain. The dye outlines the damaged areas on x-rays taken following the injection. This procedure is often suggested for patients who are considering lumbar surgery or whose pain has not responded to conventional treatments. Myelograms also enhance the diagnostic imaging of an x-ray. In this procedure, the contrast dye is injected into the spinal canal, allowing spinal cord and nerve compression caused by herniated disks or fractures to be seen on an x-ray.

- Computerized tomography (CT) is a quick and painless process used when disk rupture, spinal stenosis, or damage to vertebrae is suspected as a cause of low back pain. X-rays are passed through the body at various angles and are detected by a computerized scanner to produce two-dimensional slices (1 millimeter each) of internal structures of the back. This diagnostic exam is generally conducted at an imaging center or hospital.

- Magnetic resonance imaging (MRI) is used to evaluate the lumbar region for bone degeneration or injury or disease in tissues and nerves, muscles, ligaments, and blood vessels. MRI scanning equipment creates a magnetic field around the body strong enough to temporarily realign water molecules in the tissues. Radio waves are then passed through the body to detect the relaxation of the molecules back to a random alignment and trigger a resonance signal at different angles within the body. A computer processes this resonance into either a three-dimensional picture or a two-dimensional slice of the tissue being scanned, and differentiates between bone, soft tissues and fluid-filled spaces by their water content and structural properties. This noninvasive procedure is often used to identify a condition requiring prompt surgical treatment.

- Electrodiagnostic procedures include electromyography (EMG), nerve conduction studies, and evoked potential (EP) studies. EMG assesses the electrical activity in a nerve and can detect if muscle weakness results from injury or a problem with the nerves that control the muscles. Very fine needles are inserted in muscles to measure electrical activity transmitted from the brain or spinal cord to a particular area of the body. With nerve conduction studies the doctor uses two sets of electrodes (similar to those used during an electrocardiogram) that are placed on the skin over the muscles. The first set gives the patient a mild shock to stimulate the nerve that runs to a particular muscle. The second set of electrodes is used to make a recording of the nerve's electrical signals, and from this information the doctor can determine if there is nerve damage. EP tests also involve two sets of electrodes—one set to stimulate a sensory nerve and the other set on the scalp to record the speed of nerve signal transmissions to the brain.

- Bone scans are used to diagnose and monitor infection, fracture, or disorders in the bone. A small amount of radioactive material is injected into the bloodstream and will collect in the bones, particularly in areas with some abnormality. Scanner-generated images are sent to a computer to identify specific areas of irregular bone metabolism or abnormal blood flow, as well as to measure levels of joint disease.

- Thermography involves the use of infrared sensing devices to measure small temperature changes between the two sides of the body or the temperature of a specific organ. Thermography may be used to detect the presence or absence of nerve root compression.

- Ultrasound imaging, also called ultrasound scanning or sonography, uses high-frequency sound waves to obtain images inside the body. The sound wave echoes are recorded and displayed as a real-time visual image. Ultrasound imaging can show tears in ligaments, muscles, tendons, and other soft tissue masses in the back.

How Is Back Pain Treated?

Most low back pain can be treated without surgery. Treatment involves using analgesics, reducing inflammation, restoring proper function and strength to the back, and preventing recurrence of the injury. Most patients with back pain recover without residual functional loss. Patients should contact a doctor if there is not a noticeable reduction in pain and inflammation after 72 hours of self-care.

Although ice and heat (the use of cold and hot compresses) have never been scientifically proven to quickly resolve low back injury, compresses may help reduce pain and inflammation and allow greater mobility for some individuals. As soon as possible following trauma, patients should apply a cold pack or a cold compress (such as a bag of ice or bag of frozen vegetables wrapped in a towel) to the tender spot several times a day for up to 20 minutes. After 2 to 3 days of cold treatment, they should then apply heat (such as a heating lamp or hot pad) for brief periods to relax muscles and increase blood flow. Warm baths may also help relax muscles. Patients should avoid sleeping on a heating pad, which can cause burns and lead to additional tissue damage.

Bed rest should be limited to 1 to 2 days at most. A 1996 Finnish study found that persons who continued their activities without bed rest following onset of low back pain appeared to have better back flexibility than those who rested in bed for a week. Other studies suggest that bed rest alone may make back pain worse and can lead to secondary complications such as depression, decreased muscle tone, and blood clots in the legs. Patients should resume activities as soon as possible. At night or during rest, patients should lie on one side, with a pillow between the knees (some doctors suggest resting on the back and putting a pillow beneath the knees).

Exercise may be the most effective way to speed recovery from low back pain and help strengthen back and abdominal muscles. Maintaining and building muscle strength is particularly important for persons with skeletal irregularities. Doctors and physical therapists can provide a list of gentle exercises that help keep muscles moving and speed the recovery process. A routine of back-healthy activities may include stretching exercises, swimming, walking, and movement therapy to improve coordination and develop proper posture and muscle balance. Yoga is another way to gently stretch muscles and ease pain. Any mild discomfort felt at the start of these exercises should disappear as muscles become stronger. But if pain is more than mild and lasts more than 15 minutes during exercise, patients should stop exercising and contact a doctor.

Medications are often used to treat acute and chronic low back pain. Effective pain relief may involve a combination of prescription drugs and over-the-counter remedies. Patients should always check with a doctor before taking drugs for pain relief. Certain medicines, even those sold over the counter, are unsafe during pregnancy, may conflict with other medications, may cause side effects including drowsiness, or may lead to liver damage.

- Over-the-counter analgesics, including nonsteroidal anti-inflammatory drugs (aspirin, naproxen, and ibuprofen), are taken orally to reduce stiffness, swelling, and inflammation and to ease mild to moderate low back pain. Counter-irritants applied topically to the skin as a cream or spray stimulate the nerve endings in the skin to provide feelings of warmth or cold and dull the sense of pain. Topical analgesics can also reduce inflammation and stimulate blood flow. Many of these compounds contain salicylates, the same ingredient found in oral pain medications containing aspirin.

- Anticonvulsants—drugs primarily used to treat seizures—may be useful in treating certain types of nerve pain and may also be prescribed with analgesics.

- Some antidepressants, particularly tricyclic antidepressants such as amitriptyline and desipramine, have been shown to relieve pain (independent of their effect on depression) and assist with sleep. Antidepressants alter levels of brain chemicals to elevate mood and dull pain signals. Many of the new antidepressants, such as the selective serotonin reuptake inhibitors, are being studied for their effectiveness in pain relief.

- Opioids such as codeine, oxycodone, hydrocodone, and morphine are often prescribed to manage severe acute and chronic back pain but should be used only for a short period of time and under a physician's supervision. Side effects can include drowsiness, decreased reaction time, impaired judgment, and potential for addiction. Many specialists are convinced that chronic use of these drugs is detrimental to the back pain patient, adding to depression and even increasing pain.

Spinal manipulation is literally a hands-on approach in which trained specialists (such as chiropractors, osteopaths, and massage therapists) use leverage and a series of exercises to adjust spinal structures and restore back mobility. These specialists do not prescribe drugs or use surgery in their treatment of low back pain.

When back pain does not respond to more conventional approaches, patients may consider the following options:

- Acupuncture involves the insertion of needles the width of a human hair along precise points throughout the body. Practitioners believe this process triggers the release of naturally occurring painkilling molecules called peptides and keeps the body's normal flow of energy unblocked. Clinical studies are measuring the effectiveness of acupuncture in comparison to more conventional procedures in the treatment of acute low back pain.

- Biofeedback is used to treat many acute pain problems, most notably back pain and headache. Using a special electronic machine, the patient is trained to become aware of, to follow, and to gain control over certain bodily functions, including muscle tension, heart rate, and skin temperature (by controlling local blood flow patterns). The patient can then learn to effect a change in his or her response to pain, for example, by using relaxation techniques. Biofeedback is often used in combination with other treatment methods, generally without side effects.

- Interventional therapy can ease chronic pain by blocking nerve conduction between specific areas of the body and the brain. Approaches range from injections of local anesthetics, steroids, or narcotics into affected soft tissues, joints, or nerve roots to more complex nerve blocks and spinal cord stimulation. When extreme pain is involved, low doses of drugs may be administered by catheter directly into the spinal cord. Chronic use of steroid injections may lead to increased functional impairment.

- Traction involves the use of weights to apply constant or intermittent force to gradually pull the skeletal structure into better alignment. Traction is not recommended for treating acute low back symptoms.

- Transcutaneous electrical nerve stimulation (TENS) is administered by a battery-powered device that sends mild electric pulses along nerve fibers to block pain signals to the brain. Small electrodes placed on the skin at or near the site of pain generate nerve impulses that block incoming pain signals from the peripheral nerves. TENS may also help stimulate the brain's production of endorphins (chemicals that have pain-relieving properties).

- Ultrasound is a noninvasive therapy used to warm the body's internal tissues, which causes muscles to relax. Sound waves pass through the skin and into the injured muscles and other soft tissues.

- Minimally invasive outpatient treatments to seal fractures of the vertebrae caused by osteoporosis include vertebroplasty and kyphoplasty. Vertebroplasty uses three-dimensional imaging to help a doctor guide a fine needle into the vertebral body. A glue-like epoxy is injected, which quickly hardens to stabilize and strengthen the bone and provide immediate pain relief. In kyphoplasty, prior to injecting the epoxy, a special balloon is inserted and gently inflated to restore height to the bone and reduce spinal deformity.

In the most serious cases, when the condition does not respond to other therapies, surgery may relieve pain caused by back problems or serious musculoskeletal injuries. Some surgical procedures may be performed in a doctor's office under local anesthesia, whereas others require hospitalization. It may be months following surgery before the patient is fully healed, and he or she may suffer permanent loss of flexibility. Since invasive back surgery is not always successful, it should be performed only in patients with progressive neurologic disease or damage to the peripheral nerves.

- Discectomy is one of the more common ways to remove pressure on a nerve root from a bulging disk or bone spur. During the procedure the surgeon takes out a small piece of the lamina (the arched bony roof of the spinal canal) to remove the obstruction below.

- Foraminotomy is an operation that cleans out or enlarges the bony hole (foramen) where a nerve root exits the spinal canal. Bulging disks or joints thickened with age can cause narrowing of the space through which the spinal nerve exits and can press on the nerve, resulting in pain, numbness, and weakness in an arm or leg. Small pieces of bone over the nerve are removed through a small slit, allowing the surgeon to cut away the blockage and relieve the pressure on the nerve.

- IntraDiscal Electrothermal Therapy (IDET) uses thermal energy to treat pain resulting from a cracked or bulging spinal disk. A special needle is inserted via a catheter into the disk and heated to a high temperature for up to 20 minutes. The heat thickens and seals the disk wall and reduces inner disk bulge and irritation of the spinal nerve.

- Nucleoplasty uses radiofrequency energy to treat patients with low back pain from contained, or mildly herniated, disks. Guided by x-ray imaging, a wand-like instrument is inserted through a needle into the disk to create a channel that allows inner disk material to be removed. The wand then heats and shrinks the tissue, sealing the disk wall. Several channels are made depending on how much disk material needs to be removed.

- Radiofrequency lesioning is a procedure using electrical impulses to interrupt nerve conduction (including the conduction of pain signals) for 6 to 12 months. Using x-ray guidance, a special needle is inserted into nerve tissue in the affected area. Tissue surrounding the needle tip is heated for 90 to 120 seconds, resulting in localized destruction of the nerves.

- Spinal fusion is used to strengthen the spine and prevent painful movements. The spinal disk(s) between two or more vertebrae is removed and the adjacent vertebrae are fused by bone grafts and/or metal devices secured by screws. Spinal fusion may result in some loss of flexibility in the spine and requires a long recovery period to allow the bone grafts to grow and fuse the vertebrae together.

- Spinal laminectomy (also known as spinal decompression) involves the removal of the lamina (usually both sides) to increase the size of the spinal canal and relieve pressure on the spinal cord and nerve roots.

Other surgical procedures to relieve severe chronic pain include rhizotomy, in which the nerve root close to where it enters the spinal cord is cut to block nerve transmission and all senses from the area of the body experiencing pain; cordotomy, where bundles of nerve fibers on one or both sides of the spinal cord are intentionally severed to stop the transmission of pain signals to the brain; and dorsal root entry zone operation, or DREZ, in which spinal neurons transmitting the patient's pain are destroyed surgically.

Can Back Pain Be Prevented?

Recurring back pain resulting from improper body mechanics or other nontraumatic causes is often preventable. A combination of exercises that don't jolt or strain the back, maintaining correct posture, and lifting objects properly can help prevent injuries.

Many work-related injuries are caused or aggravated by stressors such as heavy lifting, contact stress (repeated or constant contact between soft body tissue and a hard or sharp object, such as resting a wrist against the edge of a hard desk or repeated tasks using a hammering motion), vibration, repetitive motion, and awkward posture. Applying ergonomic principles—designing furniture and tools to protect the body from injury—at home and in the workplace can greatly reduce the risk of back injury and help maintain a healthy back. More companies and homebuilders are promoting ergonomically designed tools, products, workstations, and living space to reduce the risk of musculoskeletal injury and pain.

The use of wide elastic belts that can be tightened to pull in lumbar and abdominal muscles to prevent low back pain remains controversial. A landmark study of the use of lumbar support or abdominal support belts worn by persons who lift or move merchandise found no evidence that the belts reduce back injury or back pain. The 2-year study, reported by the National Institute for Occupational Safety and Health (NIOSH) in December 2000, found no statistically significant difference in either the incidence of workers' compensation claims for job-related back injuries or the incidence of self-reported pain among workers who reported they wore back belts daily compared to those workers who reported never using back belts or reported using them only once or twice a month.

Although there have been anecdotal case reports of injury reduction among workers using back belts, many companies that have back belt programs also have training and ergonomic awareness programs. The reported injury reduction may be related to a combination of these or other factors.

Quick Tips to a Healthier Back

Following any period of prolonged inactivity, begin a program of regular low-impact exercises. Speed walking, swimming, or stationary bike riding 30 minutes a day can increase muscle strength and flexibility. Yoga can also help stretch and strengthen muscles and improve posture. Ask your physician or orthopedist for a list of low-impact exercises appropriate for your age and designed to strengthen lower back and abdominal muscles.

- Always stretch before exercise or other strenuous physical activity.

- Don't slouch when standing or sitting. When standing, keep your weight balanced on your feet. Your back supports weight most easily when curvature is reduced.

- At home or work, make sure your work surface is at a comfortable height for you.

- Sit in a chair with good lumbar support and proper position and height for the task. Keep your shoulders back. Switch sitting positions often and periodically walk around the office or gently stretch muscles to relieve tension. A pillow or rolled-up towel placed behind the small of your back can provide some lumbar support. If you must sit for a long period of time, rest your feet on a low stool or a stack of books.

- Wear comfortable, low-heeled shoes.

- Sleep on your side to reduce any curve in your spine. Always sleep on a firm surface.

- Ask for help when transferring an ill or injured family member from a reclining to a sitting position or when moving the patient from a chair to a bed.

- Don't try to lift objects too heavy for you. Lift with your knees, pull in your stomach muscles, and keep your head down and in line with your straight back. Keep the object close to your body. Do not twist when lifting.

- Maintain proper nutrition and diet to reduce and prevent excessive weight, especially weight around the waistline that taxes lower back muscles. A diet with sufficient daily intake of calcium, phosphorus, and vitamin D helps to promote new bone growth.

- If you smoke, quit. Smoking reduces blood flow to the lower spine and causes the spinal disks to degenerate.

What Research Is Being Done?

The National Institute of Neurological Disorders and Stroke, a component of the National Institutes of Health (NIH) within the U.S. Department of Health and Human Services, is the nation's leading federal funder of research on disorders of the brain and nervous system and one of the primary NIH components that supports research on pain and pain mechanisms.

Other institutes at NIH that support pain research include the National Institute of Dental and Craniofacial Research, the National Cancer Institute, the National Institute on Drug Abuse, the National Institute of Mental Health, the National Center for Complementary and Alternative Medicine, and the National Institute of Arthritis and Musculoskeletal and Skin Diseases. Additionally, other federal organizations, such as the Department of Veterans Affairs and the Centers for Disease Control and Prevention, conduct studies on low back pain.

Scientists are examining the use of different drugs to effectively treat back pain, in particular daily pain that has lasted at least 6 months. Other studies are comparing different health care approaches to the management of acute low back pain (standard care versus chiropractic, acupuncture, or massage therapy). These studies are measuring symptom relief, restoration of function, and patient satisfaction. Other research is comparing standard surgical treatments to the most commonly used standard nonsurgical treatments to measure changes in health-related quality of life among patients suffering from spinal stenosis. NIH-funded research at the Consortial Center for Chiropractic Research encourages the development of high-quality chiropractic projects. The Center also encourages collaboration between basic and clinical scientists and between the conventional and chiropractic medical communities.

Other researchers are studying whether low-dose radiation can decrease scarring around the spinal cord and improve the results of surgery. Still others are exploring why spinal cord injury and other neurological changes lead to an increased sensitivity to pain or a decreased pain threshold (where normally non-painful sensations are perceived as painful, a class of symptoms called neuropathic pain), and how fractures of the spine and their repair affect the spinal canal and intervertebral foramen (openings around the spinal roots).

Also under study for patients with degenerative disk disease is artificial spinal disk replacement surgery. The damaged disk is removed and a metal and plastic disk about the size of a quarter is inserted into the spine. Ideal candidates for disk replacement surgery are persons between the ages of 20 and 60 who have only one degenerating disk, do not have a systemic bone disease such as osteoporosis, have not had previous back surgery, and have failed to respond to other forms of nonsurgical treatment. Compared to other forms of back surgery, recovery from this form of surgery appears to be shorter and the procedure has fewer complications.

Where Can I Go for More Information?

The following organizations have information on lower back pain:

American Academy of Neurological and Orthopaedic Surgeons
2300 South Rancho Drive
Suite 202
Las Vegas, NV 89102
Phone: (702) 388-7390
Website: http://www.aanos.org

American Association of Neurological Surgeons
5550 Meadowbrook Drive
Rolling Meadows, IL 60008-3852
Toll-Free: (888) 566-2267
Website: http://www.aans.org

American Academy of Orthopaedic Surgeons (AAOS)
6300 North River Road
Rosemont, IL 60018-4262
Toll-Free: (800) 824-BONE (2663)
Phone: (847) 823-7186
Fax: (847) 823-8125
Website: http://www.aaos.org
E-mail: custserv@aaos.org

American Academy of Physical Medicine and Rehabilitation
One IBM Plaza
Suite 2500
Chicago, IL 60611-3604
Phone: (312) 464-9700
Fax: (312) 464-0227
Website: http://www.aapmr.org
E-mail: info@aapmr.org

American Academy of Family Physicians
11400 Tomahawk Creek Parkway
Leawood, KS 66211-2672
Toll-Free: (800) 274-2237
Phone: (913) 906-6000
Website: http://www.aafp.org

American Chiropractic Association
1701 Clarendon Boulevard
Arlington, VA 22209
Toll-Free: (800) 986-4636
Website: http://www.amerchiro.org

American Chronic Pain Association
P.O. Box 850
Rocklin, CA 95677
Toll-Free: (800) 533-3231
Phone: (916) 632-0922
Fax: (916) 632-3208
Website: http://www.theacpa.org
E-mail: ACPA@pacbell.net

American Pain Foundation
201 N. Charles Street
Suite 710
Baltimore, MD 21201-4111
Toll-Free: (888) 615-PAIN (7246)
Website: http://www.painfoundation.org
E-mail: info@painfoundation.org

National Institute of Arthritis and Musculoskeletal and Skin Diseases
1 AMS Circle
Bethesda, MD 20892-3675
Toll-Free: (877) 22-NIAMS (226-4267)
Phone: (301) 495-4484
TTY: (301) 565-2966
Fax: (301) 718-6366
Website: http://www.niams.nih.gov
E-mail: niamsinfo@mail.nih.gov

Chapter 6

Back Pain in Children and Teens

While back pain is very common for adults, kids are much more resilient and flexible and do not suffer the same types of back injuries to which adults are subject. In fact, medically significant back pain in children and teens is infrequently encountered, with even fewer cases in younger children.

Because children rarely suffer from back pain, any complaint by a child or teenager about acute or chronic back pain is taken very seriously by pediatricians, and usually will result in a detailed consultation that will include a review of the child's medical history and a physical exam.

Suspicious episodes of pain, or any concerning features of the pain, will result in radiological studies (such as an x-ray or MRI scan) and possibly a referral to a specialist for further examination and diagnostic tests.

The most common causes of back pain in children and teens tend to be somewhat age-dependent:

- **Younger children** are less likely to be putting their spine under the same severe stresses as older children and adults. Thus, for the most part younger children do not have medically significant back pain and their discomfort tends to be short-lived. Also, younger children tend to self-limit their activity, choosing not to repeat painful activities, which aids in their recovery if an episode of back pain does occur. At a young age, if a child has back pain there is greater concern for the possibility of a serious condition, such as a spinal tumor, growth, or an infection of the spine. Therefore, if the pain persists in a younger child despite a lack of re-injury, or if there are other symptoms suggestive of a more insidious process (infection or tumor), the child's condition will most likely be considered atypical, and therefore, further work-up and medical examination will be indicated.

- **Older children** tend to be more aggressive in their activities and sports, thereby increasing the risk of injury to the bones, nerves, and soft tissues in the spine. Teenagers are also more likely to test the limits of their bodies, often being exhorted by commercial advertising and/or peer pressure to push the envelope. At this point, compression fractures are more commonplace, and we begin to see occasional disc injuries. Older pediatric patients also can injure the joints between vertebral bones, causing painful stress injuries. Only very rarely do the nerve roots become compromised. Slightly older children can be convinced to minimize their activity to speed up healing times, but then they frequently return to the same injurious behavior that caused the initial damage. Here, older kids may also find themselves the victims of their own intermittent inactivity and suffer overuse injuries. For most injuries, the treatment of choice is usually a short period of rest with an eye towards developing and maintaining physical conditioning. Tumors and infection of the spine may occur in teens, but it is more common for back pain to be caused by sports injuries or overuse syndromes.

Scoliosis

While scoliosis (curvature of the spine) is not an uncommon diagnosis among teenagers, it is very rare that scoliosis will cause back pain. Teens with scoliosis may develop back pain, just as other teenagers, but it has not been found that people with adolescent idiopathic scoliosis are any more likely to develop back pain than the rest of the population.

Causes of Back Pain in Children and Teens

Potential Causes of Back Pain in Children and Teens

While adults can have vertebral disc injuries involving rupture, protrusion or slipping, and compression, these problems are uncommon in children. However, as kids age and their bodies mature, it becomes more likely that an injury to the spinal discs may occur and cause pain.

Causes of Back Pain that Tends to Occur in Older Children

- **Spondylolysis.** As kids' sporting events become more competitive and the activities more specialized, certain types of injuries tend to arise. Spondylolysis, a defect of the joint between vertebral bones, is commonly found in those who tend to hyperextend their backs (bend backward), such as gymnasts. This injury may actually represent a stress fracture and the period of rest and recuperation may be extensive—up to 4 to 6 weeks.

- **Spondylolisthesis.** Occasionally, further injury can be found as spondylolisthesis, a slipping of one vertebra upon another. This condition can progress through adolescence, and if it results in instability and pain it may require spinal fusion surgery at a later point.

- **Disc injuries and vertebral fractures.** Teens who tend to punish their spines through gymnastics or extreme sports (such as skateboarding, in-line skating, and vert biking) will frequently land very hard on their feet or buttocks. Either way, the force is transmitted to their vertebrae, which can result in a vertebral fracture and/or damage to the intervertebral discs. If the disc material is extruded out or herniated, the spinal cord nerve roots leaving the cord can be compressed. This causes the sensation of pain along the path of that nerve. A well-known version of this is sciatica, which presents as buttock pain radiating down the back of a leg. Conservative measures are usually the first line of treatment for this type of pain (such as physical therapy, medications, and osteopathic or chiropractic manipulation). If these treatments do not provide sufficient pain relief, patients may require surgery (e.g., a microdiscectomy or discectomy) to relieve pressure on the nerve.

Causes of Back Pain That May Occur in Younger or Older Children

- **Infection.** Of constant concern to physicians is the diagnosis of infection of the spine (discitis) in children. An infection of the spine is of great consequence and requires prompt diagnosis. Diagnosis of an infection is usually made with the assistance of a good physical exam and laboratory data. Signs of inflammation may be present (e.g., redness, swelling) even to the level of the skin. Radiographic studies are frequently normal. Treatment may consist of antibiotics if bacteria are found to be the cause of the infection. Again, prolonged rest is the primary treatment.

- **Tumor.** Another major concern for pediatricians is potential for a tumor in the spine in children. This is a very rare occurrence. As with infection of the spine, the diagnosis hinges on obtaining a good medical history, physical exam, and the suspicious nature of physicians when they cannot get an otherwise satisfactory diagnosis to explain the child's symptoms. Treatment once again depends upon the final diagnosis and the skills of several subspecialties.

Backpacks

Importantly, pediatricians are starting to see a new form of injury in school-age children and teens become more common: overuse injuries and back strain caused by carrying backpacks that are too heavy.

Often, backpacks may equal 20% to 40% of the child's own body weight (equivalent to a 150-pound adult carrying a 30- to 60-pound back pack around 5 days a week). This amount of weight understandably creates a great deal of strain on the child's spine. Additional strain is caused when children and teens carry the backpack over one shoulder, causing an uneven load on the spine.

Summary

As you may have noted, rest and careful monitoring of symptoms seems to be the answer for most diagnoses. This is because the vast majority of back pain problems in children are related to soft tissue damage (such as muscles, ligaments and tendons), which is often caused by overuse or strain.

Surgery for back pain in children is very rare, and is usually only considered for the more severe cases. If the child's pain is severe, and he or she is having difficulty functioning, then surgery may be considered.

Most importantly, a careful process of elimination of medically more significant causes of back pain (such as tumor, infection, or fracture) should always precede any therapeutic plan.

Chapter 7

Back Pain in Athletes

The lumbar spine, or lower back, is an area that is subjected to many types of stresses and forces during athletic competition. The lumbar region is susceptible to injuries and athletes will experience their share of them. The most common cause of low back injuries is acute trauma or chronic stress. All conditions affecting the lumbar spine can be aggravated by various contributing factors, such as inadequate or inappropriate conditioning, inflexibility of the hamstrings or lumbar spine, congenital abnormalities, or poor posture.

The most common injuries to the lumbar spine region are contusions, sprains, and strains. Contusions are caused by a direct blow to the low back region and usually affect the paraspinal muscles. Muscle strains and ligament sprains are common in the low back. Both types of injuries are caused by the same types of forces. Violent muscle contractions against resistance, overuse, and overstretching are the most common mechanisms resulting in sprains and strains in the soft tissues in the back.

Sprains and strains are very common injuries and will affect almost all athletes. These injuries will resolve with therapy and active rest. If an athlete chooses to ignore their back pain, a simple strain can progress to disc injuries or bony fractures. Treating these injuries at an early stage will assist the athlete in returning to competition sooner.

Treatment of lumbar injuries begins with prevention. Every athlete must be in proper physical condition prior to the season, and have worked on flexibility. Proper conditioning and flexibility will prevent most lumbar injuries from occurring. Proper conditioning should include aerobic conditioning and strength training. Proper core (abdominal and back) strengthening is very important for optimal sport performance and injury prevention. Flexibility training should concentrate on the hamstrings and gluteal muscles to prevent lumbar injuries.

Treatment after the lower back is injured begins with ice, as in any acute injury. The extent of the injury must then be determined. Many of these injuries are due to muscle spasm and can be treated quite easily. A smaller number are more serious, however. The signs and symptoms of a more serious back injury are severe pain, inability to touch the toes without severe pain, pain radiating down one or both legs, an electrical shooting pain down one or both legs, one or both legs do not seem to function properly, or the inability to run due to leg weakness.

The most common major injuries in the lumbar spine are spondylolysis and spondylolisthesis. These two injuries involve a fracture in the pars interarticularis, the area where two vertebrae form a joint. Spondylolysis is often referred to as a "scottie dog fracture," due to the shape of the bone involved. Plain film x-rays will show a fracture that appears to be the collar on a scottie dog. Spondylolisthesis results when the fracture becomes unstable and the vertebrae on top slides forward on the vertebrae below. These conditions are very common in football lineman and gymnasts. This is due to the large amount of back extension (backward bending) that these athletes must endure during participation. Both of these conditions are extremely painful and can result in life-long disability if treated improperly. It is important to consult a physician when dealing with long-term back pain to rule out these conditions.

One other area of concern with back injuries is to rule out a vertebral disc injury. The vertebral disc is located between the vertebral bodies. These structures serve as cushions and allow for smooth motion in the spine. The disc is structured like a jelly donut; there is a hard outer crust (annulus fibrosus) and a soft middle (nucleus pulposus). When long-term stress is applied to the hard outer crust, it begins to weaken and the soft middle begins to protrude. The resulting protrusion pinches on the nerve roots as they exit the vertebral column. This leads to muscle spasm and may lead to nerve damage if not treated appropriately.

Once the extent of the injury has been determined, proper rehabilitation can begin. If a physician has been consulted, remember to follow his or her suggestions before beginning any exercises. Evidence now shows complete rest is detrimental to proper healing. Active rest is the choice of sports medicine physicians and athletic trainers. Active rest involves flexibility training, cycling, walking, gentle strengthening, the use of therapeutic modalities, and/or physician prescribed anti-inflammatory and muscle relaxant medications.

Chapter 8

Neck Pain

Your head and neck region is vulnerable to many different stresses. Bad posture can cause misalignment of your neck, head, and spine. Car accidents can cause whiplash. Age and wear and tear can cause arthritis. Even activities such as gum chewing and reading in bed can cause pain. How do we avoid these potential problems? And if we can't avoid them, how can we recover as quickly as possible?

In this chapter you will learn about:

- The basic anatomy of the neck region;

- Common reasons for neck pain and headaches;

- Ways to reduce stress and the risk of injury;

- Exercises to do at home; and

- How a physical therapist can help.

Whatever the nature of your problem, physical therapy by a licensed physical therapist can often help you recover function quickly and teach you new habits to minimize the risk of further pain or injury.

Adapted from "What You Need to Know about Neck Pain," 1996, with permission from the American Physical Therapy Association. This material is copyrighted, and any further reproduction or distribution is prohibited. Reviewed by David A. Cooke, M.D., on March 20, 2004.

Anatomy of the Neck Region

One of the most flexible regions of the spine is the neck (cervical) region, which consists of vertebrae, seven shock-absorbing disks, muscles, and vertebral ligaments to hold them in place. The uppermost cervical disk connects the top of the spinal column to the base of the skull. The spinal cord, which sends nerve impulses to every part of the body, runs through a canal in the cervical vertebrae and continues all the way down the spine. The cervical nerves spread down into the arms; because of this, arm pain is sometimes traceable to a problem in the neck.

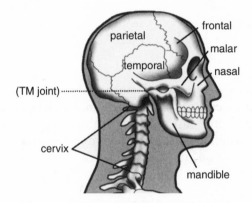

Figure 8.1. *Bones of the neck and head.*

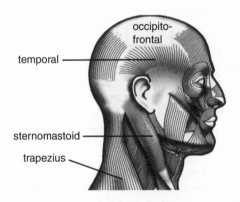

Figure 8.2. *Muscles of the neck and head.*

Possible Causes of Neck Pain and Headaches

One of the most common causes of neck pain, and sometimes headaches, is poor posture. It's easy to get into bad posture habits without even realizing it—even an activity as innocent as reading in bed can ultimately lead to pain, headaches, and more serious problems.

The basic rule is simple: Keep your neck in a neutral position whenever possible. In other words, don't bend or hunch your neck forward for long periods. Also, try not to sit in one position for a long time. If you must sit for an extended period, make sure your posture is good: Keep your head in a neutral position, make sure your back is supported, keep your knees slightly lower than your hips, and rest your arms if possible.

Reading in bed can cause neck strain—especially if you're propped up on several pillows, bending your neck forward, and trying to hold your arms out in order to support the book. If you do read in bed, make it easy on your neck: Consider purchasing one of the products specifically designed for this purpose, such as a wedge pillow to prop up the book or a portable mini desk. Finally, remember not to stay in any single position too long—our bodies are designed to move.

Your sleeping position is another possible source of neck problems. Does your pillow cause you to sleep with your neck at an angle, either too high or too low? If so, you may want to invest in a new pillow. Feather pillows are generally preferable to foam; they conform easily to the shape of the neck.

Also, remember that pillows don't last forever. After a year or so feather pillows tend to collapse and may need to be replaced. In addition, a bed that doesn't offer enough back support can also be a source of neck discomfort.

Here are some other tips to help you avoid neck strain and pain:

• Try doing stretching exercises before bed and first thing in the morning;

• Don't sleep on your stomach—this position puts great pressure on the neck; and

• Don't "over-pillow" your neck; keep your neck and spine in a neutral position.

The neutral position rule also holds true for people who spend time working at computer terminals. Again, don't bend your neck forward. Adjust your desk, monitor, and chair to a comfortable height, so that the monitor is at eye level and your knees are slightly lower than your hips. Some people find that a footstool helps in attaining this correct position. Sit close enough to the monitor so that you don't have to bend forward in order to see well. Use the chair's armrests—your arms need support. Wear your eyeglasses if necessary. Consult your physical therapist to find the setup that is right for you.

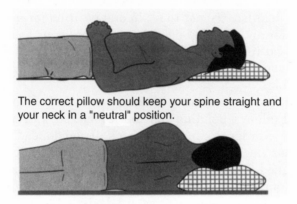

The correct pillow should keep your spine straight and your neck in a "neutral" position.

Figure 8.3. The best sleeping position to prevent neck pain.

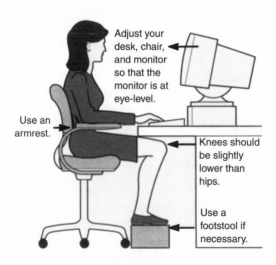

Adjust your desk, chair, and monitor so that the monitor is at eye-level.

Use an armrest.

Knees should be slightly lower than hips.

Use a footstool if necessary.

Figure 8.4. Prevent neck pain at your computer workstation.

You should also follow the neutral position rule when driving a car. Adjust the seat to bring you close enough to the pedals so that you don't have to extend your neck forward.

Proper Lifting Technique

Another cause of neck pain is poor lifting technique. People often think of the lower back as the area at risk, but the cervical region is nearly as vulnerable. Here is the correct way to lift:

- Stand up straight, close to the object.

- Bend at your hips and knees, keeping your back in the neutral position and your head and shoulders up.

- Firmly grasp the object and rise up with your hip and leg muscles.

- Keep the object close to your body. Your hips and legs absorb most of the weight, and you will put less strain on your back and neck.

- The feet should be positioned shoulder-width apart, with one foot slightly ahead of the other.

In addition, you may find that placing one foot forward and one foot back may be easier than trying to lift an object from the squatting position.

Avoiding Neck Stress

Other bad habits to avoid include:

- Shopper's tilt—carrying items on one shoulder for a long period; and
- Carrying items that are too heavy.

Shopper's tilt can be avoided by using a backpack-style bag to more evenly distribute the weight you're carrying. (Be sure to wear the backpack correctly, with both arms through the shoulder loops, or the benefit will be lost.) A variation on shopper's tilt—traveler's droop— is a familiar experience to anyone who has ever tried to lug a heavy suitcase across an airline terminal. Again, a backpack can be helpful, or consider purchasing a compact rolling suitcase with wheels and a retractable handle.

Believe it or not, simply talking on the phone can create neck problems. Some people are in the habit of cradling the telephone receiver between the shoulder and the neck. Not only does this put stress on the neck, but over a long period it can cause the cervical disks to place pressure on the nerves. If you spend a great deal of time on the phone, you might try one of the products designed to make it a more comfortable experience—neck cradles, speaker phones, or a hands-free headset.

TMJ Disorders

The TMJ—temporomandibular joint—is the joint at which the jaw is hinged to the skull. Painful TMJ problems occur in people who overuse or abuse this joint through teeth grinding, constant clenching and unclenching of the jaw, or excessive gum chewing. Sometimes people are born with a misalignment of the jaw that can bring on similar symptoms.

Because the neck and the TMJ are so closely connected, the TMJ can cause neck pain—and vice versa. In some cases a dentist may need to create an oral retainer to allow the joint to rest and let healing begin. After that, a physical therapist can help minimize the pain in the jaw or neck through a custom-designed exercise program.

Migraine Headaches

True migraine headaches are most likely the result of problems affecting the blood vessels in the head or of an allergic reaction. However, many other types of headaches can mimic migraines and are often misdiagnosed. Some of these originate in the neck or jaw, such as the TMJ disorders mentioned above.

If you don't have all the symptoms of migraines—nausea, problems with vision, and pain—get a second opinion, particularly if the pain is triggered by motion of the neck. If you don't have a true migraine, a physical therapist can help diagnose the actual source of the pain. Once an evaluation is made, your physical therapist will help you create a comfortable and appropriate home and work environment and will design a program of rest (if needed) and exercise. If the source of your headache is in the TMJ (jaw) area, your physical therapist may consult with your dentist who may create a special oral retainer in order to discourage bad habits such as teeth grinding.

Other Kinds of Headaches

Most people know from experience that emotional stress can cause headaches. These headaches can be treated in a variety of ways, from taking nonprescription pain relievers to practicing meditation. Most simple headaches will go away by themselves; however, if the headache is persistent or recurring, make sure that neck strain, poor posture, or eyestrain isn't the culprit. If your headache is severe or persists for more than a few days, it is important to seek professional attention right away. Sometimes muscles in the back of the neck can irritate nerves in the head, causing a headache. If you are having headaches, a physical therapist will first make a careful evaluation of your problem (often in consultation with a physician). After pinpointing the problem, he or she will design a program of rest, exercise, stretching, and other treatments that are very effective in eliminating the cause of your headaches.

Osteoarthritis

Osteoarthritis is inflammation of the joints caused by wear and tear. All of us experience some degree of osteoarthritis as we grow older, but the condition can also be caused by injuries. Osteoarthritis in the neck is characterized by stiffness and limited range of motion.

Physical therapy can be a great help in treating osteoarthritis. Through exercise, stretching, massage, and other therapeutic techniques, the physical therapist can gently and slowly help the patient ease the stiffness and increase range of motion.

Whiplash

Whiplash—a violent back-and-forth motion of the neck—is probably the most common traumatic injury to the neck region. It is frequently associated with automobile accidents, although it occasionally occurs in other situations (such as skiing accidents or amusement park rides). In acute cases, a device known as a cervical collar may be appropriate in order to rest the neck and calm the inflammation. Once the tissue has been rested, a physical therapy program designed to regain strength, function, and range of motion can begin.

Is It Only a Pain in the Neck?

Pain in the cervical region can cause arm pain as well as the pain in the neck. Why? In the case of the arms, it's because the nerves that branch out from the neck go all the way down into the arms and into the hands. Sometimes it's difficult to tell whether the pain is actually originating in the neck, or the arms, or both.

Symptoms in the arms include numbness, tingling, cold, aching, and pins and needles. These symptoms can be confused with carpal tunnel syndrome (CTS), a condition found in people who work at computer keyboards or perform other repetitive motion tasks for extended periods. In CTS, the nerve sheath that runs down the center of the forearm becomes inflamed and restricts the gliding movement of the nerve. It is possible, however, for a nerve impingement to start much further up the chain in the neck region. It's also possible for the nerve impingement to be taking place both in the neck and in the arm.

What to Do When Your Neck Is Hurting

When your neck hurts, and no major trauma is involved, rest is the first order of business. But don't stuff too many pillows under your neck—that will only make things worse. The goal is to keep your spine and neck in a neutral position. Make sure that the gap between the back of your neck and the bed is filled in by a pillow (or foam support) that keeps your neck in a neutral position.

You can also apply ice or heat. Many physical therapists prefer ice because of its effectiveness in reducing pain and inflammation. (To use ice, fill a plastic bag with crushed ice, place a towel over the affected area, then apply the ice-filled bag to the area.) Heat also provides relief to some people, but should be used with caution because it can sometimes make an inflamed area worse.

Apply heat or ice for 15 to 20 minutes at a time, and give yourself a 40-minute rest between applications. If you use both heat and ice, make sure to alternate between the two.

How Physical Therapy Can Help with Neck Pain and Headaches

Physical therapy always begins with a detailed history and evaluation of the problem. Your physical therapist will take many things into account, including your age, general health, occupation, and lifestyle. If major trauma or disease is involved, your physical therapist will work with you in consultation with a physician.

After a diagnosis has been made, your physical therapist may choose from a range of treatment options, including exercises for flexibility, strength, stability, and restoration of range of motion. Other options include ice, heat, electrical stimulation, traction or mobilization, and massage. Your physical therapist may also analyze your home and work environment in order to ensure that you're not reinjuring yourself.

Much evidence suggests that low-impact aerobic exercise such as swimming, walking, low-impact aerobics, and stationary bicycling may also be helpful in decreasing neck pain. A physical therapist can design a pain-free exercise program just for you.

Once your physical therapy goals are met, your physical therapist will help you continue therapy on your own with a home program designed to fit your needs. The goal of physical therapy is to return you to normal activity as quickly as possible, with the knowledge you need to minimize or eliminate your problem.

Neck and Head Pain Questions and Answers

Is arm pain, numbness, tingling, and weakness related to neck pain? Will I need surgery?

Because the nerves in the cervical region radiate down through the arms, these symptoms can sometimes be related to neck pain. While surgery is sometimes required to reduce pressure on the nerves, many cases can be treated effectively through physical therapy.

Is surgery beneficial for chronic neck pain?

Surgery may be the treatment of choice in isolated cases—for example, if you have a condition known as spinal stenosis (in which the openings for the nerve roots or spinal cord become smaller, often due to osteoarthritis). In most cases conservative treatment, including physical therapy and/or medication, is preferable.

Is it all right to take medication such as aspirin for my neck pain and headache?

Yes, although anti-inflammatories such as NSAIDs (non-steroidal anti-inflammatory drugs) or aspirin can cause stomach upset or ringing in the ears. Be aware that acetaminophen can help with pain but not inflammation. Consult your pharmacist about the medication you are taking. Do not take medication that is old or previously prescribed for someone else.

73

How long before I get better?

The nature of your injury will determine how long it takes to heal. In general, recovery from neck sprains or strains can take anywhere from a few weeks to a few months, depending on the severity of the injury, your age and ability to heal, and other factors.

Your recovery will be faster if you follow the program designed by your physical therapist. Your program will probably include exercises and other treatments designed to ensure that the neck heals properly and regains its normal range of motion. Without proper treatment, prolonged stiffness and discomfort may result.

Chapter 9

Initial Treatment for Back and Neck Disorders

Chapter Contents

Section 9.1

Preparing for Your Consultation with a Spine Doctor

Doctor visits can be intimidating and—especially when you're in pain—it can be difficult to describe your situation in a complete, concise, and accurate manner. However, it will serve you well to prepare for questions your doctor is likely to ask in advance—this way, you can avoid feeling like you didn't tell your doctor something important during the visit, and by providing complete and accurate information you can help your doctor arrive at an accurate diagnosis.

During your first visit to a spine specialist, a complete medical history will typically be taken. The physician will then review the history and related information and collect additional information during your physical exam.

If it is your first visit to the doctor, you will probably be asked several questions by the staff about payment, such as if you have insurance coverage, Medicare, if your injury is part of a worker's compensation claim, or involved in litigation or a similar situation. You may be asked if you will be able to pay for all or a part of your medical/surgical expenses if it is required.

It is important to be ready to answer the questions your doctor will ask or to fill in the details if and when asked. Basically, the better prepared you are for your doctor's visit the more productive it will be for you and for your physician.

Tips for How to Respond to the Physician's Questions

- Be prepared—read the list of questions that follow and be prepared to respond to them succinctly and accurately. Some people find it helps to write out their answers ahead of time and to write out the questions they need to ask the doctor as well.

- Be complete but brief—be sure not to leave out any important points about your situation, but try to be as concise and to the point as possible.

- Be honest—the doctor is more likely to be able to help you if you provide candid information. If some questions do not apply, cannot be answered, or are too sensitive for you, be prepared to respond if asked—why? Privacy will always be preserved but some sensitive details may be very important to your diagnosis and care.

The following list of possible questions relate to issues that are important to your spine doctor in determining the diagnosis and type of care to be recommended. Informed patients who can accurately and succinctly describe their situation to the physician play a critical role sharing in decision making for their medical care.

The following and more questions might be asked in person or on a questionnaire sheet.

- Medical/family/other history
- Details about present spine problems
- If you need surgery

Medical and Family History

Personal Medical and Health History

Basic information that your physician will probably ask for includes: your name, birthday, age, sex, marital status, and social security number, religion, race, or ethnic group.

More extensive information will be requested regarding any other health problems, such as:

- Do you have any chronic, recurrent health problems, aside from the back or neck?

- If so, what is the diagnosis and how is it treated and by whom? Give details. Who is your doctor for this or any of the other problems listed above?

For any of the above, discuss the treatment, how often, and from whom you are now being treated, such as:

- Medications taken (listing medication name, strength, daily dosage, and purpose). For example, do you take aspirin, arthritis medicine, blood thinners, or garlic tablets?

- Do you use any injections?

- Have you had trouble with prescription drugs in the past? With non-prescription drugs?

- Do you have allergies to any medications, food, etc.?

- Do you take herbal supplements or vitamins? If so, which ones and how often?

- Alcohol intake, daily or monthly, kind of alcohol? Have you ever been treated for drug or alcohol dependency?

- Have you had any recent unplanned weight loss or gain?

- How is your dietary intake?

- What surgeries have you had? When and by whom? Results? Complications?

Family History

You will probably be asked about information on your parents, siblings, children, and spouse and their health status or year and cause of death.

Specifically, you will probably be asked about:

- Any family history of diabetes, high blood pressure, or liver, lung, kidney, heart, stomach, bowel, blood, bone, joint, muscle, stroke, or nervous system disorders.

- Any arthritis in the family and age of onset—how diagnosed and how treated.

- Any history of back/neck/spine problems in family—age of onset, how diagnosed, and how treated, as well as the name of treating doctor and clinic.

Social, Occupational, and Recreational History

You may be asked a number of questions about your general background and situation, such as:

- Educational level reached

- Occupational history with length of employment

- Physical nature of the job—Working hours per week? Any illness or injury on the job? When? How diagnosed and treated? Any litigation (lawsuits or workmen's compensation issues) regarding the job? Do you have a lawyer involved?

- Does your spouse work? Details?

- Are you satisfied with your job? How do you get along with your supervisor or boss?

- How do you get along with your spouse? Children? Siblings?

- Psychological history—any diagnosis? Depression? How treated and for how long? Doctor's name and clinic? Does your spouse have any similar problems?

- How is your anger or depression, if any? Recent change?

- How well do you sleep? What do you need to get to sleep?

- Activities—what sports or hobbies do you do now, what sports or hobbies have you given up?

- Body weight now? Recent change?

- How is your energy level now? Recent change?

- Any recent infections (bladder, lung, etc.)?

- Difficulty in controlling the bowel and/or bladder?

- Past history of cancer?

Present Spine Problem

Description of Pain (and Other Symptoms)

You will probably be asked to describe your symptoms in as much detail as possible, with questions such as:

- How long have you had your present spine problem?

- What is your main spine problem? Neck, arm(s), mid back, lower back, buttock, and/or leg(s)?

- How and when did it start?

- What always makes it worse? What always makes it better (even if only a little)?

- Description of the pain, e.g., is the pain sharp, dull, hot, electrical, burning, crushing, numbing, tingling, throbbing, mixed? Other?

- When it is at its worst, what can you still do, what is it that you cannot do? What are the effects on your job? Recreation? Hobbies? Sex life? Social life? For pain, weakness, numbness, or tingling indicate what changes them, for good or bad?

- How intense is your pain right now, on average/typical, at best, and at worst on a 0-10 scale (10=intense)?

- What are the percentages of distribution of these sensations between upper and lower limbs, parts of limbs, neck and arm/hand, low back/buttock and lower legs/feet, right and left sides, day and night, and other comparisons? (Such comparisons are often difficult to evaluate by the patient but important for the doctor to know.) You will be probably be provided with front and back sketches of the human body and requested to indicate where the pain, burning, crushing, weakness, numbness, tingling, and other sensations are located.

- When is the pain best? Worst? (Includes the time of day, week, month, seasons, etc.)

Diagnostic Tests

Your physician will most likely ask for background on which diagnostic tests you have already had. If possible, it's a good idea to bring the results of any major tests you've had to your appointment (e.g., recent MRI scan of your spine). Tests that will probably be asked about include:

- Spine diagnostic tests: x-ray, CT scan, MRI scan, tomography, myelogram, ultrasound scan, radioactive bone scan, discogram, other? Which part of the spine was included, and when and where were the tests performed? What were the findings (diagnosis) from these studies?

- Have you had similar studies elsewhere of your body parts, such as heart, lungs, stomach, intestines, kidneys, other organs, or joints? Again, where and when were these performed and what were the findings (diagnosis) from these studies?

Previous Treatments

Your spine specialist will probably ask for details about which types of treatments you have already tried for your spinal condition. For example:

- What types of medications have you tried? What medications help the problem? Which ones don't help?

- What type of conservative care have you tried (osteopathic or chiropractic manipulation, physical therapy, etc.)? When, where, and by whom? Which physical therapy program? Results?

- Have you had any injections for your spine problem, such as nerve root, epidural, facet joints, other? By whom, when, and diagnosis obtained? Results? Repeat injections?

- Have you had any type of spine surgery? Have you undergone any type of chronic pain rehabilitation? What were the results?

If You Need Surgery

Expectations from Surgery

If it is determined that you might need surgery, the physician will probably ask you questions about what you expect to obtain from the surgery. For example:

- Do you expect a complete cure?

- What percentage of improvement could you live with?

- What percentage of improvement would you be happy with?

- What part of your problems would you most want to be improved?

- What things do you have trouble with now or cannot do that would you want most to be able to do?

Post-Operative Care and Arrangements

If you decide to have surgery, you should also be prepared to discuss your postoperative expectations and arrangements. For example:

- You might need extended physical therapy or rehabilitation following surgery—can you accept this?

- What home or family arrangements can be made if your treatments can be performed at home?

- When are you likely to have to return to work? To self-care?

This section has laid out a number of potential topics that your physician will probably inquire about. If you take the time to prepare for these types of questions, you will most likely find that your consultation with your doctor is much more productive and this should help get you on the road to recovery more quickly.

Section 9.2

Diagnostic Tests for Spine Problems

"Diagnosing Spine Problems," is reprinted with permission from www.allaboutbackandneckpain.com, an informational website from DePuy Spine, Inc., a Johnson & Johnson company. © 2004 DePuy Spine, Inc. All rights reserved. Some illustrations on website by Marks Creative, © 2004 www.markscreative.com.

Before your doctor can diagnose your condition and design a treatment plan, a complete history and physical exam are necessary. This will give your doctor a better idea of the cause of your condition. Then appropriate diagnostic tests may be recommended.

Complete History

Your doctor will want to get a history of your condition. This may begin by filling out a written form while you wait to see the doctor. Take time to think about everything that relates to your pain and write it down. The more information you share with your doctor, the easier your problem will be to diagnose. A physical history can give your doctor insight into when the pain began, anything that could have caused an injury, your lifestyle, physical factors that might be causing pain, and any family history of similar problems.

After reading through your written history, your physician will ask more questions that relate to the information you have given. Your doctor may want to know:

- if you have had an injury

- where you are feeling pain and how intense it is

- if the pain radiates to other parts of your body

- if and where you are feeling numbness or weakness

- what factors make the pain feel better or worse

- whether you have had this problem or something like it before

- about any recent weight loss, fever, or illness

- if you've had problems with your bladder or bowels

Physical Exam

After taking your history, your physician will give you a physical exam. This allows the doctor to rule out possible causes of pain and try to determine the source of your problem. The areas of your body that will be examined depend upon where you are experiencing pain—neck, lower back, arms, legs, etc.

- Motion of Your Spine—Is there pain when you twist, bend, or move? If so, where? Have you lost some flexibility?

- Weakness—Your muscles will be tested for strength. You might be asked to try to push or lift your arm, hand, or leg when light resistance is put against them.

- Pain—The doctor may try to determine if you have tenderness of certain areas.

- Sensory Changes—Can you feel certain sensations in specific areas of the feet or hands?

- Reflex Changes—Your tendon reflexes might be tested, such as below the kneecap and behind the ankle in the Achilles tendon.

- Motor Skills—You might be asked to walk on your heels or toes.

- Special Signs—Your doctor will also check for any red flags that could indicate something other than spinal/vertebrae problems.

Some signs of other problems include tenderness in certain areas, a fever, an abnormal pulse, chronic steroid use (leads to loss of bone mass), or rapid weight loss.

Diagnostic Tests

Diagnostic tests may be needed in order to diagnose your condition. Tests are chosen based on what your doctor suspects is causing the problem.

Part Two

Maintaining Spinal Health

Chapter 10

Your Back:
An Owner's Manual

"Stand up straight. Don't slouch. Pull your shoulders back." Well, your mother's advice was right: practicing good posture is good for your appearance and your back health.

It's estimated that 8 out of every 10 Americans suffer from back pain at least once. Although some back problems are linked to a specific disease or injury, most aches and pains develop when we ask our backs to do more than they can handle. Lifting heavy objects improperly, sitting in an awkward position, wearing high heels, or even having poor posture can all strain your back muscles. Stress and anxiety, excess weight, overuse of the back, or weak abdominal and back muscles may also play a role in your aching back.

Your back did not come with a manufacturer's warranty. You, the owner, are responsible for taking steps to prevent or lessen simple problems. This owner's manual presents basic facts about your back, and information on preventing problems and seeking further assistance. Use this information, along with your doctor's advice, to get peak performance from your back.

"Your Back: An Owner's Manual" is part of the public education brochure series, *We Care for You,* produced by the Office of Health Promotion at Baylor College of Medicine, http://www.bcm.tmc.edu/we_care/index.htm. © 2003 Baylor College of Medicine Office of Health Promotion. All rights reserved.

Standard Features

The back is a strong, yet flexible machine made up of bones, disks, nerves, muscles, and ligaments. Not only does this complex structure support your head and neck and hold you upright, it also allows you to carry heavy loads, and to walk, dance, bend, and twist. Your backbone extends from the base of the skull to the tailbone, and is formed of more than 30 individual bones called vertebrae, which encircle and protect the spinal cord and nerves. The vertebrae are connected by fibrous bands of tissue called ligaments, and separated by spongy disks that actually cushion the bones. Back muscles that are attached to the vertebrae control movement.

When to Call a Mechanic

There are two basic types of back pain: acute and chronic.

Acute pain is sudden pain that goes away quickly, usually lasting for less than three months. Most patients with acute low back problems recover spontaneously within a few days to a few weeks. If you experience acute back pain that does not resolve itself on its own within a few weeks, or if you have recurrent episodes of acute pain, see your doctor. After taking your medical history and conducting a physical exam, your doctor will determine the need for additional medical tests and diagnostic procedures such as x-rays and bone scans.

Most acute lower back pain is due to musculoskeletal strain or sprain. Poor posture, sitting at a computer, incorrect lifting, or other improper movements or activities can trigger the pain. Acute back pain can be caused by trauma from an accident or a fall, a pinched nerve (also called sciatica), or non-spinal causes, such as appendicitis, kidney disease, uterine disorders, and urinary tract infections. More rarely, acute lower back problems may be caused by an underlying spinal condition, such as a tumor, an infection, or a spinal fracture.

Back pain that lasts more than three months and impairs regular activity is **chronic**. Although most chronic back pain does not result in permanent disability, it may cause its victims to retreat from some productive and enjoyable activities.

Taking an active role in resolving your back problems can increase your chances of relief. First of all, tell your doctor about your symptoms. If your pain and/or mobility are not resolved after appropriate evaluation and conservative treatment, it may be a good idea to get a second opinion. And beware of anyone who offers you instant freedom from pain, because if it sounds too good to be true, it probably is.

Diagnosing the Problem

While the cause of back pain may frequently be unknown, doctors have classified types of back problems and can treat their symptoms.

- Traumatic injury and occupational factors may result in acute, intense pain and may lead to chronic pain.

- Degenerative disorders, such as disk hernia and osteoarthritis, usually refer to the progressive deterioration of protective discs and joints.

- Structural abnormalities may be congenital (present at birth), such as spina bifida, or acquired through long-term poor posture, such as hyperlordosis (swayback). Lateral curvature of the spine, or scoliosis, is a fairly common structural abnormality.

- Muscular or ligamentous dysfunctions appear in the form of excess tension or spasms that are usually associated with strain injuries. Strains can cause some muscles to stop working properly, while other muscles must overwork. Often the inactive muscle can be made to work normally by moving it in an unusual pattern (such as looking to the right while turning the head to the left). In many cases, the pain stops when normal muscle coordination is restored.

Tune-Ups

Acute low back pain symptoms often can be treated with nonprescription medications such as acetaminophen, aspirin, and ibuprofen. If you are still in pain, or your physical activity is still hampered, your doctor may prescribe additional medication, physical therapy, or other treatment. You should also modify activities and postures that cause or increase stress on the back.

Patients may be given a program of conditioning activities to help them return to normal activity. Although bed rest used to be prescribed for acute back pain, experts now agree that most patients with acute back pain do not require bed rest, and in fact, that bed rest for longer than four days can debilitate and weaken the patient. Surgery is not usually an effective treatment option for patients who have acute low back pain without any underlying problems.

Chronic back pain is usually treated with a combination of therapies, including:

- Medication—In the past, doctors commonly prescribed painkillers and muscle relaxants to lessen the symptoms of chronic back pain. Now most prescribe anti-inflammatory drugs like aspirin and ibuprofen, in association with other medications such as muscle relaxants and antidepressants, to reduce pain and immobility.

- Physical Therapy—The goals of physical therapy are to increase flexibility, muscular strength, endurance, and coordination. After licensed physical therapists help the patient increase flexibility, they use resistive exercises, such as weight training, to gradually strengthen muscles which may have weakened from lack of use.

- Manipulation and Traction Devices—Manipulation involves manually adjusting bones that are assumed to be dislocated; traction devices give patients short-term relief by positioning them in a way that reduces pain and muscle spasms.

- Transcutaneous Electrical Nerve Stimulation (TENS)—TENS uses a mild electrical current to temporarily relieve discomfort by interfering with nerve signals responsible for perception of pain.

- Biofeedback—Biofeedback helps patients learn to control certain body functions, such as breathing rate, to achieve maximum relaxation.

- Counseling—A psychological approach takes into account the emotional aspects of chronic pain and includes patient training in behavior change and coping skills.

- Surgery—Surgery is often a last resort for chronic back pain; unfortunately repeated surgeries usually do not provide long-term relief.

Alignment

If you've ever felt sore after sleeping in an awkward position, sitting at a desk all day, or standing for a long period of time, you've experienced the effects of poor posture. Practicing good posture will strengthen your back and lower your risk for problems and pain.

Evaluate your own standing posture by turning to the side and looking in a mirror. You should be able to draw a straight line down the side of your body starting at the tip of your shoulder, dropping through the middle of your hip, running behind your kneecap, and ending in front of your ankle bone.

To improve your alignment, try the following posture tips.

Sitting

- Sit tall, with your hips pushed back in the chair and your thighs parallel to the floor; your weight should be evenly distributed on your thighs and feet.

- To relieve swayback, occasionally place each foot on a footrest to raise the knee higher than the hip, and tilt the pelvis upward.

- At work, use a firm, straight-backed chair that has armrests and padded support for your lower back and allows your feet to rest flat on the floor (use a footrest if needed).

- Don't cross your legs or cross at the ankles only.

- Avoid bending over your desk for extended periods.

- Use a headset, speaker phone, or shoulder rest instead of cradling the phone between your ear and shoulder.

Lifting

- Always bend your knees instead of bending at the waist.

- Use your leg muscles to provide the force.

- Keep your buttocks low and your head up.

- Hold the object close to your body, and keep your back erect.

- Lift objects only chest high.

- Pivot your body using your feet and legs rather than twisting your back.

- Know your limits, and get help if the object is too heavy for you.

Standing

- Stand erect with your chin in, head up, and back straight.

- Change your posture frequently (walk, bend, or stretch) to avoid fatigue.

- Shift your weight occasionally and keep your knees slightly bent.
- If you use a heavy shoulder bag or briefcase, regularly switch it from one side of your body to the other, and lighten your load by taking out the items you don't need every day.

Driving

- Move the seat forward to keep your knees higher than your hips.
- Stop frequently on long trips to stretch and walk around.

Sleeping

- Use a firm mattress, or place a plywood board between the mattress and box springs.
- If you have back pain, sleep on your side with your knees bent and a pillow between your knees, or on your back with a pillow underneath your knees.
- Avoid sleeping on your stomach.

Preventive Maintenance: Reducing Your Risk

Regular exercise:

- strengthens bones, tendons, ligaments, and muscles in the back;
- improves muscle control and coordination;
- enhances heart and lung function;
- decreases bone loss associated with osteoporosis;
- reduces stress and depression; and
- improves your general health.

The following exercises can be helpful in preventing and/or lessening back pain. Be sure to check with your physician before starting any new exercise routine.

Relaxation Exercise

Practicing relaxation techniques can release muscle tension and give you more energy. Many bookstores have guided relaxation cassette tapes to help you. Try these simple steps to see what it's like:

- Sit in a comfortable chair, close your eyes, and place your hands in your lap. Concentrate on breathing deeply.

- Squeeze your eyes tightly, hold for a few seconds, and then release.

- Tighten your jaw and purse your lips, then relax.

- Pull your shoulders up tightly, hold, and then release.

- Tighten the muscles in your upper arms, then release.

- Clench your fists and then relax. Notice the tension running out of your fingertips.

- Take a few slow breaths.

- Contract your stomach muscles, then relax them. Do the same with your shoulder blades, back, and buttocks.

- Squeeze your knees together tightly, contracting your thighs. Hold, and then release. Contract your calf muscles, then relax. Do the same with your feet.

- Remain seated, and imagine yourself somewhere peaceful, perhaps on a raft floating on a calm blue sea.

Ofeldt Exercises

While this relatively new exercise routine from Denmark is time-consuming, it has been found to control recurrent back pain in many patients. Ask your physician for more information.

Lower Back Stretch

While sitting on the floor with your legs tucked underneath you, gently bend over from the waist until your chest touches your knees, and hold for 10 seconds. Repeat 2 to 3 times, until back muscles feel relaxed and stretched out. Remember: Don't bounce or jerk during movement.

At-Home Repairs: What You Can Do for Minor Back Problems

If you injure your back, first apply cold packs for no longer than 5 to 10 minutes at a time to help decrease the swelling and ease the pain. You can make a cold pack by putting ice in a plastic bag and wrapping it with a towel or cloth. Be sure to place a layer of cloth between the cold pack and your skin to prevent skin damage. Wait at least 30 minutes before you reapply the cold pack. Taking over-the-counter pain relievers and/or anti-inflammatory drugs also may help relieve the problem and symptoms. If you are still in significant pain or have impaired mobility after 1 to 2 days, check with your doctor to see what the next treatment steps should be. Remember that most back problems are not helped by prolonged bed rest.

Anyone who suffers from back pain, either short-term or chronic, will assure you that an ounce of prevention is worth a pound of cure. The message from both doctors and patients is clear: to get peak performance from your back, practice proper posture, exercise regularly, manage stress, and maintain a healthy weight.

Chapter 11

Tips for Preventing Back and Neck Pain

Chapter Contents

Section 11.1

How to Prevent Back Pain

© 2000 American Academy of Orthopaedic Surgeons. Reprinted with permission from *Your Orthopaedic Connection*, the patient education website of the American Academy of Orthopaedic Surgeons located at http://orthoinfo.aaos.org.

Four out of five adults will experience significant low back pain sometime during their life. Work-related back injuries are the nation's number one occupational hazard, but you could suffer back pain from activities at home and at play, too.

Are You at Risk?

You are most at risk for back pain if:

- your job requires frequent bending and lifting
- you must twist your body when lifting and carrying an object
- you must lift and carry in a hurry
- you are overweight
- you do not exercise regularly or do not engage in recreational activities
- you smoke

If you are a caregiver for an ill or injured family member, you are at greatest risk for back pain when:

- pulling the person who is reclining in bed into a sitting position
- transferring the person from the bed to a chair
- leaning over the person for long periods of time

The American Academy of Orthopaedic Surgeons has developed tips to help you reduce your risk of back pain. Whether you are lifting and moving a person or a heavy object, the guidelines are the same.

- Plan ahead what you want to do and don't be in a hurry.

- Spread your feet shoulder-width apart to give yourself a solid base of support.

- Bend your knees.

- Tighten your stomach muscles.

- Position the person or object close to your body before lifting.

- Lift with your leg muscles. Never lift an object by keeping your legs stiff while bending over it.

- Avoid twisting your body; instead, point your toes in the direction you want to move and pivot in that direction.

- When placing an object on a high shelf, move close to the shelf. Do not stand far away and extend your arms with the object in your hands.

- Maintain the natural curve of your spine; don't bend at your waist.

- When appropriate, use an assistive device such as a transfer belt, sliding board, or draw sheet to move a person.

- Do not try to lift something that is too heavy or an awkward shape by yourself. Get help.

How to Prevent Back Pain

- Use the correct lifting and moving techniques.

- Exercise regularly to keep the muscles that support your back strong and flexible.

- Don't slouch; poor posture puts a strain on your lower back.

- Maintain your proper body weight to avoid straining your back muscles.

- Keep a positive attitude about your job and home life; studies show that persons who are unhappy at work or home tend to have more back problems and take longer to recover than persons who have a positive attitude.

Section 11.2

How to Prevent Neck Pain

- Take frequent breaks. Don't sit in one place for a long time, such as your car or at your desk. Arrange some of the items in your office so that they are inconvenient. This will force you to get up, stretch, or walk around.

- Maintain good neck posture. Adjust the seat of your computer or desk chair so your hips are slightly higher than your knees— your head and neck will naturally follow in the correct position. Traveling in a car, airplane, or train? Place a small pillow or rolled towel between your neck and a headrest to keep the normal curve in your neck

- How are you sleeping? Avoid sleeping with too many pillows or falling asleep in front of the television with your head on the arm of a couch.

- On the phone a lot? Use a speakerphone or headsets—do not cradle the phone in your neck.

- Exercise. Treat your body to a consistent regimen of stretching and strengthening to balance your muscle groups. This protects your neck as well as helping your whole body. Walking at any pace is excellent exercise for your neck. The rotation of the spine provides a great natural workout for the neck muscles.

- Eat smart and drink water. Good nutrition and staying well hydrated are not only important to stay healthy, but vital in the healing process.

Chapter 12

Using Body Mechanics and Posture to Prevent Pain

Chapter Contents

Section 12.1

What Are Good Body Mechanics?

Excerpted from "Posture for a Healthy Back" © 2003 The Cleveland Clinic Foundation, 9500 Euclid Avenue, Cleveland, OH 44195, 800-223-2273 ext. 48950, www.clevelandclinic.org. Additional information is available from the Cleveland Clinic Health Information Center, 216-444-3771, or www.clevelandclinic.org/health.

What Is Good Posture?

Posture is the position in which you hold your body upright against gravity while standing, sitting, or lying down. Good posture involves training your body to stand, walk, sit, and lie in positions where the least strain is placed on supporting muscles and ligaments during movement or weight-bearing activities. Proper posture:

- Keeps bones and joints in the correct alignment so that muscles are being used properly.

- Helps decrease the abnormal wearing of joint surfaces that could result in arthritis.

- Decreases the stress on the ligaments holding the joints of the spine together.

- Prevents the spine from becoming fixed in abnormal positions.

- Prevents fatigue because muscles are being used more efficiently, allowing the body to use less energy.

- Prevents strain or overuse problems.

- Prevents backache and muscular pain.

- Contributes to a good appearance.

Proper Posture Requirements

- Good muscle flexibility
- Normal motion in the joints

- Strong postural muscles.

- A balance of muscles on both sides of the spine.

- Awareness of your own posture, plus awareness of proper posture that leads to conscious correction. With much practice, the correct posture for standing, sitting, and lying down will gradually replace your old posture.

What Contributes to Bad Posture?

- obesity

- pregnancy

- weak muscles

- high-heeled shoes

- tight muscles; decreased flexibility

- poor work environment

- poor sitting and standing habits

Body Mechanics

Body mechanics is defined as maintaining proper position during movement. Constant or repeated small stresses over a long period of time can cause faulty body mechanics and can lead to injury.

Ergonomics is the process of changing your environment to encourage good body mechanics. This can be accomplished by modifying a tool, workstation, counter height, task, or job.

The essentials of good body mechanics include:

- Learning proper posture, lifting, and carrying techniques

- Becoming aware of your body position during all activities

- Altering your habits, positions, or your environment to provide a safe and efficient work area

- Practicing good body mechanics at all times, not just when you are recovering from pain or injury

Section 12.2

Improving and Maintaining Your Posture

Adapted from "The Secret of Good Posture," 1998, with permission of the American Physical Therapy Association. This material is copyrighted, and any further reproduction or distribution is prohibited. Reviewed by David A. Cooke, M.D., on March 20, 2004.

"Stand up straight! Don't slouch!"

How many times did you hear those scolding words while growing up? Maybe more times than you would like to remember.

Behind those long-forgotten words lies a very valuable and surprisingly simple message: Good posture is important because it helps your body function at top speed. It promotes movement, efficiency, and endurance and contributes to an overall feeling of well-being.

Good posture is also good prevention. If you have poor posture, your bones are not properly aligned, and your muscles, joints, and ligaments take more strain than nature intended. Faulty posture may cause you fatigue, muscular strain, and, in later stages, pain. Many individuals with chronic back pain can trace their problems to years of faulty postural habits. In addition, poor posture can affect the position and function of your vital organs, particularly those in the abdominal region.

Good posture also contributes to good appearance; the person with good posture projects poise, confidence, and dignity.

The Anatomy of Good Posture

To have good posture, it is essential that your back, muscles, and joints be in tip-top shape.

- **Your Back.** A healthy back has three natural curves: a slight forward curve in the neck (cervical curve), a slight backward curve in the upper back (thoracic curve), and a slight forward curve in the low back (lumbar curve). Good posture actually means keeping these three curves in balanced alignment.

- **Your Muscles.** Strong and flexible muscles also are essential to good posture. Abdominal, hip, and leg muscles that are weak and inflexible cannot support your back's natural curves.

- **Your Joints.** Hip, knee, and ankle joints balance your back's natural curves when you move, making it possible to maintain good posture in any position.

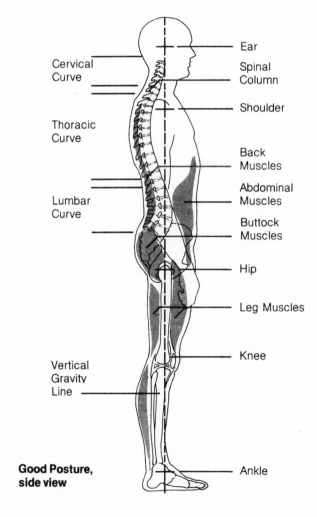

Figure 12.1. *To have good posture, it is essential that your back, muscles, and joints be in top shape.*

103

A View of Good Posture

Good posture—when you are standing—is straight vertical alignment of your body from the top of your head, through your body's center, to the bottom of your feet.

From a side view, good posture can be seen as an imaginary vertical line through the ear, shoulder, hip, knee, and ankle. In addition, the three natural curves in your back can be seen.

From a back view, the spine and head are straight, not curved to the right or left. The front view of good posture shows equal heights of shoulders, hips, and knees. The head is held straight, not tilted or turned to one side.

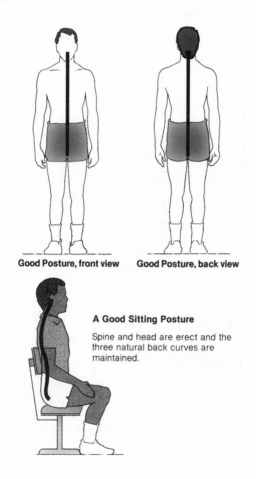

Good Posture, front view   Good Posture, back view

A Good Sitting Posture

Spine and head are erect and the three natural back curves are maintained.

Figure 12.2. Good posture for a healthy back.

Poor Posture

Poor posture distorts the body's proper vertical alignment and the back's natural curves.

Good posture only has one appearance, but poor posture comes in many unattractive styles.

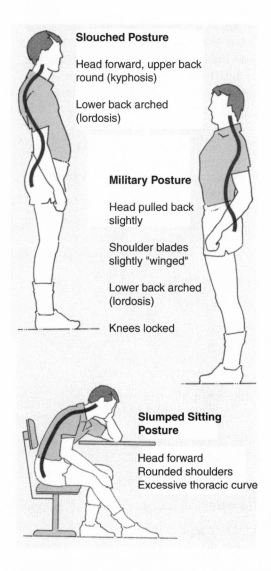

Slouched Posture

Head forward, upper back round (kyphosis)

Lower back arched (lordosis)

Military Posture

Head pulled back slightly

Shoulder blades slightly "winged"

Lower back arched (lordosis)

Knees locked

Slumped Sitting Posture

Head forward
Rounded shoulders
Excessive thoracic curve

Figure 12.3. Poor posture distorts the body's proper alignment.

Check Your Posture

The best way to check your posture is to receive a thorough postural evaluation from a physical therapist. Physical therapists have special skills to evaluate and treat postural problems.

To determine if a professional evaluation may be necessary, you can evaluate your own posture to some degree. For this you need a wall and a full-length mirror.

To check for normal curves of the spine, stand with your back to a wall, heels about three inches from the wall. Place one hand behind your neck, with the back of the hand against the wall, and the other hand behind your low back with the palm against the wall.

If there is excessive space between your back and the wall, such that you can easily move your hands forward and back more than one inch, some adjustment in your posture may be necessary to restore the normal curves of your spine.

To Check Your Posture from a Front View

Stand directly in front of a full-length mirror and answer the following questions:

Good Posture

- Is your head held straight?
- Are your shoulders level?
- Are the spaces between your arms and sides equal?
- Are your hips level?
- Do your kneecaps face straight ahead?
- Are your ankles straight?

Poor Posture

- Is your head tilted to one side or the other?
- Is one shoulder lower than the other?
- Are the spaces between your arms and sides unequal?
- Is one hip higher than the other?
- Do either of your knees turn in or out?
- Do your ankles roll in so your weight is on the inside of your feet?

To Check Your Posture from a Side View

The best way to check your posture from a side view is to have a friend photograph you in this position and to evaluate the photograph by answering the following questions:

Good Posture

- Is your head held erect?
- Is your chin parallel to the floor?
- Are your shoulders in line with your ears?
- Is your chest held moderately elevated and the upper back erect?
- Is your abdominal wall (tummy) flat?
- Does your lower back appear to have a slight forward curve?
- Are your knees straight?

Poor Posture

- Does your head slump forward?
- Does your chin tilt up with the head held back?
- Are your shoulders drooped forward or pulled back?
- Is your chest sunken in and your upper back rounded?
- Does your abdomen sag?
- Is your lower back too flat (no gentle curve) or does it curve forward into a hollow back?
- Do your knees bend forward or are they thrown backward into a locked position?

You Can Improve or Maintain Your Posture

The best way to improve or maintain your posture is to always practice good posture, when sitting, standing, or moving.

Practicing good posture is not always as easy as it sounds, especially for some of us who have forgotten what good posture feels like. The following two exercises can help bring back that good posture feeling.

Standing Position

- Stand with your back against a wall, heels about three inches from the wall and feet about six inches apart; weight should be evenly distributed.

- Place arms at your sides, palms forward.

- Keep ankles straight and kneecaps facing front.

- Keep your low back close to the wall.

- Straighten the upper back, lifting the chest and bringing shoulders back against the wall.

- Bring head back to touch the wall while keeping the chin tucked in as if a string is attached to the middle of the back of your head pulling it back.

- Pull up and in with the muscles in the lower abdomen, trying to flatten the abdomen.

- Hold position for about 10 seconds, breathing normally.

- Relax and repeat three to four times.

- Repeat entire exercise at least three times a day for optimum results.

Sitting Position

- Sit in a straight back armless chair, with both feet flat on the floor and back resting against the chair.

- Place arms at your sides, palms forward.

- Straighten the upper back, lifting the chest.

- Bring shoulders back against the chair.

- Hold head erect.

- Pull up and in with the muscles in the lower abdomen, trying to flatten the abdomen.

- Hold position for about 10 seconds, breathing normally and keeping the rest of the body relaxed.

- Relax your abdominal muscles and repeat three to four times.

- Repeat entire exercise at least three times a day.

Tips for maintaining good posture while sitting:

- Sit with back firmly against chair; chair should be low enough to allow placement of both feet on the floor with knees slightly higher than hips.

- Keep your head up and avoid leaning forward. If you work long hours at a desk or typewriter, keep your chair close to the desktop to help maintain your upright position.

- If you feel your low back arching forward while sitting, cross your legs or put your feet up on a stool.

Other Exercises You Can Do

Only after a complete postural evaluation as provided by a physical therapist can you identify your particular postural problems. At that time you may be given specific exercises to correct them.

One problem common to most people with poor posture is weakness of the lower abdominal muscles. If your lower abdomen sags and bulges, you can be sure the muscles there are weak. The best way to strengthen these muscles is to participate in an exercise that isolates and actively uses them.

Contrary to popular belief, sit ups do not always accomplish this goal. In fact, sit ups, when done improperly, often cause unnecessary strain on back muscles and may cause additional complications.

Exercise for the Lower Abdominal Muscles

- Stand comfortably.

- Clasp your hands and cup them around your lower abdomen.

- Pull up and in with the lower abdominal muscles, drawing in the lower abdomen. This step isolates and strengthens the abdominal muscles. To locate the right muscles it might help to think of hiding your tummy under your chest.

- Hold for about 10 seconds.

- Relax and repeat four to five times.

- Repeat entire exercise at least three times a day.

Good Posture for Life

Changes occur naturally in your body as you grow older. These changes can influence your posture and make it more difficult to maintain a good posture or correct a poor posture.

Some of the physical changes that occur:

- The disks between the spinal segments become less resilient and give in more readily to external forces, such as gravity and body weight.

- Muscles become less flexible.

- Compression and deterioration of the spine, commonly seen in individuals with osteoporosis, cause an increased flexed, or bent forward, posture.

- Lifestyles usually become more sedentary. Sitting for long periods of time shortens various muscles, which results in the body being pulled into poor postural positions, and stretches and weakens other muscles, which allows the body to slump.

Despite the changes that occur naturally with aging, good posture can be maintained and, for many, poor posture improved. In individuals with severe postural problems, such as poor alignments that have existed so long that structural changes have occurred, the poor posture can be kept from getting progressively worse.

In any case, all of us must consciously work at achieving and maintaining good posture as we grow older.

Tips for Maintaining Good Posture throughout Your Life

- Throughout each day, concentrate on keeping your three natural back curves in balanced alignment.

- Keep your weight down; excess weight exerts a constant forward pull on the back muscles and stretches and weakens muscles in the abdomen.

- Avoid staying in one position for long periods of time; inactivity causes muscle tension and weakness.

- Sleep on a firm mattress and use a pillow under your head just big enough to maintain the normal cervical—neck—curve. Avoid use of oversized or several pillows.

- Exercise regularly; exercise promotes strong and flexible muscles that keep you upright in a proper postural position.

- Protect your back by using good body mechanics; bend your knees when picking something up or putting it down; carry a heavy object by using two hands and keeping the load close to your waist.

- Wear comfortable and well-supported shoes. Avoid continuous use of high-heeled or platform shoes, which distort the normal shape of the foot and throw the back's natural curves out of alignment.

- Walk with good posture; keep head erect with chin parallel to the ground, allow arms to swing naturally, and keep feet pointed in the direction you are going.

Section 12.3

Sitting, Driving, Standing, Stooping, Squatting, and Kneeling to Prevent Pain

"How to Cope When You Have Low Back Pain" © 2003 The Cleveland Clinic Foundation, 9500 Euclid Avenue, Cleveland, OH 44195, 800-223-2273 ext. 48950, www.clevelandclinic.org. Additional information is available from the Cleveland Clinic Health Information Center, 216-444-3771, or www.clevelandclinic.org/health.

The following advice will benefit a majority of people with back pain. If any of the following guidelines causes an increase of pain or spreading of pain to the legs, do not continue the activity and seek the advice of a physician or physical therapist.

What Can I Do If I Have Acute Low Back Pain?

The key to recovering from acute low back pain (abrupt, intense pain that subsides after a relatively short period) is maintaining the normal curvature of the spine (hollow or lordosis). Supporting the hollow of your back will help decrease your recovery time.

For 10 to 20 days after you experience acute low back pain, follow these guidelines.

Sitting

- Sit as little as possible, and only for short periods of time (10 to 15 minutes).

- Sit with a back support (such as a rolled-up towel) at the curve of your back.

- Keep your hips and knees at a right angle (use a foot rest or stool if necessary). Your legs should not be crossed and your feet should be flat on the floor.

- Here's how to find a good sitting position when you're not using a back support or lumbar roll:

  1. Sit at the end of your chair and slouch completely.
  2. Draw yourself up and accentuate the curve of your back as far as possible. Hold for a few seconds.
  3. Release the position slightly (about 10 degrees). This is a good sitting posture.

- Sit in a high-back, firm chair with arm rests. Sitting in a soft couch or chair will tend to make you round your back and won't support the curve of your back.

- At work, adjust your chair height and work station so you can sit up close to your work and tilt it up at you. Rest your elbows and arms on your chair or desk, keeping your shoulders relaxed.

- When sitting in a chair that rolls and pivots, don't twist at the waist while sitting. Instead, turn your whole body.

- When standing up from the sitting position, move to the front of the seat of your chair. Stand up by straightening your legs. Avoid bending forward at your waist. Immediately stretch your back by doing 10 standing backbends.

Driving

- Use a back support (lumbar roll) at the curve of your back. Your knees should be at the same level or higher than your hips.

- Move the seat close to the steering wheel to support the curve of your back. The seat should be close enough to allow your knees to bend and your feet to reach the pedals.

Standing

- Stand with your head up, shoulders straight, chest forward, weight balanced evenly on both feet, and your hips tucked in.

- Avoid standing in the same position for a long time.

- If possible, adjust the height of the work table to a comfortable level.

- When standing, try to elevate one foot by resting it on a stool or box. After several minutes, switch your foot position.

- While working in the kitchen, open the cabinet under the sink and rest one foot on the inside of the cabinet. Change feet every 5 to 15 minutes.

Stooping, Squatting, and Kneeling

Decide which position to use. Kneel when you have to go down as far as a squat but need to stay that way for awhile. For each of these positions, face the object, keep your feet apart, tighten your stomach muscles, and lower yourself using your legs.

Lifting Objects

- Try to avoid lifting objects if at all possible.

- If you must lift objects, do not try to lift objects that are awkward or are heavier than 30 pounds.

- Before you lift a heavy object, make sure you have firm footing.

- To pick up an object that is lower than the level of your waist, keep your back straight and bend at your knees and hips. Do not bend forward at the waist with your knees straight.

- Stand with a wide stance close to the object you are trying to pick up and keep your feet firm on the ground. Tighten your stomach muscles and lift the object using your leg muscles. Straighten your knees in a steady motion. Don't jerk the object up to your body.

- Stand completely upright without twisting. Always move your feet forward when lifting an object.

- If you are lifting an object from a table, slide it to the edge to the table so that you can hold it close to your body. Bend your knees so that you are close to the object. Use your legs to lift the object and come to a standing position.

- Avoid lifting heavy objects above waist level.

- Hold packages close to your body with your arms bent. Keep your stomach muscles tight. Take small steps and go slowly.

- To lower the object, place your feet as you did to lift, tighten stomach muscles, and bend your hips and knees.

Reaching Overhead

- Use a footstool or chair to bring yourself up to the level of what you are reaching.

- Get your body as close as possible to the object you need.

- Make sure you have a good idea of how heavy the object is you are going to lift.

- Use two hands to lift.

Sleeping and Lying Down

- Select a firm mattress and box spring set that does not sag. If necessary, place a board under your mattress. You can also place the mattress on the floor temporarily if necessary.

- If you've always slept on a soft surface, it may be more painful to change to a hard surface. Try to do what's most comfortable for you.

- Use a back support (lumbar support) at night to make you more comfortable. A rolled sheet or towel tied around your waist may be helpful.

- Try to sleep in a position that helps you maintain the curve in your back (such as on your back with a lumbar roll or on your side with your knees slightly bent). Do not sleep on your side with your knees drawn up to your chest.

- When standing up from the lying position, turn on your side, draw up both knees and swing your legs on the side of the bed. Sit up by pushing yourself up with your hands. Avoid bending forward at your waist.

Other Helpful Tips

- Avoid activities that require bending forward at the waist or stooping.

- When coughing or sneezing, try to stand up and bend slightly back-ward to increase the curve in your spine when you cough or sneeze.

- Sleep on your side with your knees bent. You can also put a pillow between your knees.

- Try not to sleep on your stomach.

- If you sleep on your back, put pillows under your knees and a small pillow under the small of your back.

Section 12.4

High Heels and Back Problems

Women often buy footwear in a wild profusion of prints, patterns, and colors. Unfortunately, these eye-catching concoctions are rarely foot-friendly. That attractive pair of python pumps requires a balancing act on stiletto heels. And those thigh-high boots in sumptuous suede often sit upon heels the size of a dime. Once again, American women will sacrifice comfort at the altar of high fashion, donning spikes while suffering pain and discomfort. And according to the American Physical Therapy Association (APTA), high heels can lead to a lot more than just sore feet.

Women make up the majority of the 43 million Americans who experience foot problems such as bunions, calluses, and hammertoes. Prolonged wearing of high heels can lead to ankle injuries, nerve irritations (neuromas), and even back and neck problems. "Centering the body's weight on the ball of the foot instead of distributing it over the entire sole while shoving the toes into a narrow toe box may feel stylish, but it will likely cause posture problems and a host of other difficulties," said APTA member Jayne Snyder, PT, MA.

In their quest for the new look, shoemakers have pushed the heel ever higher and thinner. "The higher the heel, the worse for your body," said Snyder. "A three-inch heel creates seven times more stress on the forefoot than a one-inch heel," she explained. "This can result in a pinched nerve at the ball of the foot called a neuroma. In some cases, the bones of the foot may even shift."

The outwardly attractive effect of high heels is precisely what makes them uncomfortable and potentially hazardous. Walking in high heels forces the back to arch and the chest to thrust forward. "Basically, high heels cause the back and neck to hyperextend," said Snyder. "The body compensates by flexing, or forward bending, the hips and spine. While some women enjoy this look, they pay the price with problems of the back and neck, hips, legs, and feet."

To maintain balance in high heels, the calf, hip, and back muscles become tense. This leads to increased muscle fatigue by the end of the day and is especially true for stiletto heels that narrow to a point, because the muscles must work harder to keep balance. Also, wearing high heels causes the calf muscles to bulge, giving legs more definition and contour but contracting rear-leg ligaments. Over an extended period of time, this will cause muscle fatigue and cramping.

When only a high heel will do, keep in mind:

- Avoid wearing them for long periods of time, and stretch the muscles in the back of your leg before and after putting them on.

- "High" is a relative term. Try and set your limit at two inches.

- Pelvic tilts and calf stretches will also minimize any muscle cramping and shortening.

- Buy shoes in the afternoon or evening, as feet swell during the day.

- Change into low heels whenever you can.

- Don't go for the pointed toe. Use this rule of thumb: the higher the heel, the wider the toe box.

- Buy shoes with leather insoles to keep the foot from slipping.

- Buy a wide variety of shoes, including sneakers, oxfords, and sandals, and vary your footwear day to day.

The American Physical Therapy Association (APTA) is a national professional organization representing nearly 70,000 members. Its goal is to foster improvements in physical therapy education, research, and practice.

Chapter 13

Backpack Safety

Have you ever uttered the words, "A lot of homework won't hurt you," when battling your child over school assignments?

You might be wrong: your child's backpack may be hurting his health. Some studies have shown that as many as 30% to 50% of 15- to 16-year-olds suffer from back pain, which may be caused by a number of factors—one of them the improper use of backpacks.

"While many factors may cause back pain, such as increased level of competition in sports, poor posture while sitting, and long periods of inactivity, it is disturbing to find children carrying backpacks heavier than 15% of the body weight. Would you go on an elevator that reached the recommended safe limit? I think not, nor should children be carrying these exceedingly heavy loads," says Shelley Goodgold, PhD, associate professor of physical therapy at Simmons College in Boston, Massachusetts

There's good news, though: there are steps you can take to help your child avoid back pain and other problems associated with improperly used backpacks.

"Backpack Safety," reviewed by Richard Kruse, DO, July 2001. This information was provided by KidsHealth, one of the largest resources online for medically reviewed health information written for parents, kids, and teens. For more articles like this one, visit www.KidsHealth.org, or www.TeensHealth.org. © 2001 The Nemours Center for Children's Health Media, a division of The Nemours Foundation.

Backpack Benefits

Backpacks can be a useful tool for kids if they are used properly. Many packs come with multiple compartments that help kids stay organized while toting their books and papers from home to school and back again. Compared to shoulder bags or purses, backpacks are better because the strongest muscles in the body, the back and the abdominal muscles, support the weight of the pack. Because the weight is evenly distributed across the child's body, shoulder and neck injuries are less common than if the child carried a briefcase or purse.

What Problems Can Backpacks Cause?

The spine is made of 33 bones called vertebrae, and between the vertebrae are disks that act as natural shock absorbers.

"When a backpack is heavy, the child hyperextends (arches) the back or leans the head and trunk forward to compensate for the weight of the bag. This stresses the muscles in the neck and back, increasing the risk of fatigue and injury. Also using only one strap causes asymmetry of the spine and affects the spine's natural shock absorption abilities," Dr. Goodgold says.

Because of the heavy weight, your child might begin to develop shoulder, neck, and back pain. Most doctors and physical therapists recommend that a child carry no more than 10% to 15% of their body weight in their packs.

If your child wears his backpack on one shoulder, he may end up leaning to one side to compensate for the extra weight. He might develop lower and upper back pain and strained shoulders and neck. In addition, narrow straps that dig into the shoulders can interfere with circulation and the nervous system, and a child might develop tingling and weakness in his arms and hands.

Girls and younger kids may be especially at risk for backpack-related injuries because they are smaller and may carry loads that are heavier in proportion to their body weight. "Most studies show that girls do seem to have more back pain," says Richard Kruse, DO, an orthopedic surgeon.

Ongoing research may shed some light on the relationship between back pain and backpacks. Dr. Kruse is studying the problem of heavy backpacks and back pain in 12- to 17-year-olds.

If your child has to struggle to get his backpack on or off, has back pain, has to lean forward to carry his pack, or has numbness or weakness in the arms or legs, talk to your child's doctor or physical therapist.

Using Backpacks Safely

Despite their potential problems, backpacks can be used properly. Before you buy that backpack that your kid or teen is begging you for, consider the backpack's construction.

The safest backpacks have the following features:

- two wide, padded straps that go over the shoulders
- a padded waist or chest belt to distribute weight more evenly across the body
- multiple compartments to distribute the weight of the load
- width not greater than the child's torso

Bags that are slung over the shoulder or across the chest or only have one strap aren't as effective at distributing the weight as bags with two wide shoulder straps. You might want to consider purchasing a backpack with a metal frame (like hikers use), but check with your child's school first because many lockers won't accommodate a pack that large. You might also consider a backpack on wheels (like a flight attendant's bag), although you'll have to check with your child's school about this option as well. Many schools do not allow rolling backpacks because they can pose a tripping hazard in the hallways.

Limiting the weight of the backpack is key to preventing injuries. In a survey of physicians of the American Academy of Orthopedic Surgeons, most felt that backpack loads became a health problem when they reached 20 pounds or more. The American Physical Therapy Association recommends that children carry backpacks of no more than 15% of their body weight—but of course less is always better.

"Personally, I find 15% of my body weight much too heavy; I immediately feel pain at my shoulders and across my mid-back. Pain is a signal that something is wrong, so parents need to listen to their children. I think a 10% body weight limit is safer," Dr. Goodgold says. "No matter how well designed the backpack, children need to keep the backpack loads reasonable," she says. If your child doesn't know what 10% of his body weight feels like, use the bathroom scale to give him an idea.

Some of the responsibility for using backpacks safely rests with your child. Encourage him to use his locker or desk frequently throughout the day instead of carrying the entire day's worth of books in his backpack. Make sure your kid or teen isn't toting unnecessary items—laptops, CD players, and video games can add extra pounds to your child's pack. If your child does have to carry sports equipment or other weighty things, "heavier items should be placed closer to the back toward the body," says Dr. Kruse.

If you've noticed your child or teen seems to have a heavier pack on Fridays or Mondays, ask him about his homework planning. If your child procrastinates on homework until the weekend, he may end up with a much heavier pack, which could put him at risk for injuries.

Your child can also avoid injuries by picking up his backpack properly. As with any heavy weight, your child should bend at the knees and grab the pack with both hands when lifting a backpack to his shoulders. Another way to prevent back injury is to strengthen the stabilizing muscles of the torso, including the lower back and abdominal muscles. Weight training and yoga are two activities that can be effective in strengthening the core muscles.

Involving other parents and your child's school in solving the backpack burden might be beneficial. A few suggestions for school involvement include:

- Purchasing books on CD-ROM or putting some curriculum over the Internet, when possible

- Allowing students more time in between classes to use lockers

- Having the school purchase paperback books

- Implementing school education programs about safe backpack use

Chapter 14

Spinal Pain at Home

Chapter Contents

Section 14.1

Don't Let Housework Be a Pain in Your Back

Household chores can be a pain in the sacroiliac. Unless you're careful, routine activities around the home—washing dishes, vacuuming, even talking on the phone—can strain your back, including the sacroiliac area near the tailbone, and result in debilitating discomfort.

But you can protect your back by knowing the right way to go about such activities, according to the American Chiropractic Association (ACA).

Consider lifting. It doesn't matter whether you're picking up your child or a heavy bucket of water, you need to do it the proper way to avoid injury.

How? Bend from the knees, not the waist. As you lift, hold the item as close to your body as possible. If you have to turn to place it, step in the direction of the turn. That way, you're not twisting your body and straining your spine.

Back-Saving Tips

The American Chiropractic Association suggests the following do's and don'ts for chores and relaxation:

- When you wash dishes, open the cabinet beneath the sink, bend one knee, and put your foot on the shelf under the sink. Lean against the counter so some of your weight is supported in front.

- When ironing, raise one foot a bit. Place it on a small stool or a book to take some strain off your back.

- To vacuum, use a "fencer's stance." Put all your weight on one foot, then step forward and back with the other foot as you push the vacuum forward and back. Use the back foot as a pivot when you turn.

- While talking on the phone, don't cradle the phone between your ear and shoulder. That can lock up the spinal joints in the neck and upper back and cause pain. Instead, hold the phone with your hand or use the speakerphone.

- While watching television or relaxing, don't use the sofa arm as a pillow. The angle is much too sharp for your neck.

- Use a cold pack if your back begins to hurt. Wrap an ice pack in a towel moistened with warm water. The warmth gives way to gradual cold, which likely will alleviate the discomfort. (No ice? Try frozen veggies instead.)

- If pain persists for more than a day or two or if you experience numbness, tingling, or weakness in your arms or legs, see a doctor of chiropractic.

A doctor of chiropractic is an expert in spinal health and can help identify and treat your problem.

Section 14.2

Lifting Techniques for Home Caregivers

© 2000 American Academy of Orthopaedic Surgeons. Reprinted with permission from *Your Orthopaedic Connection,* the patient education website of the American Academy of Orthopaedic Surgeons located at http://orthoinfo.aaos.org.

If you are taking care of a spouse or family member at home, you are at greatest risk for back pain when you are:

- Pulling a person who is reclining in bed into a sitting position.

- Transferring a person from a bed to a chair.

- Leaning over a person for long periods of time.

- Always keep the person who is being moved close to your body.

- Keep your feet shoulder-width apart to maintain your balance.

- Use the muscles in your legs to lift and/or pull.

- When you lift or move a person, maintain the proper alignment of your head and neck with your spine. Maintain the natural curve of your spine; don't bend at your waist.

- Avoid twisting your body when carrying a person.

- If the person is too heavy, get help.

Sitting up in Bed

To move a person lying in bed to a wheelchair, put the chair close to the bed and lock the wheels. If the person is not strong enough to push up with his or her hands to a sitting position, place one of your arms under the person's legs and your other arm under his or her back. Move the person's legs over the edge of the bed while pivoting his or her body so the person ends up sitting on the edge of the bed. Keep your feet shoulder-width apart, your knees bent, and your back in a natural straight position.

Standing Up

If the person needs assistance getting into the chair, face the patient, place your feet shoulder-width apart, and bend your knees. Position the person's feet on the floor and slightly apart. The person's hands should be on the bed or on your shoulders. Place your arms around the person's back and clasp your hands together, Nurses, physical therapists, and others in hospitals often use lifting belts, which are fastened around a person's waist. The caregiver grasps the belt when lifting the patient. Hold the person close to you, lean back, and shift your weight.

Sitting Down

Pivot toward the chair, bend your knees and lower the person into the chair. The person should have both hands on the arms of the chair before you lower him or her down.

Chapter 15

Spinal Pain at Work

Chapter Contents

Section 15.1

Back Pain Prevention at Work

This material is excerpted from "Back Injury Prevention" with permission of AgSafe, www.agsafe.org, April 2002.

Your backbone is made up of 24 individual bones called vertebrae that are stacked on top of one another. Your vertebrae are separated by soft disks of cartilage that perform as shock absorbers for your vertebrae, and also help your back to bend, twist, and move around. Most of the support to your spine is maintained by your stomach muscles, as well as the many muscles and ligaments that run up and down the length of your back.

Prevention Is the Best Medicine

Preventing a back injury is much easier than repairing one. Because your back is critically important to your ability to walk, sit, stand, and run, it's important to take care of it. Most back pain arises from using your back improperly, so learning a few basic rules about lifting, posture, and proper exercise can help keep your back in good shape.

Exercise to Strengthen Your Back and Reduce Stress

Having strong back and stomach muscles is important to ease the work your back is put through each day. By doing simple back-toning exercises, you not only strengthen your back but also reduce stress and improve your appearance, too! Check with your doctor as to the best exercises for you.

Lose Weight

Potbellies and being overweight exerts extra force on back and stomach muscles. Your back tries to support the weight out in front by swaying backward, causing excess strain on the lower back muscles. By losing weight, you can reduce strain and pain in your back. Check with your doctor for the most sensible diet plan for you.

Maintain Good Posture

You can prevent many back pains by learning to sit, stand, and lift items correctly. When you sit down, don't slouch. Slouching makes the back ligaments, not the muscles, stretch and hurt, thus putting pressure on the vertebrae. The best way to sit is straight, with your back against the back of the chair with your feet flat on the floor and your knees slightly higher than your hips. Learn to stand tall with your head up and shoulders back.

Maintain Good Posture While You Sleep and Drive

Sleep on a firm mattress or place plywood between your box springs and mattress for good back support. If your mattress is too soft, it could result in a back sprain or swayback. Sleep on your side with your knees bent or on your back with a pillow under your knees for support. Drive with your back straight against the seat and close enough to the wheel so your knees are bent and are slightly higher than your hips.

Plan Your Lift

Lifting objects is often a mindless task, and unfortunately, many people perform their lift incorrectly resulting in unnecessary strain on their back and surrounding muscles. In order to lift correctly and reduce strain on your back, it's important to plan your lift in advance. This means to think about the weight of the object you will be moving and the distance you will be moving it. Is it bulky? Will you need help? Do you see any hazards that can be eliminated? Think about this whenever you do any lifting.

Position Yourself Correctly in Front of the Load

Once you have planned your lift, the next important step is to align yourself correctly in front of the load with your feet straddling the load—one foot slightly in front of the other for balance. Slowly squat down by bending your knees, not your back and stomach. Using both hands, firmly grab the load and bring it as close to your body as you can. This will help distribute the weight of the load over your feet and make the move easier.

Lift with Your Legs, Not Your Back

Once the load is close to your body, slowly straighten out your legs until you are standing upright. Make sure the load isn't blocking your vision as you begin to walk slowly to your destination. If you need to turn to the side, turn by moving your feet around and not by twisting at your stomach.

Set the Load Down Correctly

Once you have reached your destination, it's equally important that the load is set down correctly. By reversing the above lifting procedures you can reduce the strain on your back and stomach muscles. If you set your load on the ground, squat down by bending your knees and position the load out in front of you. If the load is set down at table height, set the load down slowly and maintain your contact with it until you are sure the load is secure and will not fall when you leave.

Get Help, If Needed

If the load is too heavy, bulky, or awkward for you to lift alone, find a friend to help you carry it. If no one is available, is it possible to break the load into two smaller loads? Or, can you locate a cart or dolly to help you move it? Look for simple solutions to help make the move easier on you and your back.

Section 15.2

Do Back Belts Really Work?

Back belts have become a common sight—we see them every day on vending machine stockers, deliverymen, and anyone else who regularly lifts heavy objects. Back belts were originally touted as an effective means of preventing back problems, but since have been said to have no effect on proper lifting techniques, making it difficult to decide whether or not to use one. A recent study once again proves the usefulness of back belts, however.

The authors of the study evaluated the effects of an elastic back belt on spine motion when lifting large and small boxes of the same weight (about 20 lbs.). Twenty-eight subjects with no prior low back pain and at least six months of manual-handling experience lifted small and large boxes with and without a back belt. The boxes were lifted from a position near the ground in front of the subjects to a position at table-height to the subject's right side.

Back belt use significantly reduced twisting of the spine when lifting large boxes. Back belts also clearly decreased spinal bending and speed of lifting when lifting both large and small boxes. Properly lifting while wearing a belt did not lead to proper lifting techniques once the belt was removed, indicating the importance of continued use.

This study supports prior research emphasizing the value of wearing back belts for manual lifting tasks; belts appear to result in slower lifts, proper squat-lift technique, and reduced torso motions. Whether or not you use a belt, always follow proper lifting techniques: lift with your legs, not with your back. If you ever need to lift moderate-to-heavy objects at work or at home, be sure to wear a back belt. It's a small price to pay, compared to costly and painful back injuries.

Reference

Giorcelli RJ, Hughes RE, Wassell JT, et al. The effect of wearing a back belt on spine kinematics during asymmetric lifting of large and small boxes. *Spine,* August 15, 2001:26(16), pp. 1794-1798.

Section 15.3

Ergonomics for Computer Workstations

National Institute of Health Office of Research Services, May 2004.
Available online at http://www.nih.gov; accessed May 2004.

Monitors

With regard to the monitor, one must take into consideration how the placement and maintenance of the monitor can affect both the eyes and the musculoskeletal system. The following suggestions can help prevent the development of eye strain, neck pain, and shoulder fatigue while using your computer workstation:

- Make sure the surface of the viewing screen is clean.

- Adjust brightness and contrast to optimum comfort.

- Position the monitor directly in front of user to avoid excessive twisting of the neck.

- Position the monitor approximately 20 to 26 inches (arm's length) from user.

- Tilt top of the monitor back 10 to 20 degrees.

- Position monitors at right angles from windows to reduce glare.

- Position monitors away from direct lighting which creates excessive glare or use a glare filter over the monitor to reduce glare.

- The top of the viewing screen should be at eye level when the user is sitting in an upright position.

Note: Bifocal wearers may need to lower monitor a couple of inches.

Adjusting Your Chair

Contrary to popular belief, sitting, which most people believe is relaxing, is hard on the back. Sitting for long periods of time can cause increased pressure on the intervertebral discs—the springy, shock-absorbing part of the spine. Sitting is also hard on the feet and legs. Gravity tends to pool blood in the legs and feet and create a sluggish return to the heart.

The following recommendations can help increase comfort for computer users:

- Practice dynamic sitting and don't stay in one static position for extended periods of time.

- When performing daily tasks, alternate between sitting and standing.

- Adjust height of backrest to support the natural inward curvature of the lower back. It may be useful to use a rolled towel or lumbar pad to support the low back. The backrest angle is set so that your hip-torso angle is 90 degrees or greater.

- Adjust height of chair so feet rest flat on floor (use footrest if necessary).

- Sit upright in the chair with the low back against the backrest and the shoulders touching the backrest.

- Thighs should be parallel to the floor and knees at about the same level as the hips. Back of knees should not come in direct contact with the edge of the seat pan (there should be 2 to 3 inches between the edge of the seat and the back of the knee).

- Don't use armrests to slouch.

- Adjust height and/or width of armrests so they allow the user to rest arms at their sides and relax/drop their shoulders while keyboarding.

- Where armrests are used, elbows and lower arms should rest lightly so as not to cause circulatory or nerve problems.

Desktops for Computer Workstations

If you are like many computer users, your computer, keyboard, and mouse are resting on your desk or a portable computer workstation. There is no specific height recommended for your desktop; however, the working height of your desk should be approximately elbow height for light duty desk work.

To allow for proper alignment of your arms, your keyboard should be approximately 1 inch to 2 inches above your thighs. Most times this requires a desk which is 25 inches to 29 inches in height (depending upon size of individual) or the use of an articulating keyboard tray.

The area underneath the desk should always be clean to accommodate the user's legs and allow for stretching.

The desktop should be organized so frequently used objects are close to the user to avoid excessive extended reaching. If a document holder is used, it should be placed at approximately the same height as the monitor and at the same distance from the eyes to prevent frequent eye shifts between the screen and reference materials.

Keyboard and Mouse

Many ergonomic problems associated with computer workstations occur in the forearm, wrist, and hand. Continuous work on the computer exposes soft tissues in these areas to repetition, awkward postures, and forceful exertions.

The following adjustments should be made to your workstation to help prevent the development of an ergonomic problem in the upper extremities:

- Adjust keyboard height so shoulders can relax and allow arms to rest at sides (an articulating keyboard tray is often necessary to accommodate proper height and distance).

- Keyboard should be close to the user to avoid excessive extended reaching.

- Forearms parallel to the floor (approximately 90 degree angle at elbow).

- Mouse should be placed adjacent to keyboard and at the same height as the keyboard (use articulating keyboard tray if necessary).

- Avoid extended and elevated reaching for keyboard and mouse. Wrist should be in neutral position (not excessively flexed or extended).

- Do not rest the hand on the mouse when you are not using it. Rest hands in your lap when not entering data.

Musculoskeletal System Exercises and Stretches

Deep Breathing

1. while standing, or in an otherwise relaxed position
2. place one hand on the abdomen and one on the chest

3. inhale slowly through the nose
4. hold for 4 seconds
5. exhale slowly through the mouth
6. repeat

Cable Stretch

1. while sitting with chin in, stomach in, shoulders relaxed, hands relaxed in lap, and feet flat on the floor, imagine a cable pulling the head upward
2. hold for 3 seconds and relax
3. repeat 3 times

Sidebend: Neck Stretch

1. tilt head to one side (ear towards shoulder)
2. hold for 15 seconds
3. relax
4. repeat 3 times on each side

Diagonal Neck Stretch

1. turn head slightly and then look down as if looking in your pocket
2. hold for 15 seconds
3. relax
4. repeat 3 times on each side

Shoulder Shrug

1. slowly bring shoulders up to the ears and hold for approximately 3 seconds
2. rotate shoulders back and down
3. repeat 10 times

Executive Stretch

1. while sitting, lock hands behind head
2. bring elbows back as far as possible
3. inhale deeply while leaning back and stretching
4. hold for 20 seconds

5. exhale and relax
6. repeat 1 time

Foot Rotation

1. while sitting, slowly rotate each foot from the ankle
2. rotate 3 times in one direction, then 3 times in the opposite direction
3. relax
4. repeat 1 time

Hand Shake

1. while sitting, drop arms to the side
2. shake hands downward gently
3. repeat frequently

Hand Massage

Note: Perform very gently!

1. massage the inside and outside of the hand using the thumb and fingers
2. repeat frequently (including before beginning work)

Finger Massage

Note: Perform very gently!

1. massage fingers of each hand individually, slowly, and gently
2. move toward nail gently
3. massage space between fingers
4. perform daily

Wrist Stretch

1. hold arm straight out in front of you
2. pull the hand backwards with the other hand, then pull downward
3. hold for 20 seconds
4. relax
5. repeat 3 times each

Chapter 16

Spinal Pain during Pregnancy

Chapter Contents

Section 16.1

Easing Back Pain during Pregnancy

What to Expect while You're Expecting

Half of all pregnant women can expect some back pain. Back pain develops for two reasons. One is simply the added weight caused by the pregnancy. Another may be that the extra weight is carried in the front of the body, shifting your center of gravity forward and putting more strain on the low back. The muscles in your back may have to work harder to support your balance.

How Can You Minimize the Discomfort?

- **Stick with your exercise program.** Find out from your doctor what abdominal and back strengthening exercises are safe for you, and how long you can maintain your regular exercise program. Swimming is an excellent way to keep fit and relieve the stress on your back from the extra weight of pregnancy.

- **Lifting.** If you have to pick something up, kneel down on one knee with the other foot flat on the floor, as near as possible to the item you are lifting. Lift with your legs, not your back, keeping the object close to your body at all times. Be careful, though—it may be easier to lose your balance while you are pregnant. Whenever possible, get assistance in lifting objects.

- **Carrying.** Two small objects (one in either hand) may be easier to handle than one large one. If you must carry one large object, keep it close to your body.

- **Sleeping.** Sleeping on your back puts 55 pounds of pressure on your back. Placing a pillow under your knees cuts the pressure in half. Lying on your side with a pillow between your knees also reduces the pressure.

How Can You Deal with the Back Pain Related to Pregnancy?

Fortunately, most back pain related to pregnancy is self-limited and will resolve. In most cases, medication is not a very good option. Do not use any medication during pregnancy without permission of your physician. Some treatment options include learning exercises to support muscles of the back and pelvis, using supportive garments that may be helpful with certain causes of back pain in pregnancy, and using spot treatments such as heat and cold. If your pain persists despite these measures, or you develop any radiating pain, numbness, tingling, or weakness in your legs, you should consult with a spine physician with expertise in women's health issues and/or pregnancy related disorders. They will be able to assist you in diagnosing and treating your specific problems.

The more you know, the better chance you have of avoiding back pain—which affects 80% of the adult population and is the second most common reason people visit their doctors. If you have back pain or want to know how to avoid it, consult a spine care specialist.

Section 16.2

Chiropractic Advice for Moms-to-Be

As many new mothers can attest, the muscle strains of pregnancy are very real and can be more than just a nuisance. The average weight gain of 25 to 35 pounds, combined with the increased stress placed on the body by the baby, may result in severe discomfort. Studies have found that about half of all expectant mothers will develop low back pain at some point during their pregnancies.[1-3] This is especially true during late pregnancy, when the baby's head presses down on a woman's back, legs, and buttocks, irritating her sciatic nerve. And for those who already suffer from low back pain, the problem can become even worse.

During pregnancy, a woman's center of gravity almost immediately begins to shift forward to the front of her pelvis. Although a woman's sacrum—or posterior section of the pelvis—has enough depth to enable her to carry a baby, the displaced weight still increases the stress on her joints. As the baby grows in size, the woman's weight is projected even farther forward, and the curvature of her lower back is increased, placing extra stress on the spinal disks. In compensation, the normal curvature of the upper spine increases, as well.

While these changes sound dramatic, pregnancy hormones help loosen the ligaments attached to the pelvic bones. But even these natural changes designed to accommodate the growing baby can result in postural imbalances, making pregnant women prone to having awkward trips and falls.

What Can You Do?

The ACA (American Chiropractic Association) recommends the following tips for pregnant women:

Exercise

- Safe exercise during pregnancy can help strengthen your muscles and prevent discomfort. Try exercising at least three times a week, gently stretching before and after exercise. If you weren't active before your pregnancy, check with your doctor before starting or continuing any exercise.

- Walking, swimming, and stationary cycling are relatively safe cardiovascular exercises for pregnant women because they do not require jerking or bouncing movements. Jogging can be safe for women who were avid runners before becoming pregnant—if done carefully and under a doctor's supervision.

- Be sure to exercise in an area with secure footing to minimize the likelihood of falls. Your heart rate should not exceed 140 beats per minute during exercise. Strenuous activity should last no more than 15 minutes at a time.

- Stop your exercise routine immediately if you notice any unusual symptoms, such as vaginal bleeding, dizziness, nausea, weakness, blurred vision, increased swelling, or heart palpitations.

Health and Safety

- Wear flat, sensible shoes. High or chunky heels can exacerbate postural imbalances and make you less steady on your feet, especially as your pregnancy progresses.

- When picking up children, bend from the knees, not the waist. And never turn your head when you lift. Avoid picking up heavy objects, if possible.

- Get plenty of rest. Pamper yourself and ask for help if you need it. Take a nap if you're tired, or lie down and elevate your feet for a few moments when you need a break.

Pregnancy Ergonomics: Your Bed and Desk

- Sleep on your side with a pillow between your knees to take pressure off your lower back. Full-length body pillows or pregnancy wedges may be helpful. Lying on your left side allows unobstructed blood flow and helps your kidneys flush waste from your body.

- If you have to sit at a computer for long hours, make your workstation ergonomically correct. Position the computer monitor so the top of the screen is at or below your eye level, and place your feet on a small footrest to take pressure off your legs and feet. Take periodic breaks every 30 minutes with a quick walk around the office.

Nutrition

- Eat small meals or snacks every four to five hours—rather than the usual three large meals—to help keep nausea or extreme hunger at bay. Snack on crackers or yogurt—bland foods high in carbohydrates and protein. Keep saltines in your desk drawer or purse to help stave off waves of morning sickness.

- Supplementing with at least 400 micrograms of folic acid a day before and during pregnancy has been shown to decrease the risk of neural tube birth defects, such as spina bifida. Check with your doctor before taking any vitamin or herbal supplement to make sure it's safety for you and the baby.

How Can Your Doctor of Chiropractic Help?

Before you become pregnant, your doctor of chiropractic can detect any imbalances in the pelvis or elsewhere in your body that could contribute to pregnancy discomfort or possible neuromusculoskeletal problems after childbirth.

Many pregnant women have found that chiropractic adjustments provide relief from the increased low-back pain brought on by pregnancy. Chiropractic manipulation is safe for the pregnant woman and her baby and can be especially attractive to those who are trying to avoid medications in treating their back pain. Doctors of chiropractic can also offer nutrition, ergonomic, and exercise advice to help a woman enjoy a healthy pregnancy.

Chiropractic care can also help after childbirth. In the eight weeks following labor and delivery, the ligaments that loosened during pregnancy begin to tighten up again. Ideally, joint problems brought on during pregnancy from improper lifting or reaching should be treated before the ligaments return to their pre-pregnancy state—to prevent muscle tension, headaches, rib discomfort, and shoulder problems.

For More Information

To find more information on prevention and wellness, or to find a doctor of chiropractic near you, go to Patient Information section on the American Chiropractic Association's website at www.acatoday.com or call (800) 986-4636.

References

1. Östgaard HC, et al. Prevalence of back pain in pregnancy. *Spine* 1991;16:549–52.

2. Berg G, et al. Low back pain during pregnancy. *Obstet Gynecol* 1988;71:71–5.

3. Mantle MJ, et al. Backache in pregnancy. *Rheumatology Rehabilitation* 1977;16:95–101.

Chapter 17

Exercises for Low Back Pain

Exercise is an important part of treating—and preventing—back pain. Your doctor will show you which exercises are right for you and tell you how often, how long, and in what order you should do them. Often, relief for back pain is a goal that can only be achieved by a team approach of physician, therapist, and patient. Your full participation is essential.

Initial Exercises

The exercises your doctor recommends as you begin treatment will help you control pain and maintain muscle tone. When done correctly, these exercises should cause little or no pain. Here are some exercises to help you begin.

Pelvic Tilt

Lie on your back with both knees bent and your feet flat on the floor. Flatten the small of your back against the floor, without pushing down with your legs. Hold for 5 seconds. Repeat 10 times.

Knee to Chest

Lie on your back with both knees bent and your feet flat on the floor. Bring one knee to your chest and hold for 10 seconds. Lower your foot to the floor and repeat with the opposite leg. Repeat 5 times. As you progress, bring one knee to your chest, then the other. Hold both knees and repeat as before.

Prone Lying

Lie on your stomach with your arms placed along your sides and head turned to one side. A small pillow under your hips and an ice pack wrapped in a towel may provide additional pain relief. Maintain this position for 3 to 5 minutes.

Prone Lying on Elbows

Lie on your stomach with your weight on your elbows and forearms and your hips on the floor. Relax your lower back for 3 to 5 minutes.

Prone Press-Up

As you progress, work up to the prone press-up. Lie on your stomach with your hands on the floor near your shoulders. Slowly push your upper body off the floor by straightening your arms, keeping your hips on the floor. Hold for 5 seconds. Repeat 10 times.

Stabilization and Strengthening Exercises

As you get stronger, the next goal is to improve back strength and function. The following exercises are designed to stabilize the spine while keeping it in a safe position.

Arm Reach

Start on your hands and knees, maintaining a straight lower back. Lift one arm straight up next to your ear. Try not to twist your body. Hold the arm parallel to the floor for 5 seconds. Return to the starting position and repeat 10 times. Then repeat with the other arm.

Leg Reach

Start on your hands and knees, maintaining a straight lower back. Extend one leg out behind you. Try not to twist your body. Hold the leg parallel to the floor for 5 seconds. Return to the starting position and repeat 10 times. Then repeat with the other leg.

Quadruped

Start on your hands and knees, maintaining a straight lower back. Lift one arm straight up next to your ear. Then extend the opposite leg out behind you. Try not to twist. Hold the arm and leg parallel to the floor for 5 seconds. Return to the starting position and repeat 10 times. Then repeat with the opposite arm and leg.

Bridging

Lie on your back with both knees bent and your feet flat on the floor. Raise your hips and your lower back from the floor, keeping your lower back straight. Hold the position for 5 seconds. Relax and repeat 10 times.

Partial Sit-Up

Lie on your back with both knees bent and your feet flat on the floor. Slowly curl your head and shoulders off the floor. Hold briefly for 1 to 2 seconds, then relax. Do 10 to 20 times.

Hip and Hamstring Stretches

Tight hip and hamstring muscles often contribute to low back pain. Exercises that stretch these muscles are an essential part of recovery and may prevent new pain from developing.

Hamstring Muscle Stretch

Lie on your back with your knees bent. Loop a towel or belt around one foot. Slowly raise and straighten your leg until you feel a stretch in your hamstrings. Hold the position for 30 seconds and release. Repeat with the other leg.

Hip Flexor Muscle Stretch

Kneel with your left foot in front of you. Slowly shift your weight forward, keeping your back straight. Lift your stomach muscles and push your left buttock toward the floor; hold for 30 seconds. Relax and return to the starting position. Repeat with the opposite leg.

Remember: This information is not intended as a substitute for medical treatment. Before starting an exercise program, consult a physician.

Chapter 18

Pilates Promotes Back Health

Pilates is an exercise program that focuses on the core postural muscles that help keep the body balanced and are essential to providing support for the spine. In particular, Pilates exercises teach awareness of neutral alignment of the spine and strengthening the deep postural muscles that support this alignment, which are important to help alleviate and prevent back pain.

The Pilates Exercise Program

Pilates is an exercise system named after its originator, Joseph Pilates. Mr. Pilates developed this system in the early 1900s to improve his health and to support the health of fellow World War I internees.

Later, he incorporated the resistance of springs into rehabilitation programs for hospitalized patients, and then translated the use of springs into machines and created the unique equipment now used in the exercise system.

Important principles of the Pilates exercise program include:

- Use of mental focus to improve movement efficiency and muscle control

- Awareness of neutral spine alignment, or proper posture, throughout the exercises

- Development of the deep muscles of the back and abdomen to support this posture

- Use of breath to promote mental focusing and centering

- Creating length, strength, and flexibility in muscles

Initially the Pilates exercise program was primarily used by professional dancers, who appreciated improved strength, balance, and flexibility. In the 1980s Pilates was rediscovered and has now become a popular form of exercise for anyone interested in its health benefits.

The exercise system is usually taught in one of two formats:

- Using the unique Pilates equipment in private, or semi-private, sessions

- Group mat classes not using equipment

Pilates Equipment

The Pilates equipment uses the resistance of springs to create effort. The principle piece of equipment is called the Reformer and consists of a sliding platform anchored at one end of its frame with springs. The platform can be moved by either pulling on ropes or pushing off from a stationary bar. Thus, exercises include the challenge of moving the platform and maintaining balance on a moving surface (if sitting or standing).

Another Pilates machine is called the Cadillac and consists of a padded platform with a cage-like frame above it. From this frame various bars or straps are attached by springs.

A third piece of equipment, the Wunda Chair, consists of a small bench-like platform with a bar attached with springs. Exercises are done by pushing on the bar while either sitting or standing on the bench, or standing or lying on the floor.

Mat Exercises

Usually taught as part of a group class, mat exercises primarily focus on strengthening the muscles of the trunk and hip and increasing the flexibility of both the spine and hips. While the scope of the mat program is limited compared to the machines, there are many mat exercises that illustrate the Pilates principles.

Lately, Pilates has merged with other movement techniques, such as yoga, or use of an exercise ball. This promotes creative integration of the Pilates principles into a greater range of exercises in the mat class setting.

Pilates Exercise and Back Pain

The important principles of Pilates are consistent with an exercise program that promotes back health. In particular, learning awareness of neutral alignment of the spine and strengthening the deep postural muscles that support this alignment are important skills for the back pain patient.

Patients with pain stemming from excessive movement and degeneration of the intervertebral disks and joints are particularly likely to benefit from a Pilates exercise program. In addition, postural asymmetries can be improved, thus decreasing wear and tear resulting from uneven stresses on the intervertebral joints and disks.

Pilates improves strength, flexibility, and suppleness of the muscles of the hip and shoulder girdle. Fluid and supported movement through these joints helps prevent unnecessary torque on the vertebral column.

The Pilates program also teaches awareness of movement habits that may stress the spine, and helps the patient change these habits to those that preserve neutral alignment. Awareness of excessive tension and the use of proper focus helps the patient use the body efficiently.

Pilates Considerations for Back Pain Patients

Before starting any new exercise system, it is always advisable to check with a physician or other healthcare provider. Before starting a Pilates exercise program, it is important to check that the potential instructor has received training in the Pilates exercise system and that he or she understands any specific back problems.

If a patient starts Pilates after physical therapy, the physical therapist should outline the exercise principles identified as particularly important for his or her rehabilitation.

Individuals with significant back problems may benefit from several one-on-one Pilates sessions with a qualified Pilates instructor. While more expensive than a group class or mat class, the time, money, and effort devoted to learning the exercises correctly can be well worth the investment, as exercises performed incorrectly can make a back problem worse. Initially, twice-a-week sessions tend to be helpful to learn the program more quickly. After that, weekly Pilates exercise sessions may be enough if the individual practices between sessions.

The principles of movement important for back health are taught in some of the simplest exercises of the Pilates system. One cannot underestimate the benefit of simple exercises that support the deep postural muscles of the trunk, awareness of neutral alignment, and supple use of the shoulders and hips. It is best to learn exercises that can be practiced at home between scheduled Pilates sessions.

Given its roots in ballet and dance, some of the movements in the Pilates system are very difficult and challenging. Many of the exercises should be avoided for individuals with significant back pain or degenerative disk disease. Remember, it is always advisable to first see a physician prior to starting any exercise program.

As a general rule, back patients should avoid exercises that push the spine into extremes of flexion or extension, or combine flexion with side bending or twisting the spine. These motions place excessive stress on the intervertebral discs. Also, it is important to avoid fatigue—either mental or physical—which is when proper form is lost and injuries more likely to occur.

The exercises in the Pilates system should be challenging (both mentally and physically) but not so difficult that they cause anyone to struggle. If an exercise causes pain—it is best to stop and tell the instructor. The exercise may be too difficult or the person may need additional help to do it correctly.

Finally, it may take awhile for the full benefits of a Pilates exercise program to be realized. Just as problems that create most back pain problems happen gradually over time, learning to use one's muscles in a way that support—rather than stress—the spine takes time and commitment.

Chapter 19

Yoga for Back Problems

Yoga is an ancient practice developed in India almost 4,000 years ago. In the last decade it has become increasingly popular in the west, and currently, about 15 million people in the United Stated do yoga.

Generally in the United States, yoga classes consist of a combination of physical exercises, breathing exercises, and meditation. Yoga has been used for thousands of years to promote health and prevent disease, and many people with back problems have found yoga to provide several benefits, including:

- Relieving pain
- Increasing strength and flexibility
- Teaching relaxation and acceptance

In recent years, researchers have become interested in studying the effects of yoga on treating disease, and studies are encouraging that yoga can be a useful part of the treatment plan for many medical conditions as varied as heart disease, carpal tunnel syndrome, epilepsy, asthma, addiction, and many neck and back problems.

"Yoga for Back Problems" by Karen P. Barr, M.D., is reprinted with permission from www.Spine-health.com. © December 2, 2003 Spine-health.com. All rights reserved. For more information, please see http://www.Spine-health.com.

Will Yoga Help Back Pain or Neck Pain?

Although no one treatment works for everyone, many aspects of yoga make it ideal for treating back pain and neck pain. For example, studies have shown that those who practice yoga for as little as twice a week for 8 weeks make significant gains in strength, flexibility, and endurance, which is a basic goal of most rehabilitation programs for back pain or neck pain.

In addition, the breathing and meditation aspects of yoga induce a "relaxation response" that has been found in many studies to assist people in decreasing their pain. Yoga has also been found to be helpful in the treatment of depression and anxiety that often accompany pain problems.

Is Yoga Possible for People Who Aren't Naturally Flexible?

Many times those who are not inherently flexible actually benefit from yoga the most. In addition, most poses can be modified for beginners so that everyone can do a version of the poses.

Yoga is more than a set of exercises to increase flexibility, however. Different skills are needed for different poses: Some help the practitioner gain strength, others challenge balance, and others train attention and concentration.

Is There Anyone Who Shouldn't Do Yoga?

Yoga can be safe for everyone, but depending on the medical condition, certain poses may need to be modified or avoided. A couple of examples include:

- Patients who have been diagnosed with advanced spinal stenosis should avoid extreme extension of the spine such as back bends.

- Patients with advanced cervical spine disease should avoid doing headstands and shoulder stands.

Most of the precautions surrounding the poses can be determined by understanding the specific medical condition, using common sense, and finding a good yoga teacher to assist.

How Do I Find a Good Yoga Teacher?

Unfortunately, yoga teacher training and certification are not strictly regulated, so it is important to talk to the instructor. Here are a few suggestions on how to evaluate a teacher:

- Inquire if the teacher has ever worked with people with spine problems.

- Ask how the person trained as a teacher, and if they have taken any additional courses on yoga and the spine. Many teachers have undergone advanced training and course work in this area.

- Some people feel more comfortable observing a class before deciding to participate. This allows one to determine if there are other people in the class at about the same level of fitness level, if the teacher takes the time during class to help individual students, and if the students in the class appear to enjoy it and leave feeling energized yet relaxed.

It is advisable to explain any medical condition to the teacher prior to class, and ask for his or her assistance in modifying poses that are too difficult or painful at first. Many teachers will also set up private lessons for beginners to allow them to learn modifications and receive more personalized instruction, after which it may be easier to transition to a group class.

Once the basic yoga poses have been learned, books and tapes can also be a valuable resource. At first, however, it is best to learn from an instructor who can observe and assist, and then use the tapes and books for home practice and additional study.

Types of Yoga

There are many different types of yoga, and it is important to choose a form that is appropriate for each individual's level of fitness, goals, and medical condition. Some of the most popular and widely available forms are briefly explained below.

Iyengar Yoga

This type of yoga focuses on proper alignment and precise movements. Props such as blocks or straps are often used as part of Iyengar yoga for those who are not as flexible or to compensate for injuries. Because of this attention to detail and the modification of poses, Iyengar yoga is often a good form of yoga for people with back pain or neck pain, as they are likely to benefit from modification to the poses.

Ashtanga Yoga

This form is commonly called power yoga because it focuses on powerful flowing movements, such as push-ups and lunges, which take strength and stamina. Ashtanga yoga may be appropriate for those who have successfully rehabilitated from a back injury and are looking for a more strenuous practice, and people who are already athletic, such as runners and cyclists, who want to add flexibility, balance, and concentration to their exercise routines.

Bikram Yoga

This form is also known as hot yoga because it is done in a very warm room. Bikram yoga is excellent for increasing flexibility because the heat helps tissues to stretch. This type of yoga is not appropriate for those with cardiovascular disease because of the strain placed on the body when vigorously exercising in the heat.

Viniyoga

This form links breath and movement in flowing exercises that are adapted to each individual. Viniyoga is often a good form of yoga for those with back problems or neck problems because it is easily adapted for each person.

There are many other schools of yoga. Before taking a class, it is a good idea to discuss with the teacher his or her philosophy and emphasis in order to find the most appropriate and personally appealing form of yoga.

Yoga can become a rewarding, lifelong activity that promotes health and maintains function as one ages. Because of the many modifications available and the different types of yoga, it can be a part of almost everyone's fitness plan, and the opportunities to advance and improve are endless.

Part Three

Chiropractic Care

Chapter 20

Chiropractic Care for Back Pain

Chiropractic is a form of health care that focuses on the relationship between the body's structure, primarily of the spine, and function. Doctors of chiropractic, who are also called chiropractors or chiropractic physicians, use a type of hands-on therapy called manipulation (or adjustment) as their core clinical procedure. While there are some differences in beliefs and approaches within the chiropractic profession, this chapter will give you a general overview of chiropractic, discuss scientific research findings on chiropractic treatment for low back pain, and suggest other sources of information.

What Is Chiropractic?

The word chiropractic combines the Greek words cheir (hand) and praxis (action) and means "done by hand." Chiropractic is an alternative medical system and takes a different approach from conventional medicine in diagnosing, classifying, and treating medical problems.

The basic concepts of chiropractic can be described as follows:

- The body has a powerful self-healing ability.

- The body's structure (primarily that of the spine) and its function are closely related, and this relationship affects health.

Excerpted from "About Chiropractic and Its Use in Treating Low-Back Pain," National Center for Complementary and Alternative Medicine, November 2003. Available online at http://www.nccam.nih.gov; accessed April 2004.

- Chiropractic therapy is given with the goals of normalizing this relationship between structure and function and assisting the body as it heals.

What Is Conventional Medicine?

Conventional medicine is medicine as practiced by holders of M.D. (Doctor of Medicine) or D.O. (Doctor of Osteopathic Medicine) degrees and by their allied health professionals, such as physical therapists, psychologists, and registered nurses. Other terms for conventional medicine include allopathy; Western, mainstream, orthodox, and regular medicine; and biomedicine.

What Is Complementary and Alternative Medicine (CAM)?

Health care practices and products that are not presently considered to be part of conventional medicine are called CAM. Complementary medicine is used together with conventional medicine. Alternative medicine is used in place of conventional medicine.

What Is the History of the Discovery and Use of Chiropractic?

Chiropractic is a form of spinal manipulation, which is one of the oldest healing practices. Spinal manipulation was described by Hippocrates in ancient Greece. In 1895, Daniel David Palmer founded the modern profession of chiropractic in Davenport, Iowa. Palmer was a self-taught healer and a student of healing philosophies of the day. He observed that the body has a natural healing ability that he believed was controlled by the nervous system. He also believed that subluxations, or misalignments of the spine (a concept that had already existed in the bonesetter and osteopathic traditions), interrupt or interfere with this "nerve flow." Palmer suggested that if an organ does not receive its normal supply of impulses from the nerves, it can become diseased. This line of thinking led him to develop a procedure to adjust the vertebrae, the bones of the spinal column, with the goal of correcting subluxations.

Some chiropractors continue to view subluxation as central to chiropractic health care. However, other chiropractors no longer view the subluxation theory as a unifying theme in health and illness or as a basis for their practice. Other theories as to how chiropractic might work have been developed.

Who Uses Chiropractic and for What Health Problems?

In 1997, it was estimated that Americans made nearly 192 million visits a year to chiropractors. Over 88 million of those visits were to treat back or neck pain. In one recent survey, more than 40 percent of patients receiving chiropractic care were being treated for back or low back problems. More than half of those surveyed said that their symptoms were chronic. Conditions commonly treated by chiropractors include back pain, neck pain, headaches, sports injuries, and repetitive strains. Patients also seek treatment of pain associated with other conditions, such as arthritis.

Low back pain is a common medical problem, occurring in up to one quarter of the population each year. Most people experience significant back pain at least once during their lifetime. Several recent reviews on low back pain have noted that in most cases acute low back pain gets better in several weeks, no matter what treatment is used. Often, the cause of back pain is unknown, and it varies greatly in terms of how people experience it and how professionals diagnose it. This makes back pain challenging to study.

What Kind of Training Do Chiropractors Receive?

Chiropractic training is a 4-year academic program consisting of both classroom and clinical instruction. At least 3 years of preparatory college work are required for admission to chiropractic schools. Students who graduate receive the degree of Doctor of Chiropractic (D.C.) and are eligible to take state licensure board examinations in order to practice. Some schools also offer postgraduate courses, including 2- to 3-year residency programs in specialized fields.

Chiropractic training typically includes:

* Coursework in anatomy, physiology, microbiology, biochemistry, pathology, nutrition, public health, and many other subjects

* The principles and practice of chiropractic

* Research methods and procedures

* Direct experience in caring for patients

The Council on Chiropractic Education, an agency certified by the U.S. Department of Education, is the accrediting body for chiropractic colleges in the United States.

What Do Chiropractors Do in Treating Patients?

If you become a chiropractic patient, during your initial visit the chiropractor will take your health history. He or she will perform a physical examination, with special emphasis on the spine, and possibly other examinations or tests such as x-rays. If he or she determines that you are an appropriate candidate for chiropractic therapy, he or she will develop a treatment plan.

When the chiropractor treats you, he or she may perform one or more adjustments. An adjustment (also called a manipulation treatment) is a manual therapy, or therapy delivered by the hands. Given mainly to the spine, chiropractic adjustments involve applying a controlled, sudden force to a joint. They are done to increase the range and quality of motion in the area being treated. Other health care professionals—including physical therapists, sports medicine doctors, orthopedists, physical medicine specialists, doctors of osteopathic medicine, doctors of naturopathic medicine, and massage therapists—perform various types of manipulation. In the United States, chiropractors perform over 90 percent of manipulative treatments.

Most chiropractors use other treatments in addition to adjustment, such as mobilization, massage, and nonmanual treatments.

Examples of Nonmanual Chiropractic Treatments

- Heat and ice
- Ultrasound
- Electrical stimulation
- Rehabilitative exercise
- Magnetic therapy
- Counseling about diet, weight loss, and other lifestyle factors
- Dietary supplements
- Homeopathy
- Acupuncture

Have Side Effects or Problems Been Reported from Using Chiropractic to Treat Back Pain?

Patients may or may not experience side effects from chiropractic treatment. Effects may include temporary discomfort in parts of the body that were treated, headache, or tiredness. These effects tend to be minor and to resolve within 1 to 2 days.

The rate of serious complications from chiropractic has been debated. There have been no organized prospective studies on the number of serious complications. From what is now known, the risk appears to be very low. It appears to be higher for cervical-spine, or neck, manipulation (e.g., cases of stroke have been reported). The rare complication of concern from low back adjustment is cauda equina syndrome, estimated to occur once per millions of treatments (the number of millions varies; one study placed it at 100 million).

For your safety, it is important to inform all of your health care providers about any care or treatments that you are using or considering, including chiropractic. This is to help ensure a coordinated course of care.

Does the Government Regulate Chiropractic?

Chiropractic practice is regulated individually by each state and the District of Columbia. Most states require chiropractors to earn continuing education credits to maintain their licenses. Chiropractors' scope of practice varies by state—including with regard to laboratory tests or diagnostic procedures, the dispensing or selling of dietary supplements, and the use of other CAM therapies such as acupuncture or homeopathy. Chiropractors are not licensed in any state to perform major surgery or prescribe drugs.

Do Health Insurance Plans Pay for Chiropractic Treatment?

Compared with CAM therapies as a whole (few of which are reimbursed), coverage of chiropractic by insurance plans is extensive. As of 2002, more than 50 percent of health maintenance organizations (HMOs), more than 75 percent of private health care plans, and all state workers' compensation systems covered chiropractic treatment. Chiropractors can bill Medicare, and over two dozen states cover chiropractic treatment under Medicaid.

If you have health insurance, check whether chiropractic care is covered before you seek treatment. Your plan may require care to be approved in advance, limit the number of visits covered, and/or require that you use chiropractors within its network.

What Has Scientific Research Found out about Whether Chiropractic Works for Low Back Pain?

For this report, the results of individual clinical trials and reviews of groups of clinical trials were examined. Sources were drawn from the National Library of Medicine's PubMed database; were published in English; and studied chiropractic techniques that were identified as such (e.g., "chiropractic manipulation") rather than some other forms of manipulation or spinal manipulation therapy—which, as noted above, may be delivered by certain other health care providers.

So far, the scientific research on chiropractic and low back pain has focused on if, and how well, chiropractic care helps in relieving pain and other symptoms that people have with low back pain. This research often compares chiropractic to other treatments.

Research Studies

The National Center for Complementary and Alternative Medicine (NCCAM) examined seven controlled clinical trials and one prospective observational study of chiropractic treatment for low back pain published between January 1994 and June 2003.

The studies all found at least some benefit to the participants from chiropractic treatment. However, in six of the eight studies, chiropractic and conventional treatments were found to be similar in effectiveness. One trial found greater improvement in the chiropractic group than in groups receiving either sham manipulation or back school. Another trial found treatment at a chiropractic clinic to be more effective than outpatient hospital treatment.

General Reviews, Systematic Reviews, and Meta-Analyses

NCCAM examined three reviews of clinical trials on chiropractic treatment for back pain, published between October 1996 and June 2003.

Overall, the evidence was seen as weak and less than convincing for the effectiveness of chiropractic for back pain. Specifically, the 1996 systematic review reported that there were major quality problems in the studies analyzed; for example, statistics could not be effectively combined because of missing and poor-quality data. The review concludes that the data "did not provide convincing evidence for the effectiveness of chiropractic." The 2003 general review states that since the 1996 systematic review, emerging trial data "have not tended to be encouraging. . . . The effectiveness of chiropractic spinal manipulation for back pain is thus at best uncertain." The 2003 meta-analysis found spinal manipulation to be more effective than sham therapy but no more or no less effective than other treatments.

Several other points are helpful to keep in mind about the research findings. Many clinical trials of chiropractic analyze the effects of chiropractic manipulation alone, but chiropractic practice includes more than manipulation. Results of a trial performed in one setting (such as a managed care organization or a chiropractic college) may not completely apply in other settings. And, researchers have observed that the placebo effect may be at work in chiropractic care, as in other forms of health care.

Are There Scientific Controversies Associated with Chiropractic?

Yes, there are scientific controversies about chiropractic, both inside and outside the profession. For example, within the profession, there have been disagreements about the use of physical therapy techniques, which techniques are most appropriate for certain conditions, and the concept of subluxations. Outside views have questioned the effectiveness of chiropractic treatments, their scientific basis, and the potential risks in subsets of patients (for example, the risks of certain types of adjustments to patients with osteoporosis or risk factors for osteoporosis, compared to patients with healthier bone structures).

Research studies on chiropractic are ongoing. The results are expected to expand scientific understanding of chiropractic. A key area of research is the basic science of what happens in the body (including its cells and nerves) when specific chiropractic treatments are given.

Is NCCAM Funding Research on Chiropractic?

Yes. For example, recent projects supported by NCCAM include:

- Comparing conventional medical care for acute back pain with an "expanded benefits" package (consisting of conventional care plus a choice of chiropractic, massage, or acupuncture)

- Finding out what happens (through measurement) in the lumbar portion of the spine after chiropractic positioning and adjustment

- Evaluating the effects of the speed of spinal adjustment on muscles and nerves

- Studying the effectiveness of chiropractic adjustment for a variety of conditions, including neck pain, chronic pelvic pain, and temporomandibular disorders (TMD) in the jaw

Definitions

Acupuncture: A health care practice that originated in traditional Chinese medicine. Acupuncture involves inserting needles at specific points on the body, in the belief that this will help improve the flow of the body's energy (or qi, pronounced "chee") and thereby help the body achieve and maintain health.

Acute pain: Pain that has lasted a short time (e.g., less than 3 weeks) or is severe.

Alternative medical system: A medical system built upon a complete system of theory and practice; these systems have often evolved apart from and earlier than the conventional medical approach used in the United States. An example from a Western culture is naturopathic medicine; from a non-Western culture, traditional Chinese medicine.

Bonesetter: A health care practitioner (not necessarily a licensed physician) whose occupation is setting fractured or dislocated bones.

Cauda equina syndrome: A syndrome that occurs when the nerves of the cauda equina (a bundle of spinal nerves extending beyond the end of the spinal cord) are compressed and damaged. Symptoms include leg weakness; loss of bowel, bladder, and/or sexual functions; and changes in sensation around the rectum or genitalia.

Chronic pain: Pain that has lasted a long time (more than 3 months).

Clinical trial: A clinical trial is a research study in which a treatment or therapy is tested in people to see whether it is safe and effective. Clinical trials are a key part of the process in finding out which treatments work, which do not, and why. Clinical trial results also contribute new knowledge about diseases and medical conditions.

Complication: A secondary disease or condition that develops in the course of a primary disease or condition, or as the result of a treatment.

Controlled clinical trial: A clinical study that includes a comparison (control) group. The comparison group receives a placebo, another treatment, or no treatment at all.

General review: An analysis in which information from various studies is summarized and evaluated; conclusions are made based on this evidence.

Hippocrates: A Greek physician born in 460 B.C. who became known as the founder of Western medicine.

Homeopathy: Also known as homeopathic medicine. It is an alternative medical system that was invented in Germany. In homeopathic treatment, there is a belief that "like cures like," meaning that small, highly diluted quantities of medicinal substances are given to cure symptoms, when the same substances given at higher or more concentrated doses would actually cause those symptoms.

Manipulation: Passive joint movement beyond the normal range of motion. The term adjustment is preferred in chiropractic.

Massage: A therapy in which muscle and connective tissue are manipulated to enhance function of those tissues and promote relaxation and well-being.

Meta-analysis: A type of research review that uses statistical techniques to analyze results from a collection of individual studies.

Mobilization: A technique, used by chiropractors and other health care professionals, in which a joint is passively moved within its normal range of motion.

Myofascial therapy: A type of physical therapy that uses stretches and massage.

Naturopathic medicine: Also known as naturopathy. It is an alternative medical system in which practitioners work with natural healing forces within the body, with a goal of helping the body heal from disease and attain better health. Practices may include dietary modifications, massage, exercise, acupuncture, minor surgery, and various other interventions.

Observational study: A type of study in which individuals are observed or certain outcomes are measured. No attempt is made to affect the outcome (for example, no treatment is given).

Orthopedist: Doctor of Medicine (M.D.) who is a surgeon specializing in disorders of the musculoskeletal system.

Osteopathic medicine: Also known as osteopathy. It is a form of conventional medicine that, in part, emphasizes diseases arising in the musculoskeletal system. There is an underlying belief that all of the body's systems work together, and disturbances in one system may affect function elsewhere in the body. Most osteopathic physicians practice osteopathic manipulation, a full-body system of hands-on techniques to alleviate pain, restore function, and promote health and well-being.

Osteoporosis: A reduction in the amount of bone mass, which can lead to breaking a bone after a minor injury, such as a fall.

Placebo: Resembles a treatment being studied in a clinical trial, except that the placebo is inactive. One example is a sugar pill. By giving one group of participants a placebo and the other group the active treatment, the researchers can compare how the two groups respond and get a truer picture of the active treatment's effects. In recent years, the definition of placebo has been expanded to include other things that could affect the results of health care, such as how a patient feels about receiving the care and what she expects to happen from it.

Prospective study: A type of research study in which participants are followed over time for the effect(s) of a health care treatment.

Randomized clinical trial: A study in which the participants are assigned by chance to separate groups that compare different treatments; neither the researchers nor the participants can choose which group. Using chance to assign people to groups means that the groups will be similar and that the treatments they receive can be compared objectively. At the time of the trial, it is not known which treatment is best. It is the patient's choice to be in a randomized trial.

Review: See general review, systematic review, or meta-analysis.

Sham: A treatment or device that is a type of placebo. An example would be positioning the patient's body and placing the chiropractor's hands in a way that mimics an actual treatment, but is not a treatment.

Subacute pain: Pain that has lasted somewhat longer than acute pain (for example, more than a few days or weeks) but is not yet chronic pain.

Systematic review: A type of research review in which data from a set of studies on a particular question or topic are collected, analyzed, and critically reviewed.

Chapter 21

Questions and Answers about Subluxation and Chiropractic Adjustment

What is a subluxation?

The word subluxation comes from the Latin words meaning "to dislocate" (luxate) and "somewhat or slightly" (sub). A subluxation means a slight dislocation (misalignment) or biomechanical malfunctioning of the vertebrae (bones of the spine). These disturbances may irritate nerve roots and blood vessels that branch off from the spinal cord between each of the vertebrae. This irritation may cause pain and dysfunction in muscle, lymphatic, and organ tissue as well as imbalance in the normal body processes.

What causes a subluxation?

A fall, injury, sudden jar, trauma, or sometimes an inherited spinal weakness can displace a vertebra. Other causes include improper sleeping conditions or habits, poor posture, occupational hazards, incorrect lifting practices, obesity, lack of rest and exercise, and stress.

How is a subluxation corrected?

Doctors of Chiropractic are specialists in neuromusculoskeletal conditions. They are trained to restore the misaligned vertebrae to their proper position in the spinal column. They do this manually, utilizing the chiropractic procedure known as spinal adjustment.

Your chiropractor, in most cases, will use his or her hands in applying corrective pressure to the spine in a specific direction and location. The manual force or thrust helps restore the alignment and mobility of the vertebrae. In some cases, the chiropractor may use instrumentation to detect subluxations and adjust the spine.

Does the adjustment hurt?

Under normal circumstances, chiropractic adjustments are painless. In cases of recent trauma, such as whiplash, mild discomfort may be experienced due to inflammation. It is also common to feel a brief sensation in the extremities immediately following an adjustment due to the sudden decompression of the affected nerve root.

Is regular chiropractic care necessary?

Regular chiropractic care may be necessary to correct spinal subluxations to help maintain sound health and fitness. Your spine is under constant strain during waking hours. Improper lifting techniques, poor posture, accidents, falls and bumps, and other causes can contribute to spinal strain. Timely adjustments can help restore the neuromusculoskeletal integrity of the spine to normalize the bodily equilibrium and increase resistance.

How old should a person be before he or she begins chiropractic care?

Chiropractic patients range in years from birth to old age. Regardless of age, the vertebrae can become misaligned. For example, the birth process may cause trauma to the neck and spine. Left uncorrected, the vertebral subluxation may disturb the delicate spinal cord and nerves that control the youngster's muscles and organs. In some cases, an uncorrected subluxation may lead to a deformity of the spinal column. An early chiropractic checkup may detect many spinal problems while they are still easily correctable.

How will the adjustment help me?

Chiropractic adjustments by themselves do not actually heal the body. When any of the 24 moveable spinal vertebrae become misaligned, a basic imbalance or disruption can occur in the nervous and blood vascular systems, which may contribute to stress in the body.

Chiropractic adjustments help eliminate that imbalance or disruption so that the body can function at its true potential.

Does an adjustment have to make a noise to be effective?

No, it is a common misconception that your joints must make a noise to be properly adjusted. However, more often than not when your vertebrae are adjusted, the smooth articular (joint) surfaces become separated, creating and then releasing a small vacuum, making a noise. This is the sound made when you crack your knuckles. Your chiropractor is concerned with the position of your vertebrae, not with the noise that may occur.

Should I go to a chiropractor if I feel fine?

Even if you feel fine, chiropractic care can help your body maintain its required level of health and fitness. Your chiropractor can recommend a preventive spinal-care program and advise you on correct posture, dietary information, and back exercises. Regular spinal checkups can help detect and prevent spinal stress due to subluxations.

Is it true that chiropractors do not prescribe medication or perform surgery?

Yes. Chiropractors do not include medication or surgery in their treatment program. Chiropractors maintain that the body has a built-in capacity to restore health within certain limits, and base their care on this principle. Occasionally, the use of medication can interfere with the body's healing mechanisms, produce side effects, create a dependence, and lead to drug-caused disease or complications. The first response in most illnesses and injuries should be conservative care. Chiropractic's principles make it possibly the safest and most appealing of the healing arts.

How does chiropractic care help the pregnant woman?

Because of the additional weight and stress on the framework of the body in pregnant women, chiropractic adjustments can help lower the incidence of pain in the low back and legs, and between the shoulder blades. In some cases, fewer headaches and problems with nausea and elimination may also result. Many chiropractors care for expectant mothers in the regular course of their daily practices. It is wise, however, to first inquire about the experience of your chiropractor in caring for pregnant women and what he or she recommends for you.

Chapter 22

Choosing a Chiropractic Practitioner

Chapter Contents

Section 22.1

Questions and Answers about Chiropractic Regulation

Why regulate health care professionals?

Regulation exists to protect the public's health, safety, and welfare. Government statute provides for a board (generally composed of both non-paid professional and consumer members) to handle regulation for each licensed profession.

Their responsibilities:

- to investigate consumer complaints;

- to oversee the general application of health care laws;

- to help update and develop regulations which better define appropriate conduct by professionals and clarify what the consumer may expect;

- to continually review required credentials for doctors to practice safely, effectively, and ethically;

- to apply appropriate disciplinary action or retraining to doctors who may have broken the public trust through violation of statute or regulation;

- to function in the global regulatory community to assist other professions or jurisdictions affected by chiropractic.

The governor usually appoints the board members for regulated professions. An appointee's term may last three to six years, with reappointment permitted for a prescribed period of time.

Where are chiropractors regulated?

Doctors of Chiropractic are licensed in all 50 states plus the District of Columbia and many U.S. territories. They are also regulated in many other countries throughout the world.

When a license is granted to a chiropractor, what does this mean to the public?

Through licensure, the board assures the public that the doctor has met certain credentialing criteria, and that he/she continues to abide by the laws and regulations of that state or province. The requirements to enter licensed chiropractic practice are defined by laws and regulations designed to protect the public's health, safety and welfare.

What credentials are required by U.S. jurisdictions?

In general, certain common criteria cross jurisdictional borders. These include:

- Pre-chiropractic education—States may require a minimum of two years in an accredited undergraduate program, which includes a prescribed science content (biology, zoology, general, or inorganic chemistry, and related laboratories). An increasing number of U.S. states require a bachelor's degree of candidates for licensure. Most candidates enrolling in chiropractic college today have their bachelor's degrees, while some may achieve it through parallel programs offered by the chiropractic college.

- Graduation from an accredited chiropractic college—All chiropractic colleges in the United States are currently accredited by the Council on Chiropractic Education (CCE), an agency recognized by the U.S. Department of Education. Most boards rely on the CCE to be certain the colleges meet both federal and professional educational standards for their programs, while several boards reserve the process of approving schools for the regulatory agency. The chiropractic college curriculum generally spans four to five years, with no less than 4,200 hours of classroom, laboratory, and clinical experience under strict supervision. Courses include differential diagnosis, anatomy, biochemistry, physiology, microbiology, pathology, gynecology, pediatrics, geriatrics, radiology, spinal analysis, and a host of other subjects.

- Rigorous examinations—Most boards rely on a four-part examination offered by the National Board of Chiropractic Examiners. This testing series covers basic sciences, clinical sciences, and clinical competency and practical skills. Boards may also require special examinations to be successfully completed by practitioners relocating from another jurisdiction, or those under review for disciplinary or impairment reasons.

- Background investigation—Boards conduct a thorough investigation into the character and credentials history for each applicant for licensure.

- Understanding of state law—This is often called the jurisprudence portion of the board's assessment of the candidate. This is important because there are some differences among jurisdictions in the type of care a chiropractor may legally provide.

What can the public expect from a doctor of chiropractic?

While the core concept of practice is based on healing without drugs or surgery, the specific scope may vary according to the laws of a specific jurisdiction. However, patients may commonly expect:

- A thorough physical examination to determine conditions which may be appropriate for chiropractic care;

- To be referred to another health care provider for conditions which are not appropriate for chiropractic care;

- To understand the type of care to be administered, and what results may be expected;

- Discussion with the doctor as the care continues, to evaluate both treatment effectiveness and projected duration;

- A clear understanding of financial arrangements;

- Appropriate, ethical care delivered in confidence, with respect for privacy and dignity.

What happens if a doctor violates these basic rights?

An essential part of the regulatory board's responsibility is to discipline and/or retrain the small fraction of doctors who step outside law and regulation.

Complaints are investigated thoroughly. If the complaint cannot be resolved satisfactorily through informal processes, formal hearings may be conducted to determine facts, severity of offense, and whether these sanctions are appropriate:

- Formal letter of reprimand

- Fine

- Probation

- Suspension

- Revocation of License

- Retraining/re-examination

- Other appropriate sanctions

Who knows if the doctor has been disciplined?

The public may contact the licensing board in each jurisdiction to determine the status of the doctor's license.

Also, the Federation of Chiropractic Licensing Boards maintains an on-line, international databank, known as CIN-BAD. This databank carries information on public actions by chiropractic regulatory agencies related to licenses of individual practitioners. It also lists doctors prohibited from receiving Medicare reimbursement due to federal sanctions imposed by U.S. Department of Health & Human Services. Members of the public may use a query form to request a search of the database.

Section 22.2

Tips on Choosing a Chiropractor

"How to Choose a Chiropractor" by G. Douglas Andersen, DC, DACBSP, CCN. Reprinted with permission from www.ChiroWeb.com. © 2002 Dynamic Chiropractic. All rights reserved.

My patients requested a list of pointers on how to find a good chiropractor when they move, and tips on how to inform their friends in cases when they suspect brainwashing.

Wellness or Maintenance Treatment

This is a good way for a chiropractor to make extra money, and a common reason many medical doctors don't refer to chiropractors. There is no scientific evidence that when you feel good chiropractic treatment can prevent or maintain anything. If you feel good and your chiropractor still wants to see you, get a second opinion before continuing care.

Questionable Diagnostics

If your chiropractor tests your muscles, notes they are weak, and diagnoses an internal problem, the DC [Doctor of Chiropractic] should refer you to an internist. On the other hand, if you have weak muscles because you are out of shape, a good chiropractor will refer you to a therapist, a gym, or design a strengthening program for you. If your muscles are weak due to a serious disease, nerve problem or serious structural problem, your DC should refer you for a second opinion with a neurologist or orthopedist. Muscle testing alone should not be the reason your chiropractor wants to continue to treat you if there is no pain.

Silly Marketing Gimmicks

Health fairs, swap meets, and shopping malls often have chiropractors giving free spinal examinations. There are a variety of gimmicks designed to procure you as a patient. The most common one is a postural analysis. If you have poor posture and no pain, a chiropractor should not want to manipulate you, but instead should design a workout or exercise program for you, or refer you to a therapist or trainer for such a program.

Treating Areas That Don't Hurt

When you receive treatment, three things happen: You get better, you get worse, or you stay the same. If you feel good, only two things can occur: You stay the same or you get worse.

If you go to a chiropractor with lower back pain, the DC should not manipulate your neck unless you also have a neck problem. There is no evidence that performing neck manipulation can help your lower back or vice versa. If your chiropractor insists on manipulating areas that don't hurt, get a second opinion before continuing care.

Excessive Supplementation

Chiropractors take many nutrition classes in school. Beware of any chiropractor who says his vitamins are the only ones that work. Beware of any chiropractor that wants to sell you large amounts of supplements without referring you to a retailer or health-food store for comparable products at a considerably lower cost.

Excessive X-Rays

Beware of any chiropractor who uses x-rays for any reason other than to rule out a fracture, dislocation, or bone disease. X-rays should only be taken if you have sustained a recent traumatic injury and are in considerable pain and discomfort; are undergoing a history and examination indicate a possible bone disease such as arthritis; or have long-standing pain in an area that has not responded or resolved with care. No person is perfectly symmetrical; no one's spine is perfectly straight and balanced. If you are pain-free and your chiropractor wants to continue treatment because of what an x-ray shows, get a second opinion before you continue care.

Excessive Visits

When a chiropractor treats you, you should feel better. It is not normal to be worse after treatment. Depending on the nature and extent of your problem, after a few visits you should notice considerable improvement. After one to four weeks, your pain should be reduced by 40 to 50 percent, depending on how severe and how extensive your original problem. Beware of any chiropractor who recommends a three, six or 12-month treatment plan based on your first or second visit.

Unwillingness to Work with Other Professionals

If you are not getting relief, you should not have to ask for a referral; your chiropractor should have already recommended one for you.

A Good Chiropractor

Good chiropractors do everything in their power to get you better as fast as possible with as few treatments as necessary. A good chiropractor will give you advice on how to avoid future problems without a costly maintenance treatment plan. A good chiropractor will only x-ray when necessary and will not use x-rays as a marketing tool to have you continue care. A good chiropractor will give you sensible nutritional advice concerning supplementation and a healthy diet without excessive pressure to purchase vitamins. A good chiropractor will have a strong working relationship with allied professionals of all specialties, including family practice physicians, orthopedists, neurologists, physiatrists, physical therapists, and athletic trainers.

Chapter 23

What to Expect at Your First Chiropractic Visit

Patients typically visit a chiropractor for the first time through a personal reference or a referral of another health care specialist. At the first visit, you can expect the chiropractor to complete a thorough chiropractic consultation that takes 60 minutes or more and includes:

- Patient history
- Physical examination
- Diagnostic studies (when indicated)
- Diagnosis
- Chiropractic treatment plan

Patient History

In preparation for your consultation with the chiropractor, you will be asked to fill out forms that provide background information about your symptoms and condition. Types of questions the chiropractor might ask include:

- When and how did the pain start?
- Where is it located?

"What to Expect at Your First Chiropractic Visit" by Peter J. Schubbe, DC, is reprinted with permission from www.Spine-health.com. © May 22, 2000 Spine-health.com. All rights reserved. For more information, please see http://www.Spine-health.com.

- Is it a result of an injury?
- What makes it better?
- What makes it worse?

You will also usually be asked to provide the chiropractor with information on family medical history, any pre-existing medical conditions or prior injuries, and previous and current health providers and treatments.

Physical Examination

Once the history has been completed, your chiropractor will perform a thorough chiropractic examination. In addition to general tests such as blood pressure, pulse, respiration, and reflexes, the chiropractic examination will include specific orthopedic and neurological tests to assess:

- Range of motion of the affected part
- Muscle tone
- Muscle strength
- Neurological integrity

Based on the above examination procedures, further chiropractic tests may be necessary to arrive at the assessment or diagnosis of the affected area (such as moving your leg in a specified manner, posture analysis, or the chiropractor manipulating your arm or leg).

Diagnostic Studies

Diagnostic studies are helpful in revealing pathologies and identifying structural abnormalities that more accurately diagnose a condition. They may or may not be necessary based upon the results of the history and chiropractic examination.

The most common diagnostic studies include:

- X-ray
- MRI (Magnetic Resonance Imaging) scan
- Laboratory tests

Many chiropractic offices can do basic x-rays, but an MRI scan and more extensive images may be referred to an outside center for which an appointment is needed.

Diagnosis

The culmination of the history, examination, and diagnostic studies is a specific diagnosis. Once the diagnosis is established, the chiropractor will determine if the condition will respond to chiropractic care.

The chiropractor will explain:

- The diagnosed condition

- The chiropractic treatment plan (or other treatments)

- The anticipated length of chiropractic care

Chiropractic Treatment Plan

Most chiropractors begin treatment during the patient's first visit, although some may wait until the next appointment. Chiropractic treatment recommendations may include some or all of the following:

- Adjustments to key joint dysfunctions

- Modalities to improve soft tissue healing and pain control (ultrasound, electrical stimulation, and traction)

- Exercises to improve muscles balance, strength, and coordination

- Patient education to improve posture and motor control

- Other treatments may be included, such as massage, heat/cold application, and nutrition education.

Importantly, at this point the chiropractor will establish specific goals for your chiropractic treatment plan.

- Short term goals—to reduce pain and restore normal joint function and muscle balance

- Long term goals—to restore functional independence and tolerance to normal activities of daily living

To reach these goals, the chiropractor will prescribe a specific number of visits. An example would be 1 to 3 visits per week for 2 to 4 weeks followed by a re-examination. At the re-examination, the chiropractor will measure the response to treatment and determine whether to:

- Continue chiropractic treatment if appropriate;

- Release you from care if your goals have been met; or

- Refer you to another health care specialist if your goals have not been fulfilled.

Chapter 24

A Parents' Guide to Chiropractic Care for Children

What is chiropractic?

Chiropractic is a conservative and natural healing art and science that concentrates on keeping people well. While chiropractic is an American science over 100 years old, its wellness practices have stood the test of time—dating back to spinal manipulations first used by Hippocrates, the Father of Healing, in the 4th century B.C.

Doctors of Chiropractic attempt to get to the root cause of a health problem rather than just treat the symptoms. They seek to maximize the natural strengths of the body and its capacity to heal itself without the use of drugs or surgery. The primary focus of chiropractic is the detection, reduction and correction of spinal misalignments and nervous system dysfunction.

Misaligned vertebrae (known as subluxations) can irritate the nerves and disrupt the body's ability to send "command center" messages through the spine to different parts of the body such as the tissue, bone, glands, and organs. All parts of the human body require proper nerve energy and a flow of information in order to function properly. If left uncorrected, a spinal malfunction can interrupt this internal communication system and cause pain, muscle, and organ dysfunction and other imbalances.

"Parents Guide to Chiropractic" is reprinted with permission from the International Chiropractors Association, www.chiropractic.org. © 2004 International Chiropractors Association. All rights reserved.

The Doctor of Chiropractic, through a procedure called adjustments, helps to restore misaligned vertebrae to a more normal position, thus allowing the nerves to properly communicate with the rest of the body and let the body heal itself—safely and naturally. Chiropractic's drugless and preventive approach to good health makes it perfectly appropriate for infants, children, and teenagers.

Is the education of a Doctor of Chiropractic on par with a medical physician?

Yes. Doctors of Chiropractic undergo a rigorous and demanding professional education equivalent to any other primary care provider. To obtain a Doctor of Chiropractic degree, they must complete several years of prerequisite undergraduate education and spend nearly the same number of classroom hours at a fully-accredited chiropractic college as physicians do in medical schools. Student doctors are thoroughly trained in the appropriate use of sophisticated diagnostic equipment including X-rays, laboratory procedures, and state of the art investigative technology. Before they can practice, Doctors of Chiropractic must pass the National Boards, similar to the Board exam of medical doctors, as well as a licensing exam for the state in which they choose to practice. Most states require the doctors to attend clinical continuing education programs for annual relicensure.

When should I take my child to a Doctor of Chiropractic?

- **When you want your child to have all the benefits of a conservative, drugless approach to health care.** Your child's first visit to the Doctor of Chiropractic can be a pleasant experience, one without painful injections and procedures, but with plenty of nurturing. A Doctor of Chiropractic should examine your child during that all-important first year of life when spinal trauma can occur during birth as well as from tumbles while learning to sit up or walk. Improper lifting and carrying of your child can also contribute to spinal stress. Your child's spine grows almost 50% in length during that first year (the equivalent of a six-footer growing to nine feet in just 12 months!) It's this kind of tremendous growth and developmental changes that makes a complete chiropractic examination so important in the early stages of your child's life.

- **When you want to give your child a head start in good health.** Doctors of Chiropractic believe it's much more important to prevent diseases than wait till some illness occurs. Through regular adjustments and counseling on proper diet, exercise, and posture, the Doctor of Chiropractic can help you raise a child whose body is structurally and functionally sound. Your child will also learn good health habits at an early age that can be very beneficial during adulthood.

- **When your child takes a fall.** Youngsters take numerous tumbles while learning to walk, riding a bike, or even while jumping or running around. But after their tears have dried, underlying injuries could go undetected—such as a misaligned vertebra during the spine's most formative period.

- **When your child takes part in athletic activities.** The sack of a young quarterback could twist a young spine. A softball pitcher could throw a vertebra out of alignment. Doctors of Chiropractic can do more than correct these problems, they can also help improve performance on and off the field by helping the body function at its optimum level, naturally without stress and without drugs.

Regular spinal exams by the Doctor of Chiropractic can provide corrective and preventive care for your son or daughter and peace of mind for you.

How safe is chiropractic for my child?

Chiropractic is one of the safest forms of health care. A baby's spine is very supple during the first few months of life and the Doctor of Chiropractic applies only a slight pressure to make spinal adjustments. Under normal circumstances, chiropractic adjustments are painless and will not hurt your child. Chiropractors do not use drugs that sometimes cause more harmful side effects than the progression of the disease itself. Drugs can also create the potential for addiction, even in young children. The Doctor of Chiropractic does not perform any invasive procedures (such as surgery) that sometimes can have irreversible side effects. These are some of the reasons why malpractice insurance rates for chiropractors are only a fraction of what physicians pay and why more than 30 million Americans choose chiropractic care for their children and themselves.

How effective is chiropractic care for children?

Doctors of Chiropractic have been providing safe and effective care or children for nearly 100 years. There are several published studies conducted by researchers in Germany, Australia, Denmark, and the United States that confirm the effectiveness of chiropractic for a variety of childhood illnesses. This body of scientific evidence is growing every day.

What if my child has a health problem that doesn't respond to chiropractic care?

Doctors of Chiropractic are trained to recognize complex health problems. Their primary obligation is the welfare of the child. When they reach their limits of skill and authority, the International Chiropractors Association's position is that "doctors in all fields of practice are ethically and morally bound to make patient referrals to practitioners in other fields of healing when such referrals are necessary to provide the highest quality of patient care."

There are so many different health care specialists today. Who is really responsible for the health of my children?

You are. As a parent, you must take responsibility for your child's health and use your best judgment as to what is most appropriate for your child. Fortunately, there are some outstanding primary health care providers to help you make your decisions, including your Doctor of Chiropractic, pediatrician, and dentist. These professionals can make up your child's personal health care team.

Do all Doctors of Chiropractic care for children? How do I choose?

Doctors of Chiropractic are licensed in all 50 states of the United States to provide chiropractic care to children and adults. A doctor who is interested in providing the best care possible will belong to a chiropractic pediatric council and take regular continuing postgraduate courses in pediatrics. Some may pursue a postgraduate degree in pediatrics. Choose a doctor with a family practice or who is referred to you by another parent. The International Chiropractors Association has a Pediatrics Council to which many doctors belong. This council regularly updates doctors with the latest in chiropractic pediatric care and encourages its members to take advanced education in chiropractic pediatrics to improve their diagnostic and clinical skills.

To find out if a doctor in your area is a member of the International Chiropractors Association Pediatrics Council, call the International Chiropractors Association at (703) 528-5000.

What if my child has a high fever, severe pain, or other serious medical problem?

Take your child immediately to the nearest emergency medical facility. When your child's condition has stabilized, then call on any of your child's health care team for help and advice. It's essential that when an emergency arises, you or anyone else responsible for your children know where to go and whom to call.

Part Four

Acute Injuries to the
Back and Neck

Chapter 25

First Aid for Spinal Injuries

Your spinal cord contains the nerves that carry messages between your brain and your body. The cord passes through your neck and back. A spinal cord injury is very serious because it can cause paralysis below the site of the injury.

Considerations

When someone has a spinal injury, additional movement may cause further damage to the nerves in the cord and can sometimes mean the difference between life and death.

If you think someone could possibly have a spinal injury, **do not** move the injured person even a little bit, unless it is absolutely necessary (like getting someone out of a burning car).

If you are in doubt about whether a person has a spinal injury, assume that he or she **does** have one.

Causes

- Bullet or stab wound
- Direct trauma to the face, neck, head, or back (e.g., car accidents)
- Diving accident
- Electric shock
- Extreme twisting of the trunk
- Sports injury (landing on head)

"Spinal/Neck Injury," © 2003 A.D.A.M., Inc. Reprinted with permission.

Symptoms

- Major blow to the head or chest, car accident, or fall from a great height

- Head held in unusual position

- Numbness or tingling that radiates down an arm or leg

- Weakness

- Difficulty walking

- Paralysis of arms or legs

- No bladder or bowel control

- Shock (with pale, clammy skin; bluish lips and fingernails; acting dazed or semi-conscious)

- Unconscious

- Stiff neck, headache, or neck pain

First Aid

The main goal is to keep the person immobile and safe until medical help arrives.

1. You or someone else should call 911.

2. Hold the person's head and neck in the position in which they were found. **Do not** attempt to reposition the neck. Do not allow the neck to bend or twist.

If the person is unresponsive:

1. Check the person's breathing and circulation. If necessary, begin rescue breathing and cardiopulmonary resuscitation (CPR).

2. **Do not** tilt the head back when attempting to open the airway. Instead, place your fingers on the jaw on each side of the head. Lift the jaw forward.

If you need to roll the person:

1. Do not roll the person over unless the person is vomiting or choking on blood or you need to check for breathing.

2. Two people are needed.

3. One person should be stationed at the head, the other at the person's side.

4. Keep the person's head, neck, and back in line with each other while you roll him or her onto one side.

Do Not

- **Do not** bend, twist, or lift the person's head or body.

- **Do not** attempt to move the person before medical help arrives unless it is absolutely necessary.

- **Do not** remove a helmet if a spinal injury is suspected.

Call Immediately for Emergency Medical Assistance

Call your local emergency number (such as 911) if there has been any injury that affects the neck or spinal cord. Keep the person absolutely immobile. Unless there is urgent danger, keep the person in the position where he or she was found.

Prevention

- Wear seat belts.

- Avoid drinking alcohol and driving.

- Avoid diving into pools, lakes, rivers and surf, particularly if you cannot determine the depth of the water, or if the water is not clear.

- Avoid motorcycles and all-terrain vehicles.

- Avoid spearing (tackling or diving into a person with your head).

Chapter 26

Neck Injuries

Chapter Contents

Section 26.1

Neck Sprain

People who are involved in motor vehicle crashes or who take hard falls in a contact sport or around the house may get a real pain in the neck. This pain can result from a ligament sprain or muscle strain.

The seven bones of the spinal column in your neck are called cervical vertebrae. They are connected to each other by ligaments, which are strong bands of tissue, like thick rubber bands.

A sprain is a stretch or tear in the ligament resulting from a sudden movement that causes the neck to extend to an extreme position. For example, in the rapid deceleration of a car crash, your head and neck can stretch far forward before stopping.

Symptoms

- Pain, especially in the back of the neck, that worsens with movement

- Pain that often peaks a day or so after the injury, instead of immediately

- Possible muscle spasms and pain in the upper regions of the shoulders

- Headache in the rear of the head

- Sore throat

- Increased irritability, fatigue, difficulty sleeping, and difficulty concentrating.

- Numbness in the arm or hand

- Stiffness or decrease in range of motion (side to side, up and down, circular)

- Tingling or weakness in the arms

Diagnosis

During the physical exam, your doctor will ask you how the injury occurred, measure range of motion, and check for any point tenderness. Your orthopaedist may request x-ray studies to look closely at the bones in your neck. This evaluation helps eliminate or identify other sources of neck pain, such as spinal fractures, dislocations, arthritis, and other serious conditions.

Treatment

All sprains or strains, no matter where they are located in the body, receive basically the same type of treatment. Usually, neck sprains, like other sprains, will gradually heal, given time and appropriate treatment. You may have to wear a soft cervical collar to help support the head and relieve pressure on the neck so the ligaments have time to heal.

Analgesics, such as aspirin or ibuprofen, can help reduce the pain and any swelling. Muscle relaxants can help ease spasms. You can apply an ice pack for 15 to 30 minutes at a time several times a day for the first two or three days after the injury. This will help reduce inflammation and discomfort. Although heat, particularly moist heat, can help loosen cramped muscles, it should not be applied too quickly.

Other treatment options include:

- Massaging the tender area

- Ultrasound

- Cervical traction

- Aerobic and isometric exercise

Most symptoms will resolve in four to six weeks. A severe injury, such as might be sustained in a motor vehicle accident, may take longer to heal completely.

Section 26.2

Stingers

What Is a Stinger?

A stinger is a sports-related injury to the nerves about the neck or shoulder. It is sometimes called a burner or nerve pinch injury, but the term stinger is most descriptive of the symptoms that the athlete experiences, including painful electrical sensations radiating through one of the arms. While the stinger is usually a spine injury, it is never a spinal cord injury. The stinger occurs most commonly in contact and collision sports, but is not as catastrophic as a spinal cord injury and does not result in paralysis in the arms and legs. A stinger is often not reported by the athlete to the coaches or the athletic trainers since the symptoms can spontaneously resolve within a short period of time. However, stingers tend to recur and if not properly diagnosed and treated can lead to persistent pain or even arm weakness, which can eventually result in extended lost playing time.

Athletes competing in various sports (most commonly football and wrestling), playing specific positions (such as defensive back, linebacker, or offensive line), or performing certain athletic maneuvers (such as tackling, blocking, or executing a take down maneuver) are at greatest risk of sustaining a stinger. The injury occurs in one of two ways: either one of the nerves off the spinal cord in the neck is compressed as the head is forced backward and toward that side; or the nerves in the neck and shoulder are over-stretched as the head is forced sideways away from the shoulder. The athlete will experience sudden and severe painful, stinging sensations in one arm, frequently lasting from seconds to minutes, occasionally hours, and less frequently days or longer. There is often associated weakness of the muscles in the shoulder and arm that are supplied by the injured nerve. The arm symptoms are usually more severe than neck pain. First-time stingers will usually go away quickly even without treatment, but there is a greater risk of recurrent injury if left untreated. Each additional stinger will likely result in continued neurologic impairment including muscle weakness. Stingers do not affect both arms at the same time, although each arm can be affected with different injuries. If both arms are symptomatic at the same time after a neck injury, a spinal cord injury is likely to have occurred, which leads to a much different treatment plan.

How Is It Diagnosed?

The diagnosis of the stinger requires the expertise of a medical professional. Ideally, the first evaluation of the athlete occurs at the time of injury at the game or match. Since these injuries are not catastrophic, the athlete often exits the field of play without assistance. A sideline evaluation will be conducted by the athletic trainer, physical therapist, and/or team physician that will include: a determination of the mechanism of the injury, the symptoms experienced by the athlete, and the physical examination findings including assessment of muscle strength. A decision will be made whether or not the athlete is medically cleared to return to that contest. Persistence of symptoms, stiffness or loss of full range of neck motion, muscle spasm, and weakness would usually keep the athlete out of competition.

Careful medical follow-up evaluations are important and necessary. These examinations should take place regularly until the athlete's condition has normalized. If the symptoms and/or neurologic findings worsen during the first few days after the injury or continue beyond 2 weeks, then further medical assessment is necessary. The physician may order specific tests such as x-ray examinations, magnetic resonance imaging (MRI), and an electromyogram (or EMG) which is designed to evaluate for nerve damage. Occasionally a stinger can result from a disk herniation in the neck. If so, this should be confirmed on the MRI.

No matter how trivial the injury may appear, in order for the physician to make the correct diagnosis and prescribe the appropriate treatment, it is very important for the athlete not to withhold information. If the injury was not witnessed by the medical personnel covering the event, then it is the responsibility of the athlete to report the injury even if the symptoms disappear quickly. In some situations, the effects of the stinger can lead to permanent nerve damage if left undiagnosed and untreated.

What Treatments Are Available?

The goals of treatment are to reduce the pain and abnormal sensations in the arm, regain the strength of weakened shoulder and arm muscles, and prevent further injuries.

There are several nonoperative options for the treatment of an acute stinger. The order in which these treatments are utilized depends largely on whether the primary complaint is pain or weakness.

Treatment for acute pain usually includes activity restriction, ice or heat, anti-inflammatory and pain medications, a cervical collar, and cervical traction. Following an acute injury, the athlete is not allowed to return to competition to allow time for recovery. Modalities such as ice and heat can be used both for comfort and to reduce inflammation. Ice is usually applied about the neck and shoulder region up to 48 hours post injury after which time heat is substituted.

Nonsteroidal anti-inflammatory medications are frequently prescribed for both reduction of swelling and inflammation as well as pain relief. Stronger analgesics (pain medications) are not usually necessary, but muscle relaxants may be utilized for a short period of time to treat muscle spasm.

A cervical collar may also be used for a short period of time to prevent further nerve root injury or irritation. Cervical traction helps to reduce pressure on the nerve root. It can be applied manually or mechanically under the guidance of a physical therapist. Often, trunk strengthening and chest-out posture correction exercises are started.

For persistent pain, cortisone injection around the injured nerve root (nerve root block) performed with x-ray guidance can be helpful to reduce inflammation of the nerve. If weakness is the main problem, then the acute treatment includes modified activities, ice or heat, and anti-inflammatory medication.

The majority of stingers are treated successfully without surgery. Surgery is only considered if the injured nerve root is found to be severely compressed by either a disk herniation or bone spur and there is severe persisting pain or worsening weakness. The two surgical options are removal of the disk (discectomy) or bone spur or discectomy followed by a fusion. In each case, the surgical decision is individualized to the athlete's symptoms and signs and the results of additional diagnostic tests.

Prevention

Many athletes who sustain a stinger are found to have substantial postural deviations that may interfere with full recovery. Some of these abnormal postures include the head jutting out too far forward from the neck and shoulders that are too rounded. These postures will cause more pressure to be placed on some of the nerve roots in the neck, making them more likely to be injured and to recover more slowly after injury.

A comprehensive physical therapy treatment program will be of value to correct the various areas of muscular and soft tissue tightness and weakness throughout the neck, upper back, and shoulder region. Trunk stabilization and chest-out posture correction exercises are usually the basis of the treatment program.

Physical therapy may also include manual therapy treatments in which the therapist provides deep tissue massage to release tight soft tissues and joint mobilization to loosen stiff spinal joints. Forceful spinal manipulation should be avoided so as not to further injure the cervical nerve root. Therapy includes specific exercises to strengthen the weak muscles of the neck, upper back, and arms. Athletes who undergo surgery must also complete a full rehabilitation program.

Return to Play

Before the athlete can return to regular athletic competition, several goals must be met. First, the athlete must be completely free of pain and weakness and must regain full range of motion of the neck. Second, the diagnostic tests such as the EMG and/or MRI should not reveal any active nerve damage or severe nerve compression. Third, the athlete must be reconditioned for the sport especially if he has not competed for awhile. Fourth, improvement in the athlete's playing technique (such as blocking and tackling) and equipment modifications should be made to protect the athlete from further injury.

In football, special pads and neck rolls can be fitted to the helmet or shoulder pads, which can help prevent re-injury. However, this type of equipment change does not replace the most important part of prevention, which is building strength and endurance of the neck and shoulder muscles. That is why athletes who have had surgery will usually take longer to return to play.

Finally, in some cases the decision to return to play must be delayed especially if the athlete has suffered several stingers in the same season. Healing is usually slower after multiple injuries. The key concern is to avoid permanent nerve damage, which could cause problems in the young athlete's personal as well as athletic life. Rarely does a history of multiple stingers signal the end of an athletic career. The sports medicine physician, working together with the athletic trainers, should provide counseling regarding how serious the injury is and discuss early or delayed return to play.

Section 26.3

Whiplash

"Whiplash Information Page" is published by the National Institute of
Neurological Disorders and Stroke (NINDS), July 1, 2001. Available
online at http://www.ninds.nih.gov; accessed May 2004.

What Is Whiplash?

Whiplash—a soft tissue injury to the neck—is also called neck
sprain or neck strain. It is characterized by a collection of symptoms
that occur following damage to the neck, usually because of sudden
extension and flexion. The disorder commonly occurs as the result of
an automobile accident and may include injury to intervertebral joints,
disks, and ligaments, cervical muscles, and nerve roots. Symptoms
such as neck pain may be present directly after the injury or may be
delayed for several days. In addition to neck pain, other symptoms
may include neck stiffness, injuries to the muscles and ligaments
(myofascial injuries), headache, dizziness, abnormal sensations such
as burning or prickling (paresthesias), or shoulder or back pain. In
addition, some people experience cognitive, somatic, or psychological
conditions such as memory loss, concentration impairment, nervous-
ness/irritability, sleep disturbances, fatigue, or depression.

Is There Any Treatment?

Treatment for individuals with whiplash may include pain medications, nonsteroidal anti-inflammatory drugs, antidepressants,
muscle relaxants, and a cervical collar (usually worn for 2 to 3 weeks).
Range of motion exercises, physical therapy, and cervical traction may
also be prescribed.

Supplemental heat application may relieve muscle tension.

What Is the Prognosis?

Generally, prognosis for individuals with whiplash is good. The neck
and head pain clears within a few days or weeks. Most patients recover

within 3 months after the injury, however, some may continue to have residual neck pain and headaches.

What Research Is Being Done?

The NINDS conducts and supports research on trauma-related disorders such as whiplash. Much of this research focuses on increasing scientific understanding of these disorders and finding ways to prevent and treat them.

Organizations

American Chronic Pain Association
P.O. Box 850
Rocklin, CA 95677
Toll-Free: (800) 533-3231
Phone: (916) 632-0922
Fax: (916) 632-3208
Website: http://www.theacpa.org
E-mail: ACPA@pacbell.net

National Chronic Pain Outreach Association, Inc.
7979 Old Georgetown Road, Suite 100
Bethesda, MD 20814-2429
Phone: (301) 652-4948
Fax: (301) 907-0745
Website: http://neurosurgery.mgh.harvard.edu/ncpainoa.htm

National Headache Foundation
820 N. Orleans, Suite 217
Chicago, IL 60610-3132
Toll-Free: (888) NHF-5552 (643-5552)
Phone: (773) 388-6399
Fax: (773) 525-7357
Website: http://www.headaches.org
E-mail: info@headaches.org

Section 26.4

Cervical Fracture

You have seven bones in your neck. These are the cervical vertebrae, which support your head and connect it to the shoulders and body. A fracture, or break, in one of the cervical vertebrae is commonly called a broken neck.

Cervical fractures usually result from high-energy trauma, such as automobile crashes or falls. Athletes are also at risk. A cervical fracture can occur if:

- A football player spears an opponent with his head.

- An ice hockey player is struck from behind and rams into the boards.

- A gymnast misses the high bar during a release move and falls.

- A diver strikes the bottom of a shallow pool.

Any injury to the vertebrae can have serious consequences because the spinal cord, the central nervous connection between the brain and the body, runs through the center of the vertebrae. Damage to the spinal cord could result in paralysis or death. Injury to the spinal cord at the level of the cervical spine can lead to temporary or permanent quadriplegia, paralyzing the entire body from the neck down.

Emergency Response

In a trauma situation, the neck should be immobilized until x-rays are taken and reviewed by a physician. Emergency medical personnel will assume that an unconscious individual has a neck injury and respond accordingly. The victim may experience shock and either temporary or permanent paralysis.

Conscious patients with an acute neck injury will usually have well-localized severe pain. They may also have pain spreading from the neck to the shoulders or arms, resulting from the vertebra compressing a nerve. There may be some bruising and swelling at the back of the neck. The physician will perform a complete neurological examination to assess nerve function and may request additional radiographic studies, such as an MRI or computed tomography (CT) scan, to determine the extent of the injuries.

Treatment

Treatment will depend on which of the seven cervical vertebrae was damaged and the kind of fracture sustained. A minor compression fracture can be treated with a cervical brace worn for six to eight weeks until the bone heals. A more complex or extensive fracture may require traction, surgery and internal fixation, two to three months in a rigid cast, or a combination of these treatments.

Improvements in athletic equipment and rule changes have reduced the number of cervical fractures over the past 20 years. You can help protect yourself and your family if you:

1. Always wear a seat belt when you are driving or a passenger in a car.

2. Never dive in a shallow pool area, and be sure that young people are properly supervised when swimming and diving.

3. Wear the proper protective equipment for your sport and follow all safety regulations, such as having a spotter and appropriate cushioning mats.

Chapter 27

Fracture of the Thoracic and Lumbar Spine

Fracture of one or more parts of the spinal column (vertebrae) of the middle (thoracic) or lower (lumbar) back is a serious injury usually caused by high-energy trauma like a car crash, fall, sports accident, or act of violence (i.e., gunshot wound). Males experience the injury four times more often than females do. The spinal cord may be injured depending on the severity of the fracture. Symptoms include:

- Moderate to severe back pain made worse by movement.

- In some cases when the spinal cord is also involved, numbness, tingling, weakness, or bowel/bladder dysfunction.

When you fracture the thoracic and lumbar spine, surgery or bracing is often necessary. Often, patients also have other life-threatening injuries. People with osteoporosis, tumors, or other underlying conditions that weaken bone can get a spinal fracture with minimal trauma or normal activities of daily living.

Emergency Treatment

Never attempt to move a person with a spinal injury because movement can cause more damage. Call 911 immediately. Rescue workers know how to properly immobilize people with injuries and safely take someone to the hospital for evaluation and treatment.

Doctor's Evaluation

After checking heart rate, breathing, and other vital signs, a doctor locates the fractured part(s) of the spine and determines the extent of damage. He or she finds out exactly how the vertebra broke (fracture pattern) and whether you have nerve (neural) injury and/or spinal instability.

The doctor considers what caused the injury, gives you a physical/neurological examination, and takes x-rays to see inside the body.

History. Every detail you can recall about what caused the injury may help the doctor. Sometimes rescue workers or other witnesses can supply more information. Did an accident eject the patient from a vehicle? Was there windshield or steering column damage? Was the person using a lap and/or shoulder seat belt? Did an airbag deploy?

Examination. The doctor carefully removes your clothing and immobilizes the body with a spine board for a complete physical examination. This may include checking for swelling, bruising, and other signs of injury to the head, chest, abdomen, and back; evaluating strength, motion, and alignment of arms and legs; feeling for tenderness on each rib and along the entire length of the spine; testing the tone and sensation of rectal muscles; and other evaluations.

You may also need a neurologic examination. This may include tests of sensory (i.e., temperature, pain, and pressure sensitivity), motor (i.e., muscle strength) and reflex (i.e., knee jerk) functions of the nervous system. If you have neurologic damage, certain tests can show whether you may recover some function (incomplete deficit) or not (complete deficit).

Imaging. X-rays of the entire spine from multiple angles may be necessary to see bone alignment and check for damage to soft tissue. Sometimes you may also need CT (computed tomography) or MRI (magnetic resonance imaging) scans to help the doctor better visualize the injury.

Classification

Doctors classify fractures of the thoracic and lumbar spine based upon pattern of injury:

- **Compression fracture:** While the front (anterior) of the vertebra breaks and loses height, the back (posterior) part of it does not. This type of fracture is usually stable and rarely associated with neurologic problems.

- **Axial burst fracture:** You lose height on both the front and back of the vertebra in this type of fracture, often caused by a fall from height in which you land on your feet.

- **Flexion/distraction (chance) fracture:** The vertebra is literally pulled apart (distraction), such as in a head-on car crash in which the upper body is thrown forward while the pelvis is stabilized by a lap seat belt.

- **Transverse process fracture:** This type of fracture results from rotation or extreme sideways (lateral) bending and usually does not affect stability.

- **Fracture-dislocation:** This is an unstable injury involving bone and/or soft tissue in which one vertebra may move off the adjacent one (displaced).

Treatment

Treatment goals include protecting nerve function and restoring alignment and stability of the spine. The doctor determines the best treatment method based upon fracture type and other factors.

Non-surgical: Doctors usually treat compression and some burst fractures without surgery. If you have a simple compression fracture, you may need to wear a hyperextension brace for sitting and standing activities for 6 to 12 weeks. You should walk and do other exercises while healing and may take medication for pain. If you have a transverse process fracture, you may need to wear a thoracolumbar corset along with doing an aerobic walking program.

Surgical: Some injuries require more aggressive treatment. You may need steroids if the spinal cord is injured. You may need surgery if you have an unstable burst fracture, flexion-distraction injury, or fracture-dislocation. Surgery realigns the spinal column and holds it together using metal plates and screws (internal fixation) and/or spinal fusion.

Chapter 28

Osteoporosis and Spinal Fractures

Introduction

Bone, the framework of the body, is made mostly of collagen (a type of protein) and a mineral called calcium phosphate. Bone is a living tissue, continually replacing itself through a process of new bone growth (formation) and old bone removal (resorption).

During childhood and teenage years, formation occurs faster than resorption. As a result, bones become larger, denser, and heavier. Then, at about age 30, resorption slowly begins to exceed formation, reducing bone mass by about 1% each year. Events such as menopause can trigger rapid bone loss. There are many other risk factors that affect bone loss; most of which can be controlled.

What Is Osteoporosis?

In osteoporosis, bone (osteo) becomes porous (porosis). As a result, bones are weakened and made brittle, becoming prone to fractures. Often referred to as a silent disease, osteoporosis may have no symptoms until a painful fracture occurs. When the osteoporosis occurs in the vertebrae of the spine, the vertebrae may collapse.

This results in severe back pain, nerve pain or dysfunction, loss of height, or spinal deformities such as kyphosis (severely stooped posture).

What Causes Osteoporosis?

Poor nutrition or lack of exercise during the bone-forming years can result in bones that are less dense than they should be. Bones that are less dense are more likely to be affected by osteoporosis. Smoking, excessive use of alcohol, lack of exercise, and poor nutrition during adulthood can cause bones to lose density.

Women with smaller, thinner bones are more prone to osteoporosis and are also adversely affected by hormonal changes. Heredity and ethnicity may also affect the chance of developing osteoporosis. Secondary osteoporosis results from other health conditions, such as hormone imbalances, arthritis and joint disease, certain medications such as steroids, and some diseases or treatments of the digestive system.

Can Osteoporosis Be Prevented?

You can prevent or slow down osteoporosis by making healthy lifestyle choices. Good nutrition, with sufficient amounts of calcium and vitamin D, are necessary for bone growth. Bones are living tissue and become stronger with exercise.

Weight-bearing exercises, done consistently, make bones stronger. These exercises may include walking, stair climbing, dancing, and tennis. Weightlifting, even if done with small weights, is beneficial. Swimming and water exercises are useful for people who can't otherwise bear weight. Not smoking and avoiding alcohol consumption reduce bone loss. Regular consumption of just 2 to 3 ounces of alcohol may be damaging to the skeleton, even in young adults.

What Are the Treatment Options for Spinal Fractures Due to Osteoporosis?

Spinal fractures that result from osteoporosis can be surgically treated, depending on the location of the fracture. Hip fractures should be treated with reconstructive surgery within 48 hours, if possible. Spinal fractures can be repaired using a procedure called kyphoplasty and percutaneous vertebroplasty.

Kyphoplasty

Kyphoplasty is a type of vertebroplasty in which the vertebral body is first prepared for the cement by using a balloon to inflate and reposition the vertebra. As the cement hardens, the vertebral body may resume a more normal shape. Kyphoplasty is minimally invasive, requiring only a very small incision in the back. A narrow tube is inserted through the incision using fluoroscopy to guide it into the correct position in the damaged vertebrae.

Using the tube as a channel, the doctor then guides a special balloon into the vertebral body.

The balloon is then carefully inflated, restoring the vertebrae to a more normal shape. It also creates a cavity in the vertebral body by compacting the soft inner bone material. The balloon is then deflated and gently removed. Special instruments are used to fill the cavity with a soft cement-like material that quickly hardens to stabilize the vertebrae.

With the vertebrae shape and height restored, the pressure on the nerves is reduced, easing the pain.

Percutaneous Vertebroplasty

Percutaneous vertebroplasty uses an epoxy cement injected into fractured vertebrae. The epoxy becomes rock-hard within minutes, yet is light and supportive. The vertebrae must be treated before total collapse. Percutaneous vertebroplasty does not necessarily restore the physiological shape of the vertebra, but does reduce further disintegration. Other injectable bone-mineral substitutes that are similar to normal bone are being tested. Percutaneous techniques (performed through the skin) derive their origins and continued success from medical advances and patients' desire for a less invasive yet effective therapy. The procedure uses a local anesthetic and the patient is able to walk around within a day.

Chapter 29

Understanding Spinal Cord Injury

A Short History of the Treatment of Spinal Cord Injury

Accounts of spinal cord injuries and their treatment date back to ancient times, even though there was little chance of recovery from such a devastating injury. The earliest is found in an Egyptian papyrus roll manuscript written in approximately 1700 B.C. that describes two spinal cord injuries involving fracture or dislocation of the neck vertebrae accompanied by paralysis. The description of each was "an ailment not to be treated."

Centuries later in Greece, treatment for spinal cord injuries had changed little. According to the Greek physician Hippocrates (460–377 B.C.) there were no treatment options for spinal cord injuries that resulted in paralysis; unfortunately, those patients were destined to die. But Hippocrates did use rudimentary forms of traction to treat spinal fractures without paralysis. The Hippocratic Ladder was a device that required the patient to be bound, tied to the rungs upside-down, and shaken vigorously to reduce spinal curvature. Another invention, the Hippocratic Board, allowed the doctor to apply traction to the immobilized patient's back using either his hands and feet or a wheel and axle arrangement.

Hindu, Arab, and Chinese physicians also developed basic forms of traction to correct spinal deformities. These same principles of traction are still applied today.

"Spinal Cord Injury: Hope Through Research," National Institute of Neurological Disorders and Stroke (NINDS), August 21, 2003. Available online at http://www.ninds.nih.gov; accessed April 2004.

In about 200 A.D., the Roman physician Galen introduced the concept of the central nervous system when he proposed that the spinal cord was an extension of the brain that carried sensation to the limbs and back. By the seventh century A.D., Paulus of Aegina was recommending surgery for spinal column fracture to remove the bone fragments that he was convinced caused paralysis.

In his influential anatomy textbook published in 1543, the Renaissance physician and teacher Vesalius described and illustrated the spinal cord in all its parts. The illustrations in his books, based on direct observation and dissection of the spine, gave physicians a way to understand the basic structure of the spine and spinal cord and what could happen when it was injured. The words we use today to identify segments of the spine—cervical, thoracic, lumbar, sacral, and coccygeal—come directly from Vesalius.

With the widespread use of antiseptics and sterilization in surgical procedures in the late nineteenth century, spinal surgery could finally be done with a much lower risk of infection. The use of x-rays, beginning in the 1920s, gave surgeons a way to precisely locate the injury and also made diagnosis and prediction of outcome more accurate. By the middle of the twentieth century, a standard method of treating spinal cord injuries was established—reposition the spine, fix it in place, and rehabilitate disabilities with exercise. In the 1990s, the discovery that the steroid drug methylprednisolone could reduce damage to nerve cells if given early enough after injury gave doctors an additional treatment option.

What Is a Spinal Cord Injury?

Although the hard bones of the spinal column protect the soft tissues of the spinal cord, vertebrae can still be broken or dislocated in a variety of ways and cause traumatic injury to the spinal cord. Injuries can occur at any level of the spinal cord. The segment of the cord that is injured, and the severity of the injury, will determine which body functions are compromised or lost. Because the spinal cord acts as the main information pathway between the brain and the rest of the body, a spinal cord injury can have significant physiological consequences.

Catastrophic falls, being thrown from a horse or through a windshield, or any kind of physical trauma that crushes and compresses the vertebrae in the neck can cause irreversible damage at the cervical level of the spinal cord and below. Paralysis of most of the body including the arms and legs, called quadriplegia, is the likely result. Automobile accidents are often responsible for spinal cord damage in the middle back (the thoracic or lumbar area), which can cause paralysis of the lower trunk and lower extremities, called paraplegia.

Other kinds of injuries that directly penetrate the spinal cord, such as gunshot or knife wounds, can either completely or partially sever the spinal cord and create lifelong disabilities.

Most injuries to the spinal cord don't completely sever it. Instead, an injury is more likely to cause fractures and compression of the vertebrae, which then crush and destroy the axons, extensions of nerve cells that carry signals up and down the spinal cord between the brain and the rest of the body. An injury to the spinal cord can damage a few, many, or almost all of these axons. Some injuries will allow almost complete recovery. Others will result in complete paralysis.

Until World War II, a serious spinal cord injury usually meant certain death, or at best a lifetime confined to a wheelchair and an ongoing struggle to survive secondary complications such as breathing problems or blood clots. But today, improved emergency care for people with spinal cord injuries and aggressive treatment and rehabilitation can minimize damage to the nervous system and even restore limited abilities.

Advances in research are giving doctors and patients hope that all spinal cord injuries will eventually be repairable. With new surgical techniques and exciting developments in spinal nerve regeneration, the future for spinal cord injury survivors looks brighter every day.

This chapter has been written to explain what happens to the spinal cord when it is injured, the current treatments for spinal cord injury patients, and the most promising avenues of research currently under investigation.

Facts and Figures about Spinal Cord Injury

- There are an estimated 10,000 to 12,000 spinal cord injuries every year in the United States.

- A quarter of a million Americans are currently living with spinal cord injuries.

- The cost of managing the care of spinal cord injury patients approaches $4 billion each year.

- 38.5 percent of all spinal cord injuries happen during car accidents. Almost a quarter, 24.5 percent, are the result of injuries relating to violent encounters, often involving guns and knifes. The rest are due to sporting accidents, falls, and work-related accidents.

- 55 percent of spinal cord injury victims are between 16 and 30 years old.

- More than 80 percent of spinal cord injury patients are men.

Source: Facts and Figures at a Glance, May 2001. National Spinal Cord Injury Statistical Center.

How Does the Spinal Cord Work?

To understand what can happen as the result of a spinal cord injury, it helps to know the anatomy of the spinal cord and its normal functions.

Spine Anatomy

The soft, jelly-like spinal cord is protected by the spinal column. The spinal column is made up of 33 bones called vertebrae, each with a circular opening similar to the hole in a donut. The bones are stacked one on top of the other and the spinal cord runs through the hollow channel created by the holes in the stacked bones.

The vertebrae can be organized into sections, and are named and numbered from top to bottom according to their location along the backbone:

- Cervical vertebrae (1–7) located in the neck

- Thoracic vertebrae (1–12) in the upper back (attached to the ribcage)

- Lumbar vertebrae (1–5) in the lower back

- Sacral vertebrae (1–5) in the hip area

- Coccygeal vertebrae (1–4 fused) in the tailbone

Although the hard vertebrae protect the soft spinal cord from injury most of the time, the spinal column is not all hard bone. Between the vertebrae are disks of semi-rigid cartilage, and in the narrow spaces between them are passages through which the spinal nerves exit to the rest of the body. These are places where the spinal cord is vulnerable to direct injury.

The spinal cord is also organized into segments and named and numbered from top to bottom. Each segment marks where spinal nerves emerge from the cord to connect to specific regions of the body. Locations of spinal cord segments do not correspond exactly to vertebral locations, but they are roughly equivalent.

- Cervical spinal nerves (C1 to C8) control signals to the back of the head, the neck and shoulders, the arms and hands, and the diaphragm.

- Thoracic spinal nerves (T1 to T12) control signals to the chest muscles, some muscles of the back, and parts of the abdomen.

- Lumbar spinal nerves (L1 to L5) control signals to the lower parts of the abdomen and the back, the buttocks, some parts of the external genital organs, and parts of the leg.

- Sacral spinal nerves (S1 to S5) control signals to the thighs and lower parts of the legs, the feet, most of the external genital organs, and the area around the anus.

The single coccygeal nerve carries sensory information from the skin of the lower back.

Spinal Cord Anatomy

The spinal cord has a core of tissue containing nerve cells, surrounded by long tracts of nerve fibers consisting of axons. The tracts extend up and down the spinal cord, carrying signals to and from the brain. The average size of the spinal cord varies in circumference along its length from the width of a thumb to the width of one of the smaller fingers. The spinal cord extends down through the upper two thirds of the vertebral canal, from the base of the brain to the lower back, and is generally 15 to 17 inches long depending on an individual's height.

The interior of the spinal cord is made up of neurons, their support cells called glia, and blood vessels. The neurons and their dendrites (branching projections that help neurons communicate with each other) reside in an H-shaped region called grey matter.

The H-shaped grey matter of the spinal cord contains motor neurons that control movement, smaller interneurons that handle communication within and between the segments of the spinal cord, and cells that receive sensory signals and then send information up to centers in the brain.

Surrounding the grey matter of neurons is white matter. Most axons are covered with an insulating substance called myelin, which allows electrical signals to flow freely and quickly. Myelin has a whitish appearance, which is why this outer section of the spinal cord is called "white matter."

Axons carry signals downward from the brain (along descending pathways) and upward toward the brain (along ascending pathways) within specific tracts. Axons branch at their ends and can make connections with many other nerve cells simultaneously. Some axons extend along the entire length of the spinal cord.

The descending motor tracts control the smooth muscles of internal organs and the striated (capable of voluntary contractions) muscles of the arms and legs. They also help adjust the autonomic nervous system's regulation of blood pressure, body temperature, and the response to stress. These pathways begin with neurons in the brain that send electrical signals downward to specific levels of the spinal cord. Neurons in these segments then send the impulses out to the rest of the body or coordinate neural activity within the cord itself.

The ascending sensory tracts transmit sensory signals from the skin, extremities, and internal organs that enter at specific segments of the spinal cord. Most of these signals are then relayed to the brain. The spinal cord also contains neuronal circuits that control reflexes and repetitive movements, such as walking, which can be activated by incoming sensory signals without input from the brain.

The circumference of the spinal cord varies depending on its location. It is larger in the cervical and lumbar areas because these areas supply the nerves to the arms and upper body and the legs and lower body, which require the most intense muscular control and receive the most sensory signals.

The ratio of white matter to grey matter also varies at each level of the spinal cord. In the cervical segment, which is located in the neck, there is a large amount of white matter because at this level there are many axons going to and from the brain and the rest of the spinal cord below. In lower segments, such as the sacral, there is less white matter because most ascending axons have not yet entered the cord, and most descending axons have contacted their targets along the way.

To pass between the vertebrae, the axons that link the spinal cord to the muscles and the rest of the body are bundled into 31 pairs of spinal nerves, each pair with a sensory root and a motor root that make connections within the grey matter. Two pairs of nerves—a sensory and motor pair on either side of the cord—emerge from each segment of the spinal cord.

The functions of these nerves are determined by their location in the spinal cord. They control everything from body functions such as breathing, sweating, digestion, and elimination, to gross and fine motor skills, as well as sensations in the arms and legs.

The Nervous Systems

Together, the spinal cord and the brain make up the central nervous system (CNS).

The CNS controls most functions of the body, but it is not the only nervous system in the body. The peripheral nervous system (PNS) includes the nerves that project to the limbs, heart, skin, and other organs outside the brain. The PNS controls the somatic nervous system, which regulates muscle movements and the response to sensations of touch and pain, and the autonomic nervous system, which provides nerve input to the internal organs and generates automatic reflex responses. The autonomic nervous system is divided into the sympathetic nervous system, which mobilizes organs and their functions during times of stress and arousal, and the parasympathetic nervous system, which conserves energy and resources during times of rest and relaxation.

The spinal cord acts as the primary information pathway between the brain and all the other nervous systems of the body. It receives sensory information from the skin, joints, and muscles of the trunk, arms, and legs, which it then relays upward to the brain. It carries messages downward from the brain to the PNS, and contains motor neurons, which direct voluntary movements and adjust reflex movements. Because of the central role it plays in coordinating muscle movements and interpreting sensory input, any kind of injury to the spinal cord can cause significant problems throughout the body.

What Happens When the Spinal Cord Is Injured?

A spinal cord injury usually begins with a sudden, traumatic blow to the spine that fractures or dislocates vertebrae. The damage begins at the moment of injury when displaced bone fragments, disk material, or ligaments bruise or tear into spinal cord tissue. Axons are cut off or damaged beyond repair, and neural cell membranes are broken. Blood vessels may rupture and cause heavy bleeding in the central grey matter, which can spread to other areas of the spinal cord over the next few hours.

Within minutes, the spinal cord swells to fill the entire cavity of the spinal canal at the injury level. This swelling cuts off blood flow, which also cuts off oxygen to spinal cord tissue. Blood pressure drops, sometimes dramatically, as the body loses its ability to self-regulate. As blood pressure lowers even further, it interferes with the electrical activity of neurons and axons. All these changes can cause a condition known as spinal shock that can last from several hours to several days.

Although there is some controversy among neurologists about the extent and impact of spinal shock, and even its definition in terms of physiological characteristics, it appears to occur in approximately half the cases of spinal cord injury, and it is usually directly related to the size and severity of the injury. During spinal shock, even undamaged portions of the spinal cord become temporarily disabled and can't communicate normally with the brain. Complete paralysis may develop, with loss of reflexes and sensation in the limbs.

The crushing and tearing of axons is just the beginning of the devastation that occurs in the injured spinal cord and continues for days. The initial physical trauma sets off a cascade of biochemical and cellular events that kills neurons, strips axons of their myelin insulation, and triggers an inflammatory immune system response. Days or sometimes even weeks later, after this second wave of damage has passed, the area of destruction has increased—sometimes to several segments above and below the original injury—and so has the extent of disability.

Changes in Blood Flow Cause Ongoing Damage

Changes in blood flow in and around the spinal cord begin at the injured area, spread out to adjacent, uninjured areas, and then set off problems throughout the body.

Immediately after the injury, there is a major reduction in blood flow to the site, which can last for as long as 24 hours and becomes progressively worse if untreated. Because of differences in tissue composition, the impact is greater on the interior grey matter of the spinal cord than on the outlying white matter.

Blood vessels in the grey matter also begin to leak, sometimes as early as 5 minutes after injury. Cells that line the still-intact blood vessels in the spinal cord begin to swell, for reasons that aren't yet clearly understood, and this continues to reduce blood flow to the injured area. The combination of leaking, swelling, and sluggish blood flow prevents the normal delivery of oxygen and nutrients to neurons, causing many of them to die.

The body continues to regulate blood pressure and heart rate during the first hour to hour-and-a-half after the injury, but as the reduction in the rate of blood flow becomes more widespread, self-regulation begins to turn off. Blood pressure and heart rate drop.

Excessive Release of Neurotransmitters Kills Nerve Cells

After the injury, an excessive release of neurotransmitters (chemicals that allow neurons to signal each other) can cause additional damage by overexciting nerve cells.

Glutamate is an excitatory neurotransmitter, commonly used by nerve cells in the spinal cord to stimulate activity in neurons. But when spinal cells are injured, neurons flood the area with glutamate for reasons that are not yet well understood. Excessive glutamate triggers a destructive process called excitotoxicity, which disrupts normal processes and kills neurons and other cells called oligodendrocytes that surround and protect axons.

An Invasion of Immune System Cells Creates Inflammation

Under normal conditions, the blood-brain barrier (which tightly controls the passage of cells and large molecules between the circulatory and central nervous systems) keeps immune system cells from entering the brain or spinal cord. But when the blood-brain barrier is broken by blood vessels bursting and leaking into spinal cord tissue, immune system cells that normally circulate in the blood—primarily white blood cells—can invade the surrounding tissue and trigger an inflammatory response. This inflammation is characterized by fluid accumulation and the influx of immune cells—neutrophils, T-cells, macrophages, and monocytes.

Neutrophils are the first to enter, within about 12 hours of injury, and they remain for about a day. Three days after the injury, T-cells arrive. Their function in the injured spinal cord is not clearly understood, but in the healthy spinal cord they kill infected cells and regulate the immune response. Macrophages and monocytes enter after the T-cells and scavenge cellular debris.

The upside of this immune system response is that it helps fight infection and cleans up debris. But the downside is that it sets off the release of cytokines—a group of immune system messenger molecules that exert a malign influence on the activities of nerve cells.

For example, microglial cells, which normally function as a kind of on-site immune cell in the spinal cord, begin to respond to signals from these cytokines. They transform into macrophage-like cells, engulf cell debris, and start to produce their own pro-inflammatory cytokines, which then stimulate and recruit other microglia to respond.

Injury also stimulates resting astrocytes to express cytokines. These "reactive" astrocytes may ultimately participate in the formation of scar tissue within the spinal cord.

Whether the immune response is protective or destructive is controversial among researchers. Some speculate that certain types of injury might evoke a protective immune response that actually reduces the loss of neurons.

Free Radicals Attack Nerve Cells

Another consequence of the immune system's entry into the CNS is that inflammation accelerates the production of highly reactive forms of oxygen molecules called free radicals.

Free radicals are produced as a by-product of normal cell metabolism. In the healthy spinal cord their numbers are small enough that they cause no harm. But injury to the spinal cord, and the subsequent wave of inflammation that sweeps through spinal cord tissue, signals particular cells to overproduce free radicals.

Free radicals then attack and disable molecules that are crucial for cell function—for example, those found in cell membranes—by modifying their chemical structure. Free radicals can also change how cells respond to natural growth and survival factors, and turn these protective factors into agents of destruction.

Nerve Cells Self-Destruct

Researchers used to think that the only way in which cells died during spinal cord injury was as a direct result of trauma. But recent findings have revealed that cells in the injured spinal cord also die from a kind of programmed cell death called apoptosis, often described as cellular suicide, that happens days or weeks after the injury.

Apoptosis is a normal cellular event that occurs in a variety of tissues and cellular systems. It helps the body get rid of old and unhealthy cells by causing them to shrink and implode. Nearby scavenger cells then gobble up the debris. Apoptosis seems to be regulated by specific molecules that have the ability to either start or stop the process.

For reasons that are still unclear, spinal cord injury sets off apoptosis, which kills oligodendrocytes in damaged areas of the spinal cord days to weeks after the injury. The death of oligodendrocytes is another blow to the damaged spinal cord, since these are the cells that form the myelin that wraps around axons and speeds the conduction of nerve impulses. Apoptosis strips myelin from intact axons in adjacent ascending and descending pathways, which further impairs the spinal cord's ability to communicate with the brain.

Secondary Damage Takes a Cumulative Toll

All of these mechanisms of secondary damage—restricted blood flow, excitotoxicity, inflammation, free radical release, and apoptosis—increase the area of damage in the injured spinal cord. Damaged axons become dysfunctional, either because they are stripped of their myelin or because they are disconnected from the brain. Glial cells cluster to form a scar, which creates a barrier to any axons that could potentially regenerate and reconnect. A few whole axons may remain, but not enough to convey any meaningful information to the brain.

Researchers are especially interested in studying the mechanisms of this wave of secondary damage because finding ways to stop it could save axons and reduce disabilities. This could make a big difference in the potential for recovery.

What Are the Immediate Treatments for Spinal Cord Injury?

The outcome of any injury to the spinal cord depends upon the number of axons that survive: the higher the number of normally functioning axons, the less the amount of disability. Consequently, the most important consideration when moving people to a hospital or trauma center is preventing further injury to the spine and spinal cord.

Spinal cord injury isn't always obvious. Any injury that involves the head (especially with trauma to the front of the face), pelvic fractures, penetrating injuries in the area of the spine, or injuries that result from falling from heights should be suspect for spinal cord damage.

Until imaging of the spine is done at an emergency or trauma center, people who might have spinal cord injury should be cared for as if any significant movement of the spine could cause further damage. They are usually transported in a recumbent (lying down) position, with a rigid collar and backboard immobilizing the spine.

Respiratory complications are often an indication of the severity of spinal cord injury. About one third of those with injury to the neck area will need help with breathing and require respiratory support via intubation, which involves inserting a tube connected to an oxygen tank through the nose or throat and into the airway.

Methylprednisolone, a steroid drug, became standard treatment for acute spinal cord injury in 1990 when a large-scale clinical trial supported by the National Institute of Neurological Disorders and Stroke showed significantly better recovery in patients who were given the drug within the first 8 hours after their injury. Methylprednisolone appears to reduce the damage to nerve cells and decreases inflammation near the injury site by suppressing activities of immune cells.

Realignment of the spine using a rigid brace or axial traction is usually done as soon as possible to stabilize the spine and prevent additional damage.

On about the third day after the injury, doctors give patients a complete neurological examination to diagnose the severity of the injury and predict the likely extent of recovery. The ASIA Impairment Scale is the standard diagnostic tool used by doctors. X-rays, MRIs, or more advanced imaging techniques are also used to visualize the entire length of the spine.

How Does a Spinal Cord Injury Affect the Rest of the Body?

People who survive a spinal cord injury will most likely have medical complications such as chronic pain and bladder and bowel dysfunction, along with an increased susceptibility to respiratory and heart problems. Successful recovery depends upon how well these chronic conditions are handled day to day.

Breathing

Any injury to the spinal cord at or above the C3, C4, and C5 segments, which supply the phrenic nerves leading to the diaphragm, can stop breathing. People with these injuries need immediate ventilatory support. When injuries are at the C5 level and below, diaphragm function is preserved, but breathing tends to be rapid and shallow and people have trouble coughing and clearing secretions from their lungs because of weak thoracic muscles. Once pulmonary function improves, a large percentage of those with C4 injuries can be weaned from mechanical ventilation in the weeks following the injury.

Pneumonia

Respiratory complications, primarily as a result of pneumonia, are a leading cause of death in people with spinal cord injury. In fact, intubation increases the risk of developing ventilator-associated pneumonia (VAP) by 1 to 3 percent per day of intubation. More than a quarter of the deaths caused by spinal cord injury are the result of VAP. Spinal cord injury patients who are intubated have to be carefully monitored for VAP and treated with antibiotics if symptoms appear.

Irregular Heartbeat and Low Blood Pressure

Spinal cord injuries in the cervical region are often accompanied by blood pressure instability and heart arrhythmias. Because of interruptions to the cardiac accelerator nerves, the heart can beat at a dangerously slow pace, or it can pound rapidly and irregularly. Arrhythmias usually appear in the first 2 weeks after injury and are more common and severe in the most serious injuries.

Low blood pressure also often occurs due to loss of tone in blood vessels, which widen and cause blood to pool in the small arteries far away from the heart. This is usually treated with an intravenous infusion to build up blood volume.

Blood Clots

People with spinal cord injuries are at triple the usual risk for blood clots. The risk for clots is low in the first 72 hours, but afterward anticoagulation drug therapy can be used as a preventive measure.

Spasm

Many of our reflex movements are controlled by the spinal cord but regulated by the brain. When the spinal cord is damaged, information from the brain can no longer regulate reflex activity. Reflexes may become exaggerated over time, causing spasticity. If spasms become severe enough, they may require medical treatment. For some, spasms can be as much of a help as they are a hindrance, since spasms can tone muscles that would otherwise waste away. Some people can even learn to use the increased tone in their legs to help them turn over in bed, propel them into and out of a wheelchair, or stand.

Autonomic Dysreflexia

Autonomic dysreflexia is a life-threatening reflex action that primarily affects those with injuries to the neck or upper back. It happens when there is an irritation, pain, or stimulus to the nervous system below the level of injury. The irritated area tries to send a signal to the brain, but since the signal isn't able to get through, a reflex action occurs without the brain's regulation. Unlike spasms that affect muscles, autonomic dysreflexia affects vascular and organ systems controlled by the sympathetic nervous system.

Anything that causes pain or irritation can set off autonomic dysreflexia: the urge to urinate or defecate, pressure sores, cuts, burns, bruises, sunburn, pressure of any kind on the body, ingrown toenails, or tight clothing. For example, the impulse to urinate can set off high blood pressure or rapid heartbeat that, if uncontrolled, can cause stroke, seizures, or death. Symptoms such as flushing or sweating, a pounding headache, anxiety, sudden high blood pressure, vision changes, or goosebumps on the arms and legs can signal the onset of autonomic dysreflexia. Treatment should be swift. Changing position, emptying the bladder or bowels, and removing or loosening tight clothing are just a few of the possibilities that should be tried to relieve whatever is causing the irritation.

Pressure Sores (or Pressure Ulcers)

Pressure sores are areas of skin tissue that have broken down because of continuous pressure on the skin. People with paraplegia and quadriplegia are susceptible to pressure sores because they can't move easily on their own.

Places that support weight when someone is seated or recumbent are vulnerable areas. When these areas press against a surface for a long period of time, the skin compresses and reduces the flow of blood to the area. When the blood supply is blocked for too long, the skin will begin to break down.

Since spinal cord injury reduces or eliminates sensation below the level of injury, people may not be aware of the normal signals to change position, and must be shifted periodically by a caregiver. Good nutrition and hygiene can also help prevent pressure sores by encouraging healthy skin.

Pain

People who are paralyzed often have what is called neurogenic pain resulting from damage to nerves in the spinal cord. For some survivors of spinal cord injury, pain or an intense burning or stinging sensation is unremitting due to hypersensitivity in some parts of the body. Others are prone to normal musculoskeletal pain as well, such as shoulder pain due to overuse of the shoulder joint from pushing a wheelchair and using the arms for transfers. Treatments for chronic pain include medications, acupuncture, spinal or brain electrical stimulation, and surgery.

Bladder and Bowel Problems

Most spinal cord injuries affect bladder and bowel functions because the nerves that control the involved organs originate in the segments near the lower termination of the spinal cord and are cut off from brain

232

input. Without coordination from the brain, the muscles of the bladder and urethra can't work together effectively, and urination becomes abnormal. The bladder can empty suddenly without warning, or become over-full without releasing. In some cases the bladder releases, but urine backs up into the kidneys because it isn't able to get past the urethral sphincter. Most people with spinal cord injuries use either intermittent catheterization or an indwelling catheter to empty their bladders.

Bowel function is similarly affected. The anal sphincter muscle can remain tight, so that bowel movements happen on a reflex basis whenever the bowel is full. Or the muscle can be permanently relaxed, which is called a flaccid bowel, and result in an inability to have a bowel movement. This requires more frequent attempts to empty the bowel and manual removal of stool to prevent fecal impaction. People with spinal cord injuries are usually put on a regularly scheduled bowel program to prevent accidents.

Reproductive and Sexual Function

Spinal cord injury has a greater impact on sexual and reproductive function in men than it does in women. Most spinal cord injured women remain fertile and can conceive and bear children. Even those with severe injury may well retain orgasmic function, although many lose some if not all of their ability to reach satisfaction.

Depending on the level of injury, men may have problems with erections and ejaculation, and most will have compromised fertility due to decreased motility of their sperm. Treatments for men include vibratory or electrical stimulation and drugs such as sildenafil (Viagra). Many couples may also need assisted fertility treatments to allow a spinal cord injured man to father children.

Once someone has survived the injury and begun to psychologically and emotionally cope with the nature of his or her situation, the next concern will be how to live with disabilities. Doctors are now able to predict with reasonable accuracy the likely long-term outcome of spinal cord injuries. This helps patients set achievable goals for themselves, and gives families and loved ones a realistic set of expectations for the future.

How Does Rehabilitation Help People Recover from Spinal Cord Injuries?

No two people will experience the same emotions after surviving a spinal cord injury, but almost everyone will feel frightened, anxious, or confused about what has happened. It's common for people to have very mixed feelings: relief that they are still alive, but disbelief at the nature of their disabilities.

Rehabilitation programs combine physical therapies with skill-building activities and counseling to provide social and emotional support. The education and active involvement of the newly injured person and his or her family and friends is crucial.

A rehabilitation team is usually led by a doctor specializing in physical medicine and rehabilitation (called a physiatrist), and often includes social workers, physical and occupational therapists, recreational therapists, rehabilitation nurses, rehabilitation psychologists, vocational counselors, nutritionists, and other specialists. A case-worker or program manager coordinates care.

In the initial phase of rehabilitation, therapists emphasize regaining leg and arm strength since mobility and communication are the two most important areas of function. For some, mobility will only be possible with the assistance of devices such as a walker, leg braces, or a wheelchair. Communication skills, such as writing, typing, and using the telephone, may also require adaptive devices.

Physical therapy includes exercise programs geared toward muscle strengthening. Occupational therapy helps redevelop fine motor skills. Bladder and bowel management programs teach basic toileting routines, and patients also learn techniques for self-grooming. People acquire coping strategies for recurring episodes of spasticity, autonomic dysreflexia, and neurogenic pain.

Vocational rehabilitation begins with an assessment of basic work skills, current dexterity, and physical and cognitive capabilities to determine the likelihood for employment. A vocational rehabilitation specialist then identifies potential work places, determines the type of assistive equipment that will be needed, and helps arrange for a user-friendly workplace. For those whose disabilities prevent them from returning to the workplace, therapists focus on encouraging productivity through participation in activities that provide a sense of satisfaction and self-esteem. This could include educational classes, hobbies, memberships in special interest groups, and participation in family and community events.

Recreation therapy encourages patients to build on their abilities so that they can participate in recreational or athletic activities at their level of mobility. Engaging in recreational outlets and athletics helps those with spinal cord injuries achieve a more balanced and normal lifestyle and also provides opportunities for socialization and self-expression.

How Is Research Helping Spinal Cord Injury Patients?

Can an injured spinal cord be rebuilt? This is the question that drives basic research in the field of spinal cord injury. As investigators try to understand the underlying biological mechanisms that either inhibit or promote new growth in the spinal cord, they are making surprising discoveries, not just about how neurons and their axons grow in the CNS, but also about why they fail to regenerate after injury in the adult CNS. Understanding the cellular and molecular mechanisms involved in both the working and the damaged spinal cord could point the way to therapies that might prevent secondary damage, encourage axons to grow past injured areas, and reconnect vital neural circuits within the spinal cord and CNS.

There has been successful research in a number of fields that may someday help people with spinal cord injuries. Genetic studies have revealed a number of molecules that encourage axon growth in the developing CNS but prevent it in the adult. Research into embryonic and adult stem cell biology has furthered knowledge about how cells communicate with each other.

Basic research has helped describe the mechanisms involved in the mysterious process of apoptosis, in which large groups of seemingly healthy cells self-destruct. New rehabilitation therapies that retrain neural circuits through forced motion and electrical stimulation of muscle groups are helping injured patients regain lost function.

Researchers, many of whom are supported by the National Institute of Neurological Disorders and Stroke (NINDS), are focused on advancing our understanding of the four key principles of spinal cord repair:

- Protecting surviving nerve cells from further damage

- Replacing damaged nerve cells

- Stimulating the regrowth of axons and targeting their connections appropriately

- Retraining neural circuits to restore body functions

A spinal cord injury is complex. Repairing it has to take into account all of the different kinds of damage that occur during and after the injury. Because the molecular and cellular environment of the spinal cord is constantly changing from the moment of injury until several weeks or even months later, combination therapies will have to be designed to address specific types of damage at different points in time.

Discoveries in Basic Research

A decade ago, researchers demonstrated a small but significant neuroprotective and anti-inflammatory effect from an adrenal corticosteroid drug called methylprednisolone if it was given within 8 hours of injury. It is the only treatment currently available to limit the extent of spinal cord injury and its risks are relatively low. Researchers continue to search for additional anti-inflammatory treatments that might prove even more effective.

Preliminary clinical trials of another compound, GM-1 ganglioside, indicate that it could be useful in preventing secondary damage in acute spinal cord injury. A large, randomized clinical trial suggested that it might also improve neurological recovery from spinal cord injury during rehabilitation.

These observations and others have led to optimism that recovery can be improved by altering cellular responses immediately after injury. Using what they know about the mechanisms that cause secondary damage—excitotoxicity, inflammation, and cell suicide (apoptosis)—researchers are creating and testing additional neuroprotective therapies to prevent the spread of post-injury damage and preserve surrounding tissue.

Some of the findings in these three different areas follow:

Stopping Excitotoxicity

When nerve cells die, they release excessive amounts of a neurotransmitter called glutamate. Since surviving nerve cells also release glutamate as part of their normal communication process, excess glutamate floods the cellular environment, which pushes cells into overdrive and self-destruction. Researchers are investigating compounds that could keep nerve cells from responding to glutamate, potentially minimizing the extent of secondary damage.

Recently, investigators tested agents called receptor antagonists that selectively block a specific type of glutamate receptor that is abundant on oligodendrocytes and neurons. These agents appear to be effective at limiting damage. Some of these receptor antagonists have already been tested in human trials as a therapy for stroke. Similar agents could enter clinical trials within several years for patients with spinal cord injury.

Controlling Inflammation

Some time within the first 12 hours after injury, the first wave of immune cells enters the damaged spinal cord to protect it from infection and clean up dead nerve cells. Other types of immune cells enter afterward. The actions of these immune cells and the messenger molecules they release, called cytokines, are the hallmarks of inflammation in the spinal cord.

Researchers have discovered that these inflammatory processes aren't entirely bad for the injured spinal cord. Although cytokines can be toxic to nerve cells because they stimulate the production of free radicals, nitric oxide, and other inflammatory substances that cause cell death, they also stimulate the production of neurotrophic factors, which are beneficial to cell repair.

Currently researchers are looking for ways to control these immune system cells and the molecules they produce by encouraging their potential for neuroprotection and reining in their neurotoxic effects. One approach being tested clinically is to exploit the ability of the PNS to mount a healing response in macrophages by injecting macrophages already stimulated by injured peripheral nerves into injured spinal cords. Recent experiments have indicated that selectively boosting the T-cell response to spinal cord injury could reduce secondary damage. Because of the possibility that these cells can also damage tissue, they must be very carefully controlled if they are to be used therapeutically.

Clinical investigators are also looking at how cooling the body protects surviving spinal cord tissue and nerve cells. Experiments have shown that cooling the body to a state of mild hypothermia (about 92 degrees Fahrenheit) for several hours immediately following the injury limits damage and promotes functional recovery. Researchers aren't yet sure why mild hypothermia is neuroprotective, but the ability of body temperature to affect many different kinds of physiological mechanisms may be one of the reasons.

Preventing Apoptosis

Days to weeks after the initial injury, apoptosis sweeps through oligodendrocytes in damaged and nearby tissue, causing the cells to self-destruct. Although genes have been identified that appear to regulate apoptosis, researchers still don't know enough to be able to specify the exact biochemical events that cause a cell to switch it on—or turn it off. Further studies are aimed at understanding these cellular mechanisms more fully. These studies will provide an opportunity to develop neural protective strategies to combat apoptotic cell death.

By understanding the process of apoptosis, researchers have been able to develop and test apoptosis-inhibiting drugs. In rodent models, animals given a drug that blocks a known apoptotic mechanism retained more ambulatory ability after traumatic spinal cord injury than did untreated animals.

Once the secondary wave of damage ends, the spinal cord is left with areas of scar tissue and fluid-filled gaps, or cysts, that axons can't penetrate or bridge. Unless these areas are reconnected by functioning nerve cells, the spinal cord remains disabled. Discovering how to bridge the gap between functioning axons and figuring out how to encourage axons to grow and make new connections could be the key to spinal cord repair.

Promoting Regeneration

Researchers are experimenting with cell grafts transplanted into the injured spinal cord that act as bridges across injured areas to reconnect cut axons, or that supply nerve cells to act as relays. Several types of cells have been studied for their potential to promote regeneration and repair, including Schwann cells, olfactory ensheathing glia, fetal spinal cord cells, and embryonic stem cells. In one group of experiments, investigators have implanted tubes packed with Schwann cells into the damaged spinal cords of rodents and observed axons growing into the tubes.

One of the limitations of cell transplants, however, is that the growth environment within the transplant is so favorable that most axons don't leave and extend into the spinal cord. By using olfactory ensheathing glia cells, which are natural migrators in the PNS, researchers have gotten axons to extend out of the initial transplant region and into the spinal cord. But it remains to be seen whether or not regenerated axons are fully functional.

Fetal spinal cord tissue implants have also yielded success in animal trials, giving rise to new neurons, which, when stimulated by growth-promoting factors (neurotrophins), extend axons that stretch up and down several segments in the spinal cord. Animals treated in these trials have regained some function in their limbs. Some patients with long-term spinal cord injuries have received fetal tissue transplants but the results have been inconclusive. In animal models, these transplants appear to be more effective in the immature spinal cord than in the adult spinal cord.

Stem cells are capable of dividing and yielding almost all the cell types of the body, including those of the spinal cord. Their potential to treat spinal cord injury is being investigated eagerly, but there are many things about stem cells that researchers still need to understand. For example, researchers know there are many different kinds of chemical signals that tell a stem cell what to do. Some of these are internal to the stem cell, but many others are external—within the cellular environment—and will have to be recreated in the transplant region to encourage proper growth and differentiation. Because of the complexities involved in stem cell treatment, researchers expect these kinds of therapies to be possible only after much more research is done.

Researchers are also looking at ways to compensate for axons that, having lost their myelin sheaths, have a decreased ability to conduct the electrical impulses essential for axonal communication. Preliminary studies with compounds known as potassium channel blockers, which block the flow of ions through the demyelinated membrane and increase the potential for messages to get through, have shown some success, but mostly in terms of reducing spasticity in muscles. Further studies might show how remyelinating axons could also improve function.

Stimulating Regrowth of Axons

Stimulating the regeneration of axons is a key component of spinal cord repair because every axon in the injured spinal cord that can be reconnected increases the chances for recovery of function.

Research on many fronts reveals that getting axons to grow after injury is a complicated task. CNS neurons have the capacity to regenerate, but the environment in the adult spinal cord does not encourage growth. Not only does it lack the growth-promoting molecules that are present in the developing CNS, it also contains substances that actively inhibit axon extension. For axon regeneration to be successful, the environment has to be changed to turn off the inhibitors and turn on the promoters.

Investigators are looking for ways to take advantage of the chemicals that drive or halt axon growth: growth-promoting and growth-inhibiting substances, neurotrophic factors, and guidance molecules.

In the developing CNS, thread-like axons grow and lengthen behind the axonal growth cone, an active tip only a few thousandths of a millimeter in diameter, which interacts with chemical signals that encourage growth and direct movement. But the environment of the adult CNS is hostile to axon growth, primarily because growth-inhibiting proteins are embedded in myelin, the insulating material around axons. These proteins appear to preserve neural circuits in the healthy spinal cord and keep intact axons from growing inappropriately. But when the spinal cord is injured, these proteins prevent regeneration.

At least three growth-inhibitory proteins operating within the axonal tract have been identified. The task of researchers is to understand how these inhibitory proteins do their job, and then discover ways to remove or block them, or change how the growth cone responds to them.

Growth-inhibiting proteins also block the glial scar near the injury site. To get past, an axon has to advance between the tangles of long, branching molecules that form the extracellular matrix. A recent experiment successfully used a bacterial enzyme to clear away this underbrush so that axons could grow.

A treatment that combines both these approaches—turning off growth-inhibiting proteins and using enzymes to clear the way—could create an encouraging environment for axon regeneration. But before trials of such a treatment can be attempted in patients, researchers must be sure that it could be controlled well enough to prevent dangerous miswiring of regenerating axons.

Neurotrophic factors (or neurotrophins) are key nervous system regulatory proteins that prime cells to produce the molecular machinery necessary for growth. Some prevent oligodendrocyte death, others promote axon regrowth and survival, and still others serve multiple functions. Unfortunately, the natural production of neurotrophins in the spinal cord falls instead of rises during the weeks after injury. Researchers have tested whether artificially raising the levels post-injury can enhance regeneration. Some of these investigations have been successful. Infusion pumps and gene therapy techniques have been used to deliver growth factors to injured neurons, but they appear to encourage sprouting more than they stimulate regeneration for long distances.

Axonal growth isn't enough for functional recovery. Axons have to make the proper connections and re-establish functioning synapses. Guidance molecules, proteins that rest on or are released from the surfaces of neurons or glia, act as chemical road signs, beckoning axons to grow in some directions and repelling growth in others.

Supplying a particular combination of guidance molecules or administering compounds that induce surviving cells to produce or use guidance molecules might encourage regeneration. But at the moment, researchers don't understand enough about guidance molecules to know which to supply and when.

Researchers hope that combining these strategies to encourage growth, clear away debris, and target axon connections could reconnect the spinal cord. Of course, all these therapies would have to be provided in the right amounts, in the right places, and at the right times. As researchers learn more and understand more about the intricacies of axon growth and regeneration, combining therapies could become a powerful treatment for spinal cord injury.

Discoveries in Clinical Research

Advances in basic research are also being matched by progress in clinical research, especially in understanding the kinds of physical rehabilitation that work best to restore function. Some of the more promising rehabilitation techniques are helping spinal cord injury patients become more mobile.

Restoring Function through Neural Prostheses and Computer Interfaces

While basic scientists strive to develop strategies to restore neurological connections between the brain and body of spinal cord injured persons, bioengineers are working to restore functional connections via advanced computer modeling systems and neural prostheses. Discovering ways to integrate devices that could mobilize paralyzed limbs requires a unique interface between electronics technology and neurobiology. A functional electrical stimulation (FES) system is one example of this kind of innovative research.

FES systems use electrical stimulators to control muscles of the legs and arms to encourage functional walking and to stimulate reaching and gripping. Electrodes are taped to the skin over nerves or surgically implanted and then controlled by a computer system under the command of the user. For example, to assist reaching, electrodes can be placed in the shoulder and upper arm and controlled by movements of the opposite shoulder. Through a computer interface, the spinal cord injured person can then trigger hand and arm movements in one arm by shrugging the opposite shoulder.

These systems are useful not just for restoring functional movements. They also help people exercise paralyzed muscle systems, which can provide significant cardiovascular benefits. So far, relatively few people utilize them because the movements are so robotic, they require extensive surgery and electrode placement, and the computer interface systems are still limited. Bioengineers are working to develop more natural interfaces.

Because the brain plans voluntary movements several seconds before the command is sent out to the muscles, people whose spinal cords no longer carry signals to their limbs might still be able to complete the planning phase in their brains but use a robotic device to carry out the command. A recent experiment used microwires implanted in the motor cortex area of the brain (in this case a monkey's brain) to record brain-wave activity, which was then relayed to a computer that analyzed the data, predicted the movement, and sent the command to a robotic arm. A device such as this could be used to control a wheelchair, a prosthetic limb, or even a patient's own arms and legs.

In the future, researchers expect that these kinds of brain-machine interfaces could be planted directly into the brain using microchips that would do the processing and transmit the results without wires. Work is already being done with hybrid neural interfaces, implantable electronic devices with a biological component that encourages cells to integrate into the host nervous system.

Retraining Central Pattern Generators

Scientists have known for years that animals' spinal cords contain networks of neurons called central pattern generators (CPG) that produce rhythmic flexing and extension of the muscles used in walking. They assumed, however, that the bipedal walking of humans was more dependent on voluntary control than on CPG activation. Therefore, scientists thought that without control from the brain, movements produced by a spinal CPG weren't likely to be useful in restoring successful walking without regulation from the brain. Current research is showing, however, that these networks can be retrained after spinal cord injury to restore limited mobility to the legs.

Using a technique called sensory patterned feedback, researchers are attempting to retrain CPG networks in spinal cord injured patients with special programs that break down walking movements into their component patterns and force paralyzed limbs to repeat them over and over again. In one of these programs, the patient is partially supported by a harness above a moving treadmill while a therapist moves the patient's legs in a stepping motion. Other researchers are experimenting with combining body weight support and electrical stimulation with actual walking rather than treadmill training.

Another technique uses an FES bicycle in which electrodes are attached to hamstrings, quadriceps, and gluteal muscles to stimulate the pedaling motion. Several studies have shown that these exercises can improve gait and balance, and increase walking speed. NINDS is currently funding a clinical trial with paraplegic and quadriplegic subjects to test the benefits of partial weight-supported walking.

Relieving Pressure through Surgery

The timing of surgical decompression (alleviating pressure on the spinal cord from fractured or dislocated vertebrae or disks) is a controversial topic. Animal studies have shown that early decompression can reduce secondary damage, but similar results haven't been reliably reproduced in human trials. Other studies have shown neurological improvement without decompression surgery, which has led some to believe that either avoiding or delaying surgery, and using pharmacologic interventions instead, is a reasonable (and noninvasive) treatment for spinal cord injuries. Additional research is needed to determine if early surgical intervention is sufficiently beneficial to offset the risk of major surgery in acute trauma.

Treating Pain

Two thirds of people with spinal cord injury report pain and a third of those rate their pain as severe. Nonetheless, both diagnosis and treatment of post-injury pain still remain a clinical challenge. There is no universally recognized scheme for classifying pain from spinal cord injury, nor is there a uniformly successful medical or surgical treatment to prevent or reduce it. The mainstays of neuropathic pain treatment are antidepressants and anticonvulsants, even though they are not uniformly effective.

Research suggests that spinal cord pain syndromes stem from the spread of secondary damage to spinal cord segments above and below the injury site. Pain can be at the level of the injury or below the level of the injury, even in areas where sensation is limited or absent. Findings indicate that at-level (junctional) pain probably results from damage to grey and white matter one or more segments above the injury site, whereas pain below the injury results from the interruption of axon pathways and the formation of abnormal connections within the spinal cord near the site of injury.

Studies suggest that functional changes in neurons, which make them hyperexcitable, could be a cause of chronic pain syndromes. Consequently, giving more aggressive treatment for spinal cord injury in the first few hours after injury could limit secondary damage and prevent or reduce the development of chronic pain afterward.

Investigators are currently testing neuroprotective and antiinflammatory strategies to calm overexcited neurons. Other studies are also looking at pharmacological options, including sodium channel blockers (such as lidocaine and mexiletine), opioids (such as alfentanil and ketamine), and a combination of morphine and clonidine. Drugs that interfere with neurotransmitters involved in pain syndromes, such as glutamate, are also being investigated. Other researchers are exploring the use of genetically engineered cells to deliver pain-relieving neurotransmitters. These treatments appear to alleviate pain in animal models and in preliminary clinical studies with terminally ill cancer patients.

Controlling Spasticity

The mechanisms of muscle spasticity after spinal cord injury are not well understood. Recent studies indicate that the loss of particular descending axonal pathways most likely results in the decreased activity of inhibitory interneurons, which causes the overreaction of motor neurons to excitatory stimuli.

Unlike treatments for post-injury pain, medical and surgical treatments for spasticity are established and highly successful. These include oral medications that act within the central nervous system (baclofen and diazepam) and one that acts directly on skeletal muscle (dantrolene). For spasticity that is resistant to drug interventions, surgical rhizotomy or myelotomy is sometimes performed to sever reflex pathways.

Investigators are currently exploring neuromodulation procedures based on preliminary results showing that electrical spinal cord stimulation below the injury can modulate spasms. Other techniques used clinically and experimentally involve implanting pump systems that continuously supply antispasmodic drugs such as baclofen.

Improving Bladder Control

A promising area of research on treatments for bladder dysfunction involves using electrical stimulation and neuromodulation to achieve bladder control. The current treatment for reflex incontinence includes a surgical procedure that cuts the sacral sensory nerve roots from S2 to S4. With the hope that a cure for spinal cord injury could be imminent, and the reluctance among men to lose any of their already compromised sexual function, few patients are willing to have these nerves cut.

Development of a sacral posterior and anterior root stimulator implant is being explored to better coordinate bladder and sphincter contractions. In preliminary studies people were able to achieve suppression of reflex incontinence and clinically useful increases in bladder volume with the use of the implanted stimulator.

Researchers hope that by combining neuromodulation for reflex incontinence with neurostimulation for bladder emptying, the bladder could be completely controlled without having to cut any sacral sensory nerves.

Understanding Changes in Sexual and Reproductive Function

Sperm count in men may or may not change due to spinal cord injury, but sperm motility often does. Researchers are investigating whether spinal cord injury causes changes in the chemical composition of semen that make it hostile to sperm viability. Preliminary studies show that the semen of men with spinal cord injury contains abnormally high levels of immunologically active leukocytes, which appear to have a negative impact on sperm motility.

Recent animal studies have revealed what appears to be a neural circuit within the spinal cord that is critical for triggering ejaculation in animal models and may play the same role in humans. Triggering ejaculation by stimulating these cells might be a better option than some of the current, more invasive methods, such as electro-ejaculation.

The Future of Spinal Cord Research

Fueled by significant federal and private funding, the past decade of spinal cord injury research has produced a wealth of discoveries that are making the repair of injured spinal cords a reachable goal. This is good news for the 10,000 to 12,000 Americans every year who sustain these traumatic injuries.

Because spinal cord injuries happen predominantly to people under the age of 30, the human cost is high. Major improvements in emergency and acute care have improved survival rates but have also increased the numbers of individuals who have to cope with severe disabilities for the rest of their lives. The cost to society, in terms of health care costs, disability payments, and lost income, is disproportionately high compared to other medical conditions.

Considering the biological complexity of spinal cord injury, discovering successful ways to repair injuries and create rehabilitative strategies that significantly reduce disabilities is not an easy task. Researchers, many of them supported by the NINDS, are actively developing innovative research strategies aimed at making the kinds of exciting new discoveries that will translate into better clinical care and better lives for all.

Information Resources

For information on other neurological disorders or research programs funded by the National Institute of Neurological Disorders and Stroke, contact the Institute's Brain Resources and Information Network (BRAIN) at:

BRAIN
P.O. Box 5801
Bethesda, MD 20824
Toll-Free: (800) 352-9424
Website: http://www.ninds.nih.gov

A number of private organizations offer services and information for those with spinal cord injury and their families, including:

Christopher Reeve Paralysis Foundation/ Paralysis Resource Center
500 Morris Avenue
Springfield, NJ 07081
Toll-Free: (800) 225-0292
Phone: (973) 379-2690
Fax: (973) 912-9433
Website: http://www.christopherreeve.org
E-mail: info@crpf.org; research@crpf.org

Daniel Heumann Fund for Spinal Cord Research
6516 Truman Lane, Suite #100
Falls Church, VA 22043-1821
Phone: (703) 442-8797
Fax: (703) 448-6914
Website: http://www.heumannfund.org
E-mail: dannycuse@aol.com

Geoffrey Lance Foundation for SCI Research and Support
132 S. 10th Street, #375 Main
c/o Regional SCI Center of Delaware Valley
Philadelphia, PA 19107
Phone: (877) GLANCE1 (452-6231)
Fax: (215) 955-5152
Website: http://www.geofflance.com
E-mail: info@geofflance.com

Miami Project to Cure Paralysis/Buoniconti Fund

P.O. Box 016960
R-48
Miami, FL 33101-6960
Phone: (305) 243-6001
Toll-Free: (800) STANDUP (782-6387)
Fax: (305) 243-6017
Website: http://www.themiamiproject.org
E-mail: mpinfo@miamiproject.med.miami.edu

National Spinal Cord Injury Association

6701 Democracy Blvd., #300-9
Bethesda, MD 20817
Toll-Free: (800) 962-9629
Phone: (301) 214-4006
Fax: 301-881-9817
Website: http://www.spinalcord.org
E-mail: info@spinalcord.org

Paralyzed Veterans of America (PVA)

801 18th Street, NW
Washington, DC 20006-3517
Toll-Free: (800) 424-8200
Phone: (202) USA-1300 (872-1300)
Fax: (202) 785-4452
Website: http://www.pva.org
E-mail: info@pva.org

Spinal Cord Society

19051 County Highway 1
Fergus Falls, MN 56537
Phone: (218) 739-5252
Phone: (218) 739-5261
Fax: (218) 739-5262
Website: http://members.aol.com/scsweb

Glossary

agonist—a drug capable of combining with a receptor and initiating action.

antagonist—a drug that opposes the effects of another by physiological or chemical action or by a competitive mechanism.

apoptosis—also called programmed cell death. A form of cell death in which a programmed sequence of events leads to the elimination of old, unnecessary, and unhealthy cells.

arrhythmia—an abnormal heart rhythm. The heartbeats may be too slow, too rapid, too irregular, or too early.

astrocyte—a type of glial cell responsible for neurotransmission and neuronal metabolism.

autonomic dysreflexia—a potentially dangerous complication of spinal cord injury in which blood pressure rises to dangerous levels. If not treated, autonomic dysreflexia can lead to stroke and possibly death.

axial traction—the application of a mechanical force to stretch the spine; used to relieve pressure by separating vertebral surfaces and stretching soft tissues.

axon—the long, thin extension of a nerve cell that conducts impulses away from the cell body.

axonal growth cone—dynamic structures present at the tip of developing and regenerating axons that respond to chemical cues for growth and direction.

central pattern generators (CPG)—neural circuits that produce self-sustaining patterns of behavior independent of their sensory input. Researchers have found evidence of a locomotor CPG in the spinal cord that synchronizes muscle activity during alternating stepping of the legs and feet.

cervical—the part of the spine in the neck region.

coccygeal—the part of the spine at the bottom of the spinal column, above the buttocks.

cytokine—a small protein released by immune cells that has a specific effect on the interactions between cells, or communications between cells, or on the behavior of cells.

dendrite—a short arm-like protuberance from a neuron. Dendrite is from the Greek for "branched like a tree."

disk—shortened terminology for an intervertebral disk, a disk-shaped piece of specialized tissue that separates the bones of the spinal column.

electroejaculation—a technique that uses an electric probe to stimulate ejaculation.

embryonic stem cells—undifferentiated cells from the embryo that have the potential to become a wide variety of specialized cell types.

excitotoxicity—a neurological process that is the result of the release of excessive amounts of the neurotransmitter glutamate.

extracellular matrix—the material found around cells composed of structural proteins, specialized proteins, and proteoglycans.

fetal spinal cord cells—cells used by scientists to derive undifferentiated embryonic stem cells for transplant into the damaged spinal cord.

free radicals—highly reactive chemicals that attack molecules and modify their chemical structure.

functional electrical stimulation (FES)—the therapeutic use of low-level electrical current to stimulate muscle movement and restore useful movements such as standing or stepping; also called functional neuromuscular stimulation.

glia—supportive cells in the brain and spinal cord. Glial cells are the most abundant cell types in the central nervous system. There are three types: astrocytes, oligodendrocytes, and microglia.

glutamate—an excitatory neurotransmitter.

growth-inhibiting proteins—protein molecules that inhibit axon regeneration.

guidance molecules—molecules that guide axons to their target. Some guidance molecules attract certain axons while repelling others.

hypothermia—abnormally low body temperature.

interneurons—neurons with axons that remain within the spinal cord.

intubation—the process of putting a tube into a hollow organ or passageway, often into the airway.

ligament—a tough band of connective tissue that connects various structures such as two bones.

lumbar—the part of the spine in the middle back, below the thoracic vertebrae and above the sacral vertebrae.

macrophage—a type of white blood cell that engulfs foreign material. Macrophages are key players in the immune response to foreign invaders such as infectious microorganisms Macrophages also release substances that stimulate other cells of the immune system.

methylprednisolone—a steroid drug used to improve recovery from spinal cord injury.

microglia—glial cells that function as part of the immune system in the brain and spinal cord.

monocyte—a white blood cell that has a single nucleus and can engulf foreign material. Monocytes emigrate from blood into the tissues of the body and evolve into macrophages.

myelin—a structure of cell membranes that forms a sheath around axons, insulating them and speeding conduction of nerve impulses.

myelotomy—a surgical procedure that cuts into the spinal cord.

neural prostheses—prosthetic devices that can respond to signals from the brain.

neurogenic pain—generalized pain that results from nervous system malfunction.

neuromodulation—a series of techniques employing electrical stimulation or the administration of medication by means of devices implanted in the body. These techniques allow the treatment of a range of disorders including certain forms of pain, spasticity, tremor, and urinary problems.

neuron—also known as a nerve cell; the structural and functional unit of the nervous system. A neuron consists of a cell body and its processes: an axon and one or more dendrites.

neurostimulation—the act of stimulating neurons with electrical impulses delivered via electrodes attached to the brain.

neurotransmitter—a chemical released from neurons that transmits an impulse to another neuron, muscle, organ, or other tissue.

neurotrophic factors—proteins responsible for the growth and survival of neurons.

neutrophil—a type of white blood cell that engulfs, kills, and digests microorganisms.

oligodendrocyte—a type of nerve cell in the brain and spinal cord that surrounds and insulates axons.

olfactory ensheathing glia—non-myelinating glial cells that ensheath olfactory axons within both the PNS and CNS portions of the primary olfactory pathway. They are being used in experiments to build bridges between damaged areas of the spinal cord.

paralysis—the inability to control movement of a part of the body.

paraplegia—a condition involving complete paralysis of the legs.

pressure sore (also known as a pressure ulcer or bed sore)—a reddened area or open sore caused by unrelieved pressure on the skin over bony areas such as the hipbone or tailbone.

quadriplegia—a condition involving complete paralysis of the legs and partial or complete paralysis of the arms.

receptor—a structure on the surface or interior of a cell that selectively receives and binds to a specific substance.

regeneration—repair, regrowth, or restoration of tissues; opposite of degeneration.

rhizotomy—an operation to disconnect specific nerve roots in order to stop severe spasticity.

sacral—refers to the part of the spine in the hip area.

Schwann cell—the cell of the peripheral nervous system that forms the myelin sheath.

spasticity—increased tone in muscles of the arms and legs (due to lesions of the upper motor neurons).

spinal shock—a temporary physiological state that can occur after a spinal cord injury in which all sensory, motor, and sympathetic functions of the nervous system are lost below the level of injury. Spinal shock can lower blood pressure to dangerous levels and cause temporary paralysis.

stem cell—special cells that have the ability to grow into any one of the body's more than 200 cell types. Unlike mature cells, which are permanently committed to their fate, stem cells can both renew themselves and create cells of other tissues.

synapse—a specialized junction between two nerve cells. At the synapse, a neuron releases neurotransmitters that diffuse across the gap and activate receptors situated on the target cell.

T-cell—an immune system cell that produces substances called cytokines, which stimulate the immune response.

thoracic—the part of the spine at the upper-back to midback level.

vertebrae—the 33 hollow bones that make up the spine.

Chapter 30

Adapting to
Spinal Cord Injury

What Is Adjustment?

Adjustment is defined as adapting to a new condition. Everyone makes adjustments during their lifetime. Some of the conditions that you adjust to may be planned and you have time to think about how you are going to react to the situation. For example, you may have to make adjustments in your work hours when you start a new job. Other events may be a surprise, and you are forced to adjust to an unplanned event.

After Spinal Cord Injury

A spinal cord injury (SCI) is one of the most devastating of all traumatic events. It results in a loss of some or all of an individual's sensation and movement. It is common for individuals who are newly injured to have health problems. Plus, it takes time to build enough strength to be able to fully participate in daily activities.

Individuals who are newly injured will likely experience grief. This is a period of mourning that is similar to that following the death of a loved one. The difference is that you are grieving the loss of your sense

Phil Klebine, Linda L. Lindsey, and Patricia A. Rivera. InfoSheet #20 on "Adjustment to Spinal Cord Injury" is produced by the University of Alabama at Birmingham Department of Physical Medicine and Rehabilitation along with the University of Alabama at Birmingham Model Spinal Cord Injury System of Care (http://www.spinalcord.uab.edu/). © 2001 University of Alabama at Birmingham Board of Trustees.

of touch along with your ability to walk or use your hands. You will likely experience many different thoughts and feelings after injury. Some may seem extreme and others mild. There is no step-by-step grieving process, but some thoughts and feelings are common after injury.

Denial/Disbelief

You may first react to your injury as if nothing happened. You may refuse to accept that your loss of feeling and movement is permanent. Instead, you may see the injury as an illness similar to a cold or flu that will soon pass with time.

Sadness

Obviously, no one is happy to be injured. It does not matter what your level of injury. Extreme sadness is common after injury because you have experienced a great personal loss. Sadness is that down, or blue feeling that you have when something bad happens. However, it is important that you not confuse sadness with depression.

Depression is a medical condition that requires professional treatment. You may be depressed if you have symptoms such as extreme sadness, inactivity, difficulty in thinking and concentrating, a significant increase or decrease in your appetite and/or time spent sleeping, and feelings of dejection, hopelessness or worthlessness. You may even have thoughts about suicide if you have depression.

Anger

Some people react to their injury with strong feelings of displeasure. You might lash out verbally or want to become physically violent towards others. You may feel angry toward yourself if your actions resulted in your injury. You may even feel anger toward God or someone else for causing your injury.

Bargaining

At some time following your injury, you may begin to admit to yourself that you have a serious condition. However, you may still want to hold onto the belief that your injury is not permanent. You may act as if you accept your injury as "the way things are," but your acceptance may come with the belief that you will be rewarded for your prayers and hard work in therapy and eventually recover from your injury at some point in the foreseeable future.

Acceptance

Grieving usually ends as you come to accept a realistic view of your current condition and find meaning in your life. You begin to think about your future as an individual with SCI and set goals to pursue in life.

Adjustment to SCI

Individuals who adjust well to unexpected events generally lead healthy, active, and happy lives after their injury. Individuals who do not adapt well to unexpected events tend to be less healthy, less active, and unhappier after their injury. You basically experience two primary issues of adjustment to spinal cord injury.

1. When you are first injured, it takes time to get used to your life after injury. Some people grieve longer than others, so the adjustment period is different for everyone. It may take as much as a year for you to accept the realities of your injury.

2. You will also experience a continued process of adjusting to the unique issues that occur in your every day life as a person with SCI.

Problems Adjusting to SCI

If you have been injured for a year or more and have not come to accept your injury, it is a good idea to look into other areas to find out whether or not you are having problems adjusting to SCI. You may find it hard to believe upon first thought, but what happens to you is not as important as what you are thinking when something happens to you. Your thinking directly influences how you feel and react to events that occur in your life. This concept is the basis for Rational Emotive Behavior Therapy (REBT). Many counselors and psychologists teach REBT as a way to help people with and without SCI gain a healthy view of their lives.

You can use Figure 30.1 as your step-by-step guide showing how events in your life can trigger a "chain reaction" that can have a negative impact on your overall well being.

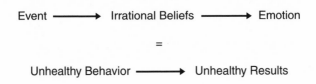

Figure 30.1. *Events in your life can negatively affect well being.*

Event

An event is something that happens to you. It can be something as small as misplacing the keys to your car or something as devastating as a spinal cord injury.

Irrational Beliefs

Anytime an event occurs in your life, you start to talk to yourself about that event. This self-talk is based on what you know or what you believe to be true. For example, a person who gets a promotion at work might think, "I earned it!"

There are times when this self-talk is based on completely false or partially false assumptions about an event. If you do not know all the facts involved in the event, your self-talk may be based on wrong information or a series of unrealistic, irrational beliefs about the event. Some examples of self-talk based on irrational beliefs are:

- my life is over because I can never live my life and be happy after a spinal cord injury; and

- I must be able to walk or must be able to use my hands if I am ever again going to be happy.

Although these irrational beliefs are common for individuals who are newly injured, many persons with SCI continue to hold onto these types of unrealistic, irrational beliefs long after their injury. The longer you hold onto such beliefs, the more likely it is that you are not adjusting well to your injury. You may have even adopted other false assumptions that are limiting your acceptance of your injury. Although there are countless possibilities for self-talk, some other examples of irrational beliefs are:

- because of my injury, it is now impossible for me to ever work or have a family;

- I am less of a person because of my injury;

- no one will accept, respect, or love a person with SCI;

- people should feel sorry for me and do things for me because my life has been unfair; and

- everyone will take advantage of me because I cannot defend myself.

Emotion

As you can see in Figure 30.1, what you are feeling, or your emotional response, depends on your self-talk. For example, individuals who are newly injured may think that their life is over because they cannot live with a spinal cord injury. This unrealistic self-talk may lead to extreme feelings such as anger, fear, and/or other emotional responses. If you have been injured for a year or more, you may feel sad, lonely, hopeless, or worthless if you continue to hold onto irrational beliefs such as "no one can possibly accept, respect, or love a person with SCI."

It is also important to know that feelings are neither good nor bad. It is normal to feel excited at times and sad at times. You may feel both sad and excited at the same time. Because your self-talk might be different from another person, you may feel differently than others about the same event.

Unhealthy Behavior

If your feelings are based on irrational beliefs, you can follow Figure 30.1 to see that your reactions to your feelings may result in behavior that is bad for your overall health and happiness. For example, you may not see the need to take proper care of your bladder or skin if you feel worthless. You may isolate yourself from others and avoid spending time with family and participating in other enjoyable activities.

Individuals with a history of alcohol and/or substance abuse may return to their old pattern of self-destructive behavior. Others may start drinking or taking drugs. Either way, substance abuse is unhealthy behavior. People who abuse alcohol will deny there is a problem, but it is estimated that individuals with SCI abuse alcohol at about twice the rate of the general population.[1]

Do you have a problem with substance abuse?

1. Have you ever felt you should cut down on your drinking or drug use?

2. Have people annoyed you by criticizing your drinking or drug use?

3. Have you ever felt bad or guilty about your drinking or drug use?

4. Have you ever taken a drink or taken drugs first thing in the morning as an eye opener to steady your nerves or get rid of a hangover?

Professionals often ask these four questions (CAGE Questionnaire) to help identify persons with a drinking problem. If you answered "yes" to one of the above questions, it is a warning sign that you may have a problem with alcohol abuse. If you believe that you or a member of your family has a problem with alcohol or substance abuse, seek help! Ask a family member, doctor, or clergy to help you find help.

Unhealthy Results

Unhealthy behavior almost always leads to unhealthy results. When you neglect your personal care, you put yourself at greater risk for developing a wide range of health problems such as respiratory complications, urinary tract infection, and pressure sores. These problems can limit your ability to participate in activities. In some extreme cases, you may die. Substance abuse can complicate existing medical problems or lead to other health problems. Substance abuse can also lead to other injuries and a loss of personal relationships.

Healthy Adjustment to SCI

No matter what the event, you know that it triggers self-talk. These ideas, thoughts, and/or beliefs lead to your feelings. Your behavior and the results of your behavior are guided by your feelings.

One of the biggest keys to adjusting to spinal cord injury is personal motivation. Individuals who are newly injured are often motivated to attend therapy sessions out of a desire to gain strength and function. You probably have a strong belief that your paralysis is only temporary, and you will soon return to your old, "normal" self. This hope is a common reaction after an injury. Unfortunately, it is far more likely for individuals to recover function based on their level and completeness of injury. In fact, only a few people actually fully recover from their injury. This does not mean that all hope is lost for a full or partial recovery. Almost all individuals with SCI continue to hope that they will walk again one day. However, a cure for paralysis may or may not come in your lifetime. A healthy approach to this reality is to move forward with your life after injury with the continued hope that advances in medicine will one day lead to a cure. In other words, do not wait on a cure to proceed with your life!

People who adjust well to life after injury are usually motivated to meet personal goals. These goals are different for everyone and often change throughout life. For example, your goal today may be to get a job, and you may want to have children in the future. Research shows that people with SCI who are goal-oriented are less likely to be depressed and more likely to obtain some acceptance of their disability than persons who are not goal-oriented.[2]

However, it is up to you to find purpose in your life and the motivation to achieve your goals. It may help to think about what you wanted out of your life before you were injured. For example, you may have once strived for good health, an enjoyable job, and a loving family. There is no reason that you cannot continue to strive for the same things now that you have a spinal cord injury.

Replacing Irrational Beliefs with Rational Beliefs

Once you have motivation for change and set your personal goals, you may find it easier to identify unrealistic, unfounded information and false assumptions. You can help yourself avoid irrational beliefs by not:

- using words like always, never, no one, everyone and other "all-or-nothing" words.

- over exaggerating (making something small into something big or something big into something impossible).

- focusing only on negatives and ignoring the positives.

- thinking things "should" or "must" be a certain way.

- trying to predict the future.

It does not matter what your level of injury, you can challenge your irrational beliefs and replace your false assumptions with information that is based on fact. It is up to you to take time to learn the facts about living with SCI. An individual who is newly injured may want information on bladder or bowel management. An individual who has been injured for a year or more may want information on employment or sexuality.

When you are looking for educational information, only rely on information that comes from a knowledgeable source on issues of SCI. For example, most rehabilitation facilities offer patient education classes for individuals who are newly injured. In fact, you may have been given an informational booklet to take home with you from the rehabilitation center. You can also easily get educational information on the Internet. Websites such as the National Spinal Cord Injury Association (www.spinalcord.org) and SPINALCORD Injury Information

Network (www.spinalcord.uab.edu) have information indexed by topics. These websites are great starting points for anyone looking for information to assist in everyday living with SCI. You may have access to the Internet at home, school, work, or your local library.

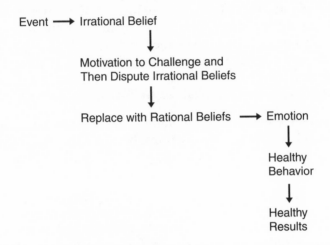

Figure 30.2. Use your skills to dispute and replace irrational beliefs.

Now you can use Figure 30.2 to help you develop the skills to dispute and replace your irrational beliefs. When you challenge your beliefs, it is important to ask yourself what evidence you have to support your beliefs. Is there evidence to disprove your belief? You can then learn to recognize those beliefs that are based on false assumptions. For example:

- "My life is over because I can never live or be happy after a spinal cord injury." Individuals who are newly injured often use this irrational belief as a way to deny the possibility that their injury is permanent. Individuals who have been injured for over a year may use this statement as a reason to do nothing. To dispute this assumption, you focus on the word "never." It is similar to words such as "always," "everyone," "no one," and "must." This is "all-or-nothing" thinking. By using these words you are not allowing yourself to believe that there are other possibilities. According to the National Spinal Cord Statistical Center's "Facts and Figures at a Glance," there are about 243,000 people in the United States alone who are currently living with SCI. You are ignoring the fact that many, if not most, of the people living with SCI are happy.

"Although I hope that my injury is not permanent and I fully recover, I know that many people are happy and living many years with all levels of injury." This type of rational self-talk is supporting your hope for recovery, but it also supports the fact that you can be happy and live with or without an injury. You are recognizing the fact that other people with the same level of injury are alive and happy.

- "Because of my injury, it is now impossible for me to ever work or have a family." This is a false assumption that many people hold onto long after injury. There are some individuals with SCI, family members, friends, and others in the community that wrongly believe that "no one" with SCI can work, especially those individuals with high levels of injury. They may wrongly believe that you cannot get married or have children because you have physical limitations. You may even find it hard to imagine that you can work, or your family and friends may try to discourage you from becoming a parent, especially if you need help with your own care. These are all false assumptions that you can challenge with facts.

"Although I have an injury and physical limitations to what I can do, I can put myself in a position to work and have a family if that is what I want." This rational self-talk acknowledges the fact that you have an injury. In reality you may have physical limitations that prevent you from doing some jobs, which may include the same job that you did before your injury. For example, if you were a construction worker before your injury, it is not likely that you can return to that job if you have a high level injury. However, this fact does not mean that you cannot work. With job retraining and support from your family, friends, and employer, you may find there are a number of jobs that you can do. As far as having a family, you might about people who are married and have children before their injury. It is irrational to think that people who are spouses and parents suddenly become "bad" spouses or "useless" parents simply because they become injured. The facts are to the contrary. Individuals with SCI continue to be loving, caring, supportive spouses and parents, no matter what their levels of injury. This fact also applies to people who want to have a family after injury. Although you may need to find ways to get things done, you need not base your desire to have a family solely on your physical limitations.

Emotion

Once you challenge your irrational beliefs and replace them with beliefs that are based on facts, you will likely feel differently. Instead of feeling sad, you might feel hopeful about your future. Instead of feeling worthless, you might begin to feel that you have value as a person, spouse, parent, and an employee.

Healthy Behavior

When you begin thinking more rationally and experiencing a change in your feelings, you will usually act differently. If you have set goals for yourself, you may make plans on how you intend to reach your goals. You might then take better care of yourself so that you can reach your goals. This is healthy behavior! It is the action that you take to improve your life.

Different people have their own way of getting things done. You may find that you can no longer get things done the same way as before your injury. It may be necessary to ask someone for help when you need it, but you may want to hold onto your irrational belief that you "must" do "everything" on your own. When you challenge this irrational belief, you may realize that people, both with and without SCI, help each other in many ways. This help may be as little as one person opening a door for another person. Some people simply get more help than others. When you ask for help, you are simply finding ways to overcome obstacles and get things done.

It may be necessary for you to find other ways to get things done. UAB [University of Alabama at Birmingham] is among the leaders in SCI research. In their studies of individuals with SCI and their family caregivers, evidence shows that good problem solving behavior can help individuals with SCI avoid medical problems and reach their goals.

Healthy Results

Hopefully, you will notice that healthier behavior leads to healthier results. When you take care of your health, you give yourself more of an opportunity to get out in the community and participate in enjoyable activities. You can solve the problems that prevent you from doing those things that you desire. You may soon discover that you are living a healthier, happier, and more satisfying life. It may take time, but you can reach your goals.

Family Adjustment to SCI

As an individual with SCI, it is important to recognize that your injury also has a tremendous impact on your family. Although they may not have to adjust to losing the use of their hands or ability to walk, your family may experience a loss of the way their life was before your injury. For example, they may have to adjust to the role of caregiver. They may need to work to help with family finances. All of the changes that they face can lead to added stress and anxiety.

Family members also grieve after injury. They may ask questions to try and understand the full impact of the injury and to help ease their feelings of sadness and fear. As your family comes to accept the injury, they face issues of adjustment similar to those you may experience.

Children are naturally curious and adjust to events by asking questions. They ask questions because they make few assumptions about how the injury impacts their life. Therefore, children adjust rather quickly to an injury if their questions are answered in a clear, honest manner.

Problems in Family Adjustment to SCI

As an adult family member, you may have difficulty with adjustment if you have your own irrational beliefs about life after injury. For example, you may hold the false assumption that individuals with SCI cannot work. You may hold the unrealistic idea that "no one" with SCI can or "should" have children. You may hold the irrational belief that you "must" do everything for your loved one who is injured.

Your actions as a family member are reflected in what you say and do around your loved one. If your actions are based on irrational beliefs, you may be unknowingly acting with less than supportive behavior. For example, if you continue to do things for your loved one that he/she can do, your actions may be encouraging your loved one to be overly dependent on others. You may also be reinforcing your loved one's false assumptions that individuals with SCI should be pitied or felt sorry for because life has treated them unfairly. You may be enabling your loved one to engage in destructive behavior if you ignore or deny the possibility of a problem with substance abuse. Plus, it is also likely that your irrational beliefs will influence your own feelings, which may then lead to unhealthy behavior and unhealthy results. If you experience prolonged feelings of stress and anxiety, you may be putting yourself at risk for serious health problems such as disease or stroke if you do not adjust your views of life after injury.

Healthy Family Adjustment to SCI

If you are a family member, healthy family adjustment is, essentially, taking care of you. For example, you can take time away from your loved one to do those things that you enjoy. You can help minimize your stress and anxiety by working to replace your own false assumptions, unrealistic ideas, and irrational beliefs. You can start by learning the facts about SCI. Then, challenge your irrational beliefs with evidence to dispute your beliefs. Finally, replace your false information with facts. Hopefully, you will soon discover that you too are living a healthier, happier, and more satisfying life.

Conclusion

No matter if you have a spinal cord injury or not, you have control over your life by choosing how you want to think about your situation. You can be happy and more hopeful about your life, but it will only happen when you work to make it happen. Your thoughts, feelings, and behavior do not change overnight. It takes time to grieve your loss and come to accept the realities of the injury. Then, you face a continued process of adjusting to everyday issues of living with SCI. If you avoid false assumptions, unrealistic ideas, and irrational beliefs, you will give yourself more opportunities to reach your goals and have the life that you desire.

Resources

1. Aging with SCI: Alcohol Abuse, a Modular Educational Tract (MET) produced and available at Craig Hospital. Call 303-789-8202 or go to www.craighospital.org for a copy.

2. Elliott TR, Uswatte G, Lewis L, Palmatier A (2000). Goal instability and adjustment to physical disability. *Journal of Counseling Psychology,* 47(2). 251–265.

This article is intended to help individuals with SCI and their families help themselves through the process of adjustment to the unique conditions that follow traumatic injury. This model is to be used as a guide through the process of adjustment—not for the treatment of any physical, emotional, and/or behavioral condition(s).

Part Five

Chronic Disorders Associated with Back and Neck Pain

Chapter 31

Ankylosing Spondylitis

Ankylosing spondylitis (AS) is the main rheumatic disease in a group of conditions called the spondyloarthropathies (SpA). Collectively, they are referred to as spondylitis.

Although AS primarily affects the mobility of the spine, it rarely affects the entire spine. Sometimes other areas of the body such as the eyes and or small joints of the hands and feet can be involved, but there are treatments available to reduce symptoms.

It is helpful to remember that even if you have mild symptoms, which you are able to manage quite well, it is important to see your rheumatologist once a year to ensure that the condition is not progressing.

Symptoms

The early symptoms of ankylosing spondylitis (AS) can vary from person to person. Most often, the symptoms begin slowly over the course of several months, however, some people describe the pain and muscle spasms as suddenly appearing, almost overnight. Many people notice that the fatigue, muscle spasms, and poor sleep quality when symptoms first appear can cause activities that were once enjoyable and easy to suddenly become exhausting and difficult to accomplish. Early diagnosis is essential. Here are important telltale symptoms to look out for: Symptoms include:

The information in this chapter is reprinted with permission from the Spondylitis Association of America, www.spondylitis.org. © 2003 Spondylitis Association of America. All rights reserved.

- Gradual onset of back pain and stiffness over a period of weeks or months

- Duration of symptoms longer than 3 months

- Early morning stiffness, which is improved by a warm shower or light exercise

- Sometimes the pain is located in other areas of the body, such as the buttocks or the neck.

- Average age, 26 years; gender, male or female

The pain is usually first felt in the low back, but may eventually be present throughout the whole spine or felt down the back of the buttocks and thighs (sciatic-like pain). Areas of the body where inflammation is most likely to develop are the central parts of the skeleton, i.e., the spine and pelvis. Anecdotally, the pain in women can first show in places other than the lower back. The neck is reported to be vulnerable to the first signs of pain and stiffness in some women. In children, the symptoms almost never appear first in the spine, but pain is usually felt in the heel or knee.

Iritis is an inflammation that can sometimes show up as a first symptoms of AS.

Diagnosis

Clues to Diagnosis

X-ray changes are considered to be important in the definitive diagnosis of AS. However, this poses a problem in that plain x-rays don't show anything for many years after the first symptoms are felt. That is why it is important for your rheumatologist to be very astute in recognizing clues that can quickly lead to a diagnosis of AS before x-rays of the pelvic area show any changes.

Detailed Clinical History of Symptoms and Physical Examination

Rheumatologists are trained to recognize the symptoms of AS. Typically, early morning stiffness that gets better after a warm shower, deep buttock pain in the night, possibly bouts of iritis (inflammation of the eye), and other clues should tip your doctor off to a possible diagnosis of AS.

HLA-B27 Gene Test Is Not Diagnostic of AS

A very high percentage of people with AS test positive for this gene—depending upon ethnicity. HLA-B27 is a perfectly normal gene found in 8% of the general population. Generally speaking, no more than 2% of people born with this gene will eventually get spondylitis. The gene itself does not cause spondylitis, but people with HLA-B27 are more susceptible to getting it. Occasionally, a test for HLA-B27 will be done, particularly if your doctor isn't quite sure that you have AS.

Treatment

If you, a family member, or friend has been diagnosed with ankylosing spondylitis (AS), it is important to know that there is a lot that can be done to reduce its effects. As with other chronic conditions, the more you learn, the better off you will be. It is also helpful to build a good relationship with your medical team. Even those people with mild symptoms can benefit from seeing a rheumatologist at least annually, so that he or she can check to make sure that you are doing well. Complications can sometimes occur and it is better to catch them early on.

What Is Important?

A treatment plan includes medications to help reduce the pain and stiffness caused by AS; this paves the way so that a daily exercise program can be adopted. Some people do not need to take medication, but this is not usually the norm. Good posture techniques are critical to put less strain on the body.

Additional Aids to Improved Quality of Life

Additional symptom management tools include: heat for stiffness, ice for swelling, hot baths and warm showers, ultrasound or gentle massage therapy, electrical stimulators for pain (transcutaneous electrical nerve stimulation [TENS]), and avoiding excess calories and obesity to lessen body weight stress on joints. Much can be done to help.

Medications

Many types of medications are effective in managing the symptoms of ankylosing spondylitis (AS) and related diseases (spondyloarthropathies or SpA), sometimes collectively called spondylitis.

Recent Developments

The United States Food and Drug Administration (FDA) recently approved the Tumor-Necrosis- Factor alpha (TNF) blocker etanercept (brand name Enbrel), the first biological medicine approved for the treatment of ankylosing spondylitis in the U.S.. The FDA based its decision on a study conducted at California-based Stanford University, which showed that at 24 weeks, 58 percent of those treated with twice-weekly etanercept injections maintained a significant improvement in measures of pain, function, and inflammation (greater than 20 percent improvement), as compared 23 percent of those patients on the placebo. The study's principal investigator, John Davis, M.D., noted that this is the first treatment to show improvement in range of motion in ankylosing spondylitis patients.

Non-Steroidal Anti-Inflammatories (NSAIDs)

Non-steroidal anti-inflammatories (NSAIDs) are the most commonly used medications to treat AS. For many people they can be effective in reducing the pain and stiffness associated with these conditions. However, they can sometimes cause heartburn, gastritis, and even bleeding. It is important to talk to your doctor about the possible side effects of any medication that you are being prescribed. Sometimes is it necessary to take medication that is designed to neutralize or prevent the production of gastric acid when you are taking NSAIDs. Some of these are called antacids or H2 blockers.

There are also medications that can coat the stomach, such as Carafate. Another type of medication can help to restore the lost gastric mucus caused by NSAIDs. They may also cause less common additional side effects that include: fluid retention, headaches, dizziness, and even confusion. Increasing evidence suggests that the new class of NSAIDs, the cyclooxygenase-2 specific inhibitors, or COX-2 inhibitors, sold under various brand names, may reduce the risk of these gastrointestinal problems. There is still some controversy among medical experts as to whether these drugs reduce gastrointestinal complications, but evidence seems to point in this direction.

When NSAIDs Are Not Enough

In severe spondylitis when NSAIDs do not sufficiently control the pain and stiffness and other symptoms, additional medications can be tried. However, it is important to give the NSAIDs sufficient time to be effective—this can take up to several weeks for some NSAIDs. If you are considering changing medications, remember to ask your doctor about the potential benefits and side effects before you and your doctor decide whether the change in treatment is right for you.

Sulfasalazine

Sulfasalazine is one type of medication that can be helpful to some people with severe disease. It is known to effectively control not only pain and joint swelling from arthritis of the small joints, but also the intestinal lesions in inflammatory bowel disease. Side effects can include headaches, abdominal bloating, nausea, and oral ulcers. Rarely, someone being prescribed this medication can develop bone marrow suppression, which is why it is important for your doctor to regularly monitor your blood count.

Methotrexate

Methotrexate can also be effective in controlling the symptoms of severe spondylitis in some people, particularly those with psoriatic arthritis and reactive arthritis (Reiter syndrome). It has the added benefit of controlling the skin rash of psoriasis. Side effects include bone marrow suppression, with lowering of the blood counts, oral ulcers, nausea, gastritis or peptic laceration, and liver toxicity. Use of this medication requires frequent monitoring of the blood counts and liver profile. The vitamin folic acid is often prescribed to combat the thinning hair and mouth ulcers associated with methotrexate.

Corticosteroids

Corticosteroids, such as prednisone, can be effective in relieving the inflammation associated with spondyloarthropathies, but the side effects of long-term use (weight gain, osteoporosis, etc.) can be very severe. They are sometimes prescribed for short periods of time. The use of corticosteroid injections into inflamed joints can also provide temporary relief of the pain and swelling of arthritis or bursitis. But because of the concern of rupture of the Achilles tendon, such injections are rarely, if ever used to treat Achilles tendonitis. Similarly, their usefulness in plantar fasciitis (inflamed heals) is not clear.

Chapter 32

Cauda Equina Syndrome

Back pain is a common experience, and in many instances a herniated disk is the cause. This condition can almost always be treated conservatively, at least initially. But back pain can be a symptom of a serious condition that is not well known and is often misdiagnosed. Cauda equina syndrome is a severe neurologic disorder that usually results from a herniated disk. But, unlike with a herniated disk alone, cauda equina syndrome can be a medical emergency. It can lead to incontinence and even permanent paraplegia. Though rare, occurring in only 1 to 2 percent of patients undergoing surgery for a herniated lumbar disk, cauda equina syndrome can be devastating if left untreated.

What Is Cauda Equina Syndrome?

Cauda equina is Latin for horse's tail, which is an apt physical description of the cauda equina. The cauda equina is the sack of nerve roots with a common covering at the end of the spinal cord. The spinal cord ends at the upper portion of the lumbar spine. The individual nerve roots at the end of the spinal cord that provide motor and sensory function to the legs and the bladder continue along in the spinal canal. The cauda equina is the continuation of these nerve roots in the lumbar region.

Cauda equina syndrome most commonly results from a massive disk herniation in the lumbar region. A disk herniation occurs when one of the soft flexible disks that functions as an elastic shock absorber between the bones of the spinal column herniates or displaces from its normal position. The herniation occurs after the disk begins to break down with aging and can be precipitated by stress or a mechanical problem in the spine. The result is that the softer, center portion of the disk pushes out and causes pressure on the nerve roots in the lumbar spine. Cauda equina syndrome is caused by this compression on the nerve roots.

Cauda equina syndrome is accompanied by a range of symptoms, the severity of which depend on the degree of compression and the precise nerve roots that are being compressed. Symptoms include severe low back pain, urinary or bowel incontinence, motor weakness or sensory loss in both legs, and saddle anesthesia (unable to feel anything in the body areas that would sit on a saddle).

Diagnosis

Cauda equina syndrome is difficult to diagnose. It is rare and its symptoms mimic those of other conditions. Besides a herniated disk, other conditions with similar symptoms to cauda equina syndrome include peripheral nerve disorder, spinal cord compression, and irritation or compression of the nerves after they exit the spinal column and travel through the pelvis, a condition known as lumbosacral plexopathy.

Another difficulty in diagnosing cauda equina syndrome is that its symptoms may vary in intensity and evolve slowly over time. Also, an x-ray will often not be helpful in detecting the cause of the syndrome.

How then is a physician to know to look for cauda equina syndrome?

Physicians need to be aware of certain red flags that indicate cauda equina syndrome. Red flags in someone with back pain include saddle anesthesia, recent onset of bladder dysfunction (such as urinary retention or incontinence), bowel incontinence, and motor weakness in the lower extremity. The presence of these symptoms warns of cauda equina compression.

Red flags also may be present in a patient's history. Recent trauma, a history of cancer, or a severe infection may predispose a person to cauda equina syndrome. Any of these diseases can involve the disks or the bones of the lumbar spine and result in cauda equina syndrome. Other conditions that may rarely lead to cauda equina syndrome include osteoporotic vertebral fractures and spinal stenosis.

Besides the classic red flag symptoms, physicians suspecting the syndrome look for reflex abnormalities such as the loss or diminution of reflexes, sensory abnormality in the legs, bladder or rectum, and muscle weakness or wasting in the legs.

MRI (magnetic resonance imaging) or myelograms are diagnostic tools valuable in discovering cauda equina syndrome. MRI uses energy from a powerful magnet to produce cross-sectional images of the back. The MRI is especially helpful in detecting damage or disease of soft tissue such as disks. A myelogram is a liquid dye injected into the spinal column. A myelogram can show pressure on the cauda equina from herniated disks and other conditions.

The incidence of cauda equina syndrome is not related to sex or race. It occurs primarily in adults, though trauma-related cauda equina syndrome is not age specific.

Treatment

Treatment of cauda equina syndrome is necessary to restore bladder and bowel function. Treatment also can prevent further weakness in the lower extremities. Left untreated, cauda equina syndrome can result in paraplegia.

Those experiencing any of the red flag syndromes should seriously consider seeing a neurosurgeon, who provides the operative and non-operative management of neurological disorders. Prompt surgery is the best treatment for patients with cauda equina syndrome. Treating patients within 48 hours after the onset of the syndrome provides a significant advantage in improving sensory and motor deficits as well as urinary and rectal function. But even patients who undergo surgery after the 48-hour ideal time frame may experience significant improvement, too. Although short-term recovery of bladder function may lag behind reversal of lower extremity motor deficits, the function may continue to improve years after surgery. Following surgery, drug therapy coupled with intermittent self-catheterization can help lead to slow but steady recovery of bladder and sphincter function.

Although steroids have proven useful in the treatment of spinal cord injury and some physicians advocate steroids for cauda equina syndrome, no evidence suggests that they are useful in treatment of cauda equina compression. In fact, some physicians point to the potential risks of high-dose steroid use and do not advocate their use to treat cauda equina syndrome.

Chapter 33

Cervical Spine Disorders

Chapter Contents

Section 33.1

What Are Cervical Spine Disorders?

You have probably been referred to see a neurosurgeon because of pain in your neck or shoulder or perhaps tingling or numbness in your arms. You may also have experienced some weakness when using your arms or hands.

You may be wondering if there is a chance that everything will return to normal or whether the surgery that may have been talked about is very risky. These questions and concerns can be addressed by your neurosurgeon, who is a physician trained in the surgical treatment of disorders of the nervous system.

He or she will ask a number of questions and then perform a neurological examination. Following a review of any x-rays or other diagnostic tests you may have brought with you, additional tests may be ordered if further information is needed. Finally, he or she will propose a course of treatment, which may or may not involve surgery.

The decisions regarding your care should be reached after discussions between you, your family and your neurosurgeon. This information will help educate you about the issues involved in your care.

Understanding the Problem

Your neck is part of a long flexible column extending through most of your body often referred to as the spinal column, or backbone. The neck region of the spinal column (the cervical spine) consists of seven bones (vertebrae) shaped like building blocks, which are separated from one another by shock absorbing pads (intervertebral disks).

These disks allow the spine to move freely and act as shock absorbers during activity. Attached to the back of each vertebral body is an arch of bone that forms a continuous hollow longitudinal space much like a tube that runs the whole length of your back. This space is the spinal canal, through which runs the spinal cord and nerve bundles. The spinal cord is surrounded by fluid (cerebrospinal fluid) and three layers of protective membrane: the dura, the pia, and the arachnoid.

At each vertebral level a pair of spinal nerves exit through small openings called foramina (one to the left and one to the right). These nerves serve the muscles, skin, and tissues of the body and thus provide sensation and movement to all parts of the body. The delicate spinal cord and nerves are further supported by strong muscles and ligaments that are attached to the vertebrae.

Cervical Disk Disease

With age, injury, poor posture, or diseases such as arthritis there can be damage to the bone or joints of the cervical spine. The cervical disks may become worn out and abnormal growths (bone spurs) may form as a result of repetitive movement of the disk. Sudden movement or injury such as whiplash may cause the disk to slip or herniate. The herniated disk or bone spurs may narrow the spinal canal through which the spinal cord runs or the small openings (foramina) through which spinal nerves exit.

What Problems Might You Experience?

Pressure on a nerve by a herniated (slipped) disk or a bone spur may irritate the nerve resulting in pain in the neck and arm, incoordination, or numbness or weakness in the arm, forearm, or fingers. Pressure on the spinal cord in the neck (cervical) region can be a very serious problem because virtually all of the nerves to the rest of the body have to pass through the neck to reach their final destination (arms, chest, abdomen, legs); therefore, the function of many important organs is potentially at risk.

Initially, the symptoms of cervical disk disease may be limited to neck pain and later arm pain; weakness or numbness may also occur along with difficulty walking or incoordination of the legs. Further progression may lead to severe impairment or even paralysis.

Diagnosis

Your doctor will document your symptoms and find out the extent to which these symptoms affect your life. The physical examination will include an assessment of sensation, strength, and reflexes in various parts of your body to help pinpoint which nerves or what parts of your spinal cord are affected.

Your doctor may then order studies to confirm the diagnosis and determine more precisely the nature and extent of the disease process. These studies may include:

- **X-rays:** A simple x-ray will show the bones of the neck and determine if there is significant wear and tear or disease of the bone. It will also show whether the bones are lined up properly.

- **Myelogram:** The myelogram is an x-ray with a special dye that highlights the spinal cord and nerves. The dye is usually injected into the spine with a needle and then the x-rays are obtained.

- **Computed Tomography (CT):** A CT (also known as CAT scan) of the spine is a computerized map of an x-ray of the neck. The CT will show the anatomy of the neck in more detail and from different angles. It will also better define the relationship of the disk or bone spurs to the spinal cord and nerves. The CT may be done in conjunction with a myelogram of the neck to provide additional information.

- **Magnetic Resonance Imaging (MRI):** The MRI uses a powerful magnetic field rather than x-rays to produce a detailed anatomical picture of the neck and the structures within it. During the study you will hardly feel that anything is going on.

- **Electromyogram and Nerve Conduction Studies (EMG/ NCS):** Unlike the previous tests, which help your doctor determine anatomy and structure, these tests primarily study how the nerve and muscles are actually working together. This information can assist in determining which nerves or muscles are functioning abnormally.

Treatment

Cervical disk disease does not always mean that you require surgery. In fact, many of your symptoms can be relieved by nonsurgical management.

Your doctor may prescribe medications to reduce the pain or inflammation and allow time for healing to occur. Bed rest, reduction of physical activity, or a cervical collar may also be prescribed. The collar provides support for the spine, reduces mobility, and may reduce the pain and irritation.

To further relieve the pressure on the nerves in your neck your doctor may prescribe a cervical traction device. This device is attached to your head and pulls up on it using a pulley system and weights. It is usually applied a few times a day and can be used while sitting or lying in bed.

What Kind of Surgery May Be Helpful?

There are several operations that may be used to treat cervical disk disease. The selection of which operation and the determination of when to perform the operation depend on many factors, which obviously differ for each patient and doctor combination. However, some general factors include the kind of disk disease you have (herniated disk or bone spurs), whether there is pressure on the spinal cord or spinal nerve, the presence of one or more areas of disease within the cervical spine, and if the spine is dislocated in addition to pressure on the cord or nerves.

Other factors are determined by your age, how long you have had the disease, other medical problems, previous operations on the neck, and so on.

The particular combination of these and other factors will determine the choice of surgical treatment.

Anterior Cervical Discectomy

This operation is performed on the neck to relieve pressure on one or more nerve roots or on the spinal cord. The procedure is performed from the front, or anterior, approach. Discectomy means to remove the disk.

Surgery for anterior cervical discectomy is performed with the patient under general anesthesia lying on his or her back. The surgeon may place a traction device to pull on the neck. During the course of the operation x-rays may be obtained to assist the surgeon in the surgery.

The surgeon will make an incision in the front of your neck; if only one disk is to be removed it will typically be a small horizontal incision in the crease of the skin. If the operation is to be more extensive, the incision may be oblique (slanted) or longer.

The soft tissues within the neck are separated to allow the surgeon to reach the front of the spine, following which the intervertebral disk and bone spurs are removed. An operating microscope may be used to better display the area while part of the disk is removed with forceps. Other instruments such as a drill or bone-cutting instruments may be used to enlarge the disk space. This will help the surgeon to relieve any pressure on the nerve or spinal cord due to bone spurs or the ruptured (herniated) disk.

Sometimes the space between the vertebrae is refilled with a small piece of bone (fusion). The bone may be yours (for example, from your hip bone) or it may be taken from a bone bank. In time, the vertebrae may fuse, or join together. In addition to the piece of bone, some surgeons may place a metal plate at the fusion site to strengthen it.

The neck incision is closed in several layers. Skin suture material may need to be removed or the surgeon may use absorbing sutures and strips of tape, which you can later remove by yourself.

Historically and statistically, there are few surgical risks with anterior cervical discectomy; however, some risk is unavoidable and the unexpected may occur resulting in complications.

Although every precaution will be taken to avoid complications, common risks possible with surgery are: infection, excessive bleeding (hemorrhage) and an adverse reaction to anesthesia. Other risks possible with anterior cervical discectomy include: stroke; injury to the recurrent laryngeal nerve, which causes hoarseness and may or may not be permanent; and injury to the involved nerve root(s) or the spinal cord, both of which can cause varying types and degrees of paralysis.

The process of informed consent is designed to make you familiar and comfortable with the reasonable expectations and foreseeable risks. Your surgeon and anesthesiologist will discuss these with you and assist you in your decision making.

Cervical Corpectomy

This operation is an extension of the discectomy procedure. Also using an anterior approach, the surgeon removes a part of the vertebral body to relieve pressure on the spinal cord. One or more vertebral bodies may be removed including the adjoining disks. The incision is generally longer. The space between the vertebrae is filled using a piece of bone (fusion) and maybe a metal plate. Because more bone is removed, the recovery process for the fusion to heal and the neck to become stable again is usually longer than with anterior cervical discectomy.

Cervical Laminectomy and Discectomy

This operation is performed through a vertical incision in the back of the neck, generally in the middle. Through this opening the surgeon will use an instrument (a retractor) to pull aside the strong muscles of the neck and expose the arch of bone (lamina) that forms the spinal canal. A drill and bone cutting instruments are used to remove the bone around the spinal cord (laminotomy) or the bone around the nerve opening (foraminotomy). Once the nerve is located, it is moved gently aside and an incision is made on the outside covering of the disk through which the disk material is then removed.

Recovery after Surgery

Following surgery, you will be taken to the recovery room for a short while and then spend a few days in a hospital room. When you awake you may have a collar or brace around your neck or a drainage tube coming out of your neck. Typically, the drainage tube is removed in a day or two.

If you had an anterior cervical discectomy or corpectomy, your throat may be slightly sore. If a piece of bone was taken from your hip, the area of incision is usually sore. Your physician will give you appropriate medication to address these problems. Fortunately, most of them are temporary.

Intravenous (IV) fluids will be ordered during the early recovery period.

Discharge from the Hospital

Your length of stay in the hospital will be determined by your progress and by your home situation. When you are ready to leave the hospital you will be provided with instructions regarding your brace, care of your incision(s), and physical activity.

Generally, you will wear a brace for a few weeks, but this is variable and it may be much longer. Usually you have to keep it on continuously, but your doctor may allow you to take it off for short periods. It is unlikely that you will be allowed to drive, lift heavy objects, or engage in contact sports or vigorous physical activity for a while. Keep your incision clean and dry and report any signs of drainage or inflammation promptly to your doctor.

Unless instructed otherwise, you may take a shower after surgery. This should be done with a dressing in place to protect the incision.

Practice good posture and body mechanics even during routine daily tasks. It is normal to have some pain, especially in the incision area; pain in the neck or arms is also not unusual, and is caused by inflammation of the previously compressed nerve. It will slowly lessen as the nerve heals. Medication may also help. Discomfort is normal while you gradually return to normal activity, but pain is a signal to stop what you are doing or proceed more slowly.

Follow-Up

Your doctor will see you in the office after surgery and examine your incision. He or she may remove skin sutures and will evaluate nerve and muscle function. X-rays may be ordered to check on the fusion of the bone graft. Physical therapy may be recommended.

Numbness or tingling sensations are often the last symptoms to leave. Your doctor will help determine when you can return to work and with what limitations.

Driving a motor vehicle will be possible once your doctor determines that you have recovered full coordination and are experiencing minimal pain and that your neck is stable.

The Role of the Neurosurgeon

If you are perceiving problems in your cervical spine caused by pressure on the nerves, a neurosurgeon is the appropriate medical professional to direct your treatment. Although his or her primary concerns will be diagnosis, interpretation of test results (when necessary), and surgery, you will most likely have other medical professionals involved in your treatment as well, such as anesthesiologists, physical therapists, and other specialists.

Neurological surgery is the medical specialty concerned with the diagnosis and treatment of disorders of the nervous system, the brain, or the spinal cord. Neurosurgeons treat patients with injuries to the head, spinal cord, or nerves; patients with a stroke or in danger of a stroke due to clogged arteries in the neck; patients with tumors or malformations of the brain or spinal cord; as well as patients with back or neck pain associated with a slipped disk.

Neurosurgeons undergo six to eight years of rigorous training following medical school. After successfully completing this training, two years of medical practice and a written examination, neurosurgeons can become board certified.

Section 33.2

Cervical Radiculopathy

Usually, when something hurts, you don't have to look far to find the source of the pain. But an injury near the root of a nerve could result in pain at the end of the nerve, where sensation is felt. For example, an injury to the vertebrae or disks in your neck (your cervical vertebrae) could result in pain, numbness, or weakness in your shoulder, arm, wrist, or hand. That's because the nerves that extend out from between the cervical vertebrae provide sensation and trigger movement in these areas. This condition is called cervical radiculopathy.

Causes of Cervical Radiculopathy

Several conditions can put pressure on nerve roots in the neck. The most common causes for cervical radiculopathy are:

- **Herniated cervical disk.** In this situation, the outer layer (annulus) of the disk cracks and the gel-like center (nucleus) breaks through. This causes the disk to protrude, putting pressure on the nerve that exits the spinal column at that point.

- **Spinal stenosis.** Sometimes, the space in the center of the vertebrae narrows and squeezes the spinal column and nerve roots.

- **Degenerative disk disease.** As we age, the water content in our body cells diminishes and other chemical changes occur that can cause the disk to shrink. Without sufficient cushioning, the vertebrae may begin to press against each other, pinching the nerve or forming bony spurs.

Diagnosis and Treatment

Your physician will give you a careful examination and ask about your symptom history. You may be asked to extend and rotate your neck and/or arm to reproduce the pain symptoms. An x-ray will usually show any degenerative disk problems. Sometimes your physician may request an MRI (magnetic resonance image) or a CT scan (computed tomography) using a colored dye to outline the nerves. Initial treatment is usually conservative and aims to reduce the pain by easing the pressure on the nerves. The treatment consists of three parts: rest, medication, and physical therapy.

- **Rest.** You may have to take it easy for a few days or wear a soft cervical collar to limit motion and relieve irritation on the nerves.

- **Medication.** Your doctor may prescribe a non-narcotic pain medicine and anti-inflammatory drug to relieve any swelling.

- **Physical therapy.** After muscle spasms subside, your orthopaedic surgeon may prescribe a cervical traction device or other types of physical therapy such as heat or cold therapies, electrical stimulation, or isometric and stretching exercises.

If conservative treatment doesn't relieve your pain over the course of 6 to 12 weeks, surgery may be an option. The surgical procedure will depend on the underlying condition. Your orthopaedic surgeon will discuss the options with you. In most cases, surgery not only relieves the pain, but also improves functioning and movement of the affected areas.

Chapter 34

Degenerative Disk Disease

Introduction

Disks are the cartilage that lies between the bony vertebral bodies of the spine.

Since motion occurs in this area, these are considered a joint. As a natural phenomenon of the aging process, disks lose their water content and degenerate. Concurrently, tears occur in the outer lining of the disk (the annulus).

In adults, the annulus has nerve fibers whereas the center of a disk does not. A tear in this outer annulus can be quite painful. Although these degenerative processes are part of the natural aging of the spine, the disks of some people degenerate much more quickly than others. Also, for reasons as yet unknown, some individuals experience much more pain from these degenerative changes than others.

The symptoms of degenerative disk disease typically follow one of three courses:

- a significant injury followed by sudden and unexpected back pain;

- a trivial injury accompanied by significant back pain; and

- a gradual onset and worsening of midline low back pain.

What Treatment Options Are Available for Degenerative Disk Disease?

Artificial Disk Replacement

The Cedars-Sinai Institute for Spinal Disorders is the first West Coast center to perform artificial disk replacement procedures as part of a Federal Drug Administration clinical trial. When performing artificial disk replacement (ADR) for degenerative disk disease, the doctor inserts a small prosthetic (artificial) disk comprising a polyethylene core that slides between two metal end plates. The end plates are attached to the vertebral body with anchoring teeth built along the rim of the end plates.

The prosthetic disks replace the injured disks, helping to relieve chronic back pain. The polyethylene core allows movement of the spine, unlike fusions which prevent normal movement.

The disk is made of the same material used in artificial hips and knees.

Bone Morphogenic Protein (BMP)

Pinpointed bone growth and formation is vital to the supporting structures of the spine. Bone morphogenic protein (BMP) is a substance that stimulates bone growth and can be based on and matched to properly identified material from the patient. Material such as BMP can be used to produce a spinal fusion without the additional pain of using the patient's own bone for this purpose. BMP can be implanted to allow support for the structure of the spine in a way that bone grafts have difficulty doing. BMP relies on the patient's own genetic makeup to provide safe, effective bone growth for the patient.

Replacement of Nucleus Pulposus

If you imagine the disk as a jelly doughnut, the annulus fibrosis (a ring of cartilage between the vertebrae) is the doughnut and the nucleus pulposus (a gel-like material inside the annulus) is the jelly. If you have a herniated disk, it's as if the jelly is squeezed out of the doughnut. Research is currently underway to create artificial replacement materials, such as hydrogels and various polymers, for the nucleus pulposus when all or part of it is removed. The objective of implanting replacement material is to maintain or restore the physiologic (normal functional) height of the intervertebral disk space, as well as the mobility and the mechanical function of the spine.

Repair of Annulus Fibrosis

Minimally invasive surgery is available for annular tears. Micro-discectomy is a procedure in which a small incision is made in the back and part of the nucleus that is putting pressure on the nerve is removed. Annular tears can also be treated with intradiscal electro-thermal therapy (IDET). IDET applies heat to the fibers in the an-nulus, which puts a seal on the tissue and allows it to heal.

Gene Therapy

Current treatments for many spine problems require bone grafts. Unfortunately, up to 40 percent of spinal fusions may fail to form adequate bone. In 1997 a gene was discovered that induces bone growth. Cell culture and early animal studies suggest the gene is key to the body's ability to build new bone. The technology to grow new bone has enormous potential. Although not available yet, local gene therapy for spine fusion is poised to move from bench research to the operating room.

Chapter 35

Lordosis

What Is It?

Lordosis is a disorder defined by an excessive inward curve of the spine. It differs from the spine's normal curves at the cervical, thoracic, and lumbar regions, which are, to a degree, either kyphotic or lordotic. The spine's natural curves position the head over the pelvis and work as shock absorbers to distribute mechanical stress during movement.

Lordosis can be found in all age groups. It primarily affects the lumbar spine, but does occur in the neck (cervical). When found in the lumbar spine, the patient may appear swayback, the buttocks appear more prominent, and in general the person may have an exaggerated posture. A lumbar lordosis can be painful and sometimes affects movement.

Certain disease processes can adversely affect the structural integrity of the spine and contribute to lordosis. Some common causes include achondroplasia, discitis, kyphosis, obesity, osteoporosis, and spondylolisthesis.

- Achondroplasia is an inherited bone growth disorder that may cause a type of dwarfism.

- Discitis is inflammation of intervertebral disk space.

Reprinted with permission from John Regan, M.D., Co-Director, Cedars-Sinai Institute for Spinal Disorders, Los Angeles, California. For additional information about spinal disorders and treatments, visit Dr. Regan's website at http://www.spinesource.com. © 2004 John Regan. All rights reserved.

- Kyphosis (e.g., humpback) may force the low back to compensate for the imbalance created by a curve occurring at a higher level of the spine (e.g., thoracic).

- Obesity may cause some overweight people to lean backward to improve balance. This has a negative impact on posture.

- Osteoporosis is a bone density disease that may cause vertebrae to lose strength, compromising the spine's structural integrity.

- Spondylolisthesis occurs when one vertebra slips forward in relation to an adjacent vertebra, usually in the lumbar spine.

Not every lordosis requires medical treatment. However, when the curve is rigid (fixed), medical evaluation is warranted.

Diagnosis

Physical Examination

A thorough physical examination reveals a lot about the health and general fitness of the patient. The physician will want to know when the curvature was first noticed, past progression, and other related symptoms the patient experiences. The exam provides a baseline from which the physician can measure the patient's progress during treatment. The physical exam may include:

- Palpation determines spinal abnormalities by feel.

- Range of motion measures the degree to which a patient can perform movement of flexion, extension, lateral bending, and spinal rotation. Asymmetry is also noted.

Neurologic Evaluation

A neurological evaluation includes an assessment of the following symptoms: pain, numbness, paresthesias (e.g., tingling), extremity sensation and motor function, muscle spasm, weakness, and bowel/bladder changes.

Radiographic Evaluation

The patient stands to reveal the entire length of the spine when posterior/anterior (or back and front) and lateral (side) x-rays are taken. Side bending anterior/posterior x-rays are sometimes used to evaluate spinal flexibility. An MRI may be ordered if the spinal cord has been compromised (or suspected).

Further, the Cobb Angle Method may be used to measure the lordotic curve in degrees using a standard full-length anterior/posterior x-ray. Conservative treatment measures may include:

- Analgesics and anti-inflammatory medication may be prescribed.

- Physical therapy, which enables the patient to build strength, flexibility, and increase range of motion. The therapist may provide a customized home exercise program.

- Bracing may be used control curve progression in adolescents.

- Reduction of body weight to ideal weight.

- Surgery may be considered if the lordotic curve is severe with neurologic involvement.

Surgery

Surgical intervention is considered if the lordotic curve is severe, when neurologic involvement exists, or when conservative treatment has failed to provide relief.

A spine surgeon decides which surgical procedure and approach (anterior/posterior, front or back) is best for the patient. His or her decisions are based on the patient's medical history, symptoms, and radiographic findings.

A variety of surgical treatment options are utilized. You should discuss what is best for your condition with your spine surgeon.

Recovery

Whether the treatment course is conservative or surgical, it is important to closely follow the physician and/or physical therapist's instructions. Discuss any concerns about activity restrictions. They will be able to suggest safe alternatives.

Physical therapy may be incorporated into the treatment plan to build strength, flexibility, and increase range of motion. The therapist may provide the patient a customized home exercise program.

If the patient undergoes surgery, written instructions and prescriptions for necessary medication are given prior to release from the hospital. The patient's care continues during follow-up visits with their surgeon.

Chapter 36

Kyphosis

Chapter Contents

Section 36.1

What Is Kyphosis?

Introduction

The 33 vertebrae in the human spine are uniquely aligned to efficiently support the body. The gentle curves (as seen from the side of the spine) help the muscles support the body with minimal effort. The alignment also provides openings for the nerves originating in the spinal cord to pass out of the spinal column to their destinations. When a vertebra is not in alignment, many problems may occur.

What Is Kyphosis?

Kyphosis is a deformity of the spine that results in a segment of the spine curving (flexing) more than is normal. Because the vertebrae are no longer stacked properly, the muscle and nerve functions are disturbed. Symptoms include pain and impaired nerve function, which can develop slowly or rapidly and may get worse over a period of time. When excessive, this abnormal flexing may result in a hunchback.

What Causes Kyphosis?

Kyphosis is caused by the deformity of the vertebra. Kyphosis that occurs in children is usually due to abnormal development (congenital or during adolescent growth) or poor posture. In adults, kyphosis may be caused by fractures to the spine, injury, tumors, infection, or osteoporosis (deterioration of the bone).

Can Kyphosis Be Prevented?

Not all causes of kyphosis can be prevented, but certain actions may reduce the possibility of developing kyphosis. These actions include good posture, good nutrition, consistent and sensible exercise, avoiding smoking, proper lifting, and accident prevention.

What Surgical Treatment Options Exist for Kyphosis?

Kyphoplasty for Osteoporotic Fractures

Kyphoplasty is a surgical procedure that treats kyphosis caused by fractures of the vertebral body caused by osteoporosis or bone diseases such as multiple myeloma. The surgery is minimally invasive, requiring only a very small incision in the back. A narrow tube is inserted through the incision using fluoroscopy to guide it into the correct position in the damaged vertebrae. Using the tube as a channel, the doctor then guides a special balloon into the vertebral body.

The balloon is then carefully inflated, restoring the vertebrae to a more normal shape. The balloon also creates a cavity in the vertebral body by compacting the soft inner bone material.

The balloon is then deflated and gently removed. Special instruments are then used to fill the cavity with a soft cement-like material that quickly hardens to stabilize the vertebrae. With the vertebrae shape and height restored, the pressure on the nerves is reduced, easing the pain.

Fusion with Bone Graft

Spinal fusion is a welding process by which two or more of the vertebrae that make up the spinal column are fused together with bone grafts and internal devices such as metal rods. The surgery eliminates motion between vertebrae segments. Spinal fusion may be used to treat abnormal curvatures such as scoliosis or kyphosis.

Bone is the most commonly used material to help promote fusion. Generally, small pieces of bone are placed into the space between the vertebrae to be fused. Sometimes larger solid pieces of bone are used to provide immediate structural support. Bone may come from the patient (autogenous bone) or a bank of bone harvested from other individuals (allograft bone). After the fusion procedure has been performed, the adjacent spinal segments are held immobile to allow fusion to progress. Immobilization is achieved through internal fixation devices or external bracing or casting. Both forms of immobilization may be necessary at times.

Fusion with Instrumentation

Normally, each vertebrae moves with respect to the one above and below it, allowing the spine to bend and rotate. A fusion means to fuse the two vertebrae so that they cannot move on one another. Spinal instrumentation is often used to help provide stability for the spine after vertebrae have been fused together. Common types of instrumentation include:

- Anterior cervical plates, which can be applied to the front of the spine.

- Posterior cervical plates, which can be placed on the side of the spine.

- Posterior cervical wiring, which can be placed around the spinous processes or the facet joints in the posterior cervical spine.

- Post-operative cervical braces. Because of their relatively small size, the cervical spine is well suited for postoperative braces.

Section 36.2

Scheuermann's Kyphosis

Kyphosis is a curving of the spine that causes a bowing of the back, which leads to a hunchback or slouching posture.

Causes, Incidence, and Risk Factors

Kyphosis is a spinal deformity that can result from trauma, developmental problems, or degenerative disease. Kyphosis can occur at any age, although it is rare at birth.

Adolescent kyphosis, also known as Scheuermann's disease, results from the wedging together of several consecutive vertebrae (bones of the spine). The cause of Scheuermann's disease is unknown.

In adults, kyphosis can be a result of osteoporotic compression fractures (fractures caused by osteoporosis), degenerative disease (such as arthritis), or spondylolisthesis (slipping of one vertebra forward on another).

Other causes of kyphosis include the following:

- infection (such as tuberculosis)
- neurofibromatosis
- connective tissue disorders
- muscular dystrophy
- spina bifida (a birth defect involving incomplete formation of part of the spine)
- disk degeneration
- certain endocrine diseases
- Paget's disease
- polio
- tumors

Kyphosis can also be seen in association with scoliosis (an abnormal sideways curvature of the spine seen in children and adolescents). Risk factors are related to the causes.

Symptoms

- mild back pain
- fatigue
- tenderness and stiffness in the spine
- round back appearance
- difficulty breathing (in severe cases)

Signs and Tests

Physical examination by a health care provider confirms the abnormal curvature of the spine. The doctor will also look for any neurologic changes (weakness, paralysis, or changes in sensation) below the level of the curve.

A spine x-ray will be done to document the severity of the curve and allow serial measurements to be performed.

Occasionally, pulmonary function tests may be used to assess whether the kyphosis is affecting breathing.

If there is any question of a tumor, infection, or neurologic symptoms, then an MRI may be ordered.

Treatment

Treatment depends on the cause of the disorder:

- Congenital kyphosis requires corrective surgery at an early age.

- Scheuermann's disease is initially treated with a brace and physical therapy.

- Occasionally surgery is needed for large (greater than 60 degrees), painful curves.

- Multiple compression fractures from osteoporosis can be left alone if there is no neurologic problems or pain, but the osteoporosis needs to be treated to help prevent future fractures. For debilitating deformity or pain, surgery is an option.

- Kyphosis secondary to infection or tumor needs to be treated more aggressively, often with surgery and medications.

Treatment for other types of kyphosis depends on the cause. Surgery may be necessary if neurological symptoms develop.

Expectations (Prognosis)

Adolescents with Scheuermann's disease tend do well even if they need surgery, and the disease stops once they stop growing. If the kyphosis is due to degenerative joint disease or multiple compression fractures, correction of the defect is not possible without surgery, and improvement of pain is less reliable.

Complications

- disabling back pain
- neurological symptoms including leg weakness or paralysis
- decreased lung capacity
- round back deformity

Prevention

Treating and preventing osteoporosis can prevent many cases of kyphosis in the elderly. Early diagnosis and bracing of Scheuermann's disease can reduce the need for surgery, but there is no way to prevent the disease.

Chapter 37

Osteoarthritis: Degenerative Spinal Joint Disease

What Is Osteoarthritis?

Osteoarthritis is the most common type of arthritis, especially among older people. Sometimes it is called degenerative joint disease or osteoarthrosis.

Osteoarthritis is a joint disease that mostly affects the cartilage. Cartilage is the slippery tissue that covers the ends of bones in a joint. Healthy cartilage allows bones to glide over one another. It also absorbs energy from the shock of physical movement. In osteoarthritis, the surface layer of cartilage breaks down and wears away. This allows bones under the cartilage to rub together, causing pain, swelling, and loss of motion of the joint. Over time, the joint may lose its normal shape. Also, bone spurs—small growths called osteophytes—may grow on the edges of the joint. Bits of bone or cartilage can break off and float inside the joint space. This causes more pain and damage.

People with osteoarthritis usually have joint pain and limited movement. Unlike some other forms of arthritis, osteoarthritis affects only joints and not internal organs. For example, rheumatoid arthritis—the second most common form of arthritis—affects other parts of the body besides the joints. It begins at a younger age than osteoarthritis, causes swelling and redness in joints, and may make people feel sick, tired, and (uncommonly) feverish.

"Osteoarthritis," National Institute of Arthritis and Musculoskeletal and Skin Diseases (NIAMS), NIH Pub. No. 02-4617, July 2002. Available online at http://www.niams.nih.gov; accessed March 2004.

Who Has Osteoarthritis?

Osteoarthritis is one of the most frequent causes of physical disability among adults. More than 20 million people in the United States have the disease. By 2030, 20 percent of Americans—about 70 million people—will have passed their 65th birthday and will be at risk for osteoarthritis. Some younger people get osteoarthritis from joint injuries, but osteoarthritis most often occurs in older people. In fact, more than half of the population age 65 or older would show x-ray evidence of osteoarthritis in at least one joint. Both men and women have the disease. Before age 45, more men than women have osteoarthritis, whereas after age 45, it is more common in women.

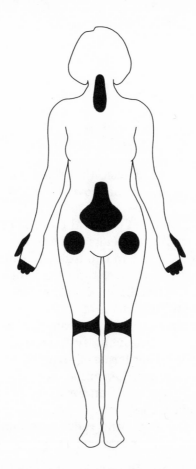

Figure 37.1. Osteoarthritis most often occurs at the ends of the fingers, thumbs, neck, lower back, knees, and hips.

How Does Osteoarthritis Affect People?

Osteoarthritis affects each person differently. In some people, it progresses quickly; in others, the symptoms are more serious. Scientists do not know yet what causes the disease, but they suspect a combination of factors, including being overweight, the aging process, joint injury, and stresses on the joints from certain jobs and sports activities.

Osteoarthritis hurts people in more than their joints: their finances and lifestyles also are affected.

Financial effects include:

- The cost of treatment
- Wages lost because of disability

Lifestyle effects include:

- Depression
- Anxiety
- Feelings of helplessness
- Limitations on daily activities
- Job limitations
- Trouble participating in everyday personal and family joys and responsibilities

Despite these challenges, most people with osteoarthritis can lead active and productive lives. They succeed by using osteoarthritis treatment strategies, such as the following:

- Pain relief medications
- Rest and exercise
- Patient education and support programs
- Learning self-care and having a good attitude

Osteoarthritis Basics: The Joint and Its Parts

Most joints—the place where two moving bones come together—are designed to allow smooth movement between the bones and to absorb shock from movements like walking or repetitive movements. The joint is made up of:

- Cartilage: a hard but slippery coating on the end of each bone.

- Joint capsule: a tough membrane sac that holds all the bones and other joint parts together.

- Synovium: a thin membrane inside the joint capsule.

- Synovial fluid: a fluid that lubricates the joint and keeps the cartilage smooth and healthy.

- Ligaments, tendons, and muscles: tissues that keep the bones stable and allow the joint to bend and move. Ligaments are tough, cord-like tissues that connect one bone to another. Tendons are tough, fibrous cords that connect muscles to bones. Muscles are bundles of specialized cells that contract to produce movement when stimulated by nerves.

How Do You Know If You Have Osteoarthritis?

Usually, osteoarthritis comes on slowly. Early in the disease, joints may ache after physical work or exercise. Osteoarthritis can occur in any joint. Most often it occurs at the hands, knees, hips, or spine.

Hands: Osteoarthritis of the fingers is one type of osteoarthritis that seems to have some hereditary characteristics; that is, it runs in families. More women than men have it, and they develop it especially after menopause. In osteoarthritis, small, bony knobs appear on the end joints of the fingers. They are called Heberden nodes. Similar knobs, called Bouchard nodes, can appear on the middle joints of the fingers. Fingers can become enlarged and gnarled, and they may ache or be stiff and numb. The base of the thumb joint also is commonly affected by osteoarthritis. Osteoarthritis of the hands can be helped by medications, splints, or heat treatment.

Knees: The knees are the body's primary weight-bearing joints. For this reason, they are among the joints most commonly affected by osteoarthritis. They may be stiff, swollen, and painful, making it hard to walk, climb, and get in and out of chairs and bathtubs. If not treated, osteoarthritis in the knees can lead to disability. Medications, weight loss, exercise, and walking aids can reduce pain and disability. In severe cases, knee replacement surgery may be helpful.

Hips: Osteoarthritis in the hip can cause pain, stiffness, and severe disability. People may feel the pain in their hips, or in their groin, inner thigh, buttocks, or knees. Walking aids, such as canes or walkers, can reduce stress on the hip. Osteoarthritis in the hip may limit moving and bending. This can make daily activities such as dressing and foot care a challenge. Walking aids, medication, and exercise can help relieve pain and improve motion. The doctor may recommend hip replacement if the pain is severe and not relieved by other methods.

Spine: Stiffness and pain in the neck or in the lower back can result from osteoarthritis of the spine. Weakness or numbness of the arms or legs also can result. Some people feel better when they sleep on a firm mattress or sit using back support pillows. Others find it helps to use heat treatments or to follow an exercise program that strengthens the back and abdominal muscles. In severe cases, the doctor may suggest surgery to reduce pain and help restore function.

How Do Doctors Diagnose Osteoarthritis?

No single test can diagnose osteoarthritis. Most doctors use a combination of the following methods to diagnose the disease and rule out other conditions:

Clinical history: The doctor begins by asking the patient to describe the symptoms, and when and how the condition started. Good doctor-patient communication is important. The doctor can give a better assessment if the patient gives a good description of pain, stiffness, and joint function, and how they have changed over time. It also is important for the doctor to know how the condition affects the patient's work and daily life. Finally, the doctor also needs to know about other medical conditions and whether the patient is taking any medicines.

Physical examination: The doctor will check the patient's general health, including checking reflexes and muscle strength. Joints bothering the patient will be examined. The doctor will also observe the patient's ability to walk, bend, and carry out activities of daily living.

X-rays: Doctors take x-rays to see how much joint damage has been done. X-rays of the affected joint can show such things as cartilage loss, bone damage, and bone spurs. But there often is a big difference between the severity of osteoarthritis as shown by the x-ray and the degree of pain and disability felt by the patient. Also, x-rays may not show early osteoarthritis damage, before much cartilage loss has taken place.

Other tests: The doctor may order blood tests to rule out other causes of symptoms. Another common test is called joint aspiration, which involves drawing fluid from the joint for examination.

It usually is not difficult to tell if a patient has osteoarthritis. It is more difficult to tell if the disease is causing the patient's symptoms. Osteoarthritis is so common—especially in older people—that symptoms seemingly caused by the disease actually may be due to other medical conditions. The doctor will try to find out what is causing the symptoms by ruling out other disorders and identifying conditions that may make the symptoms worse. The severity of symptoms in osteoarthritis is influenced greatly by the patient's attitude, anxiety, depression, and daily activity level.

How Is Osteoarthritis Treated?

Most successful treatment programs involve a combination of treatments tailored to the patient's needs, lifestyle, and health. Osteoarthritis treatment has four general goals:

- Improve joint care through rest and exercise.

- Maintain an acceptable body weight.

- Control pain with medicine and other measures.

- Achieve a healthy lifestyle.

Osteoarthritis treatment plans often include ways to manage pain and improve function. Such plans can involve exercise, rest and joint care, pain relief, weight control, medicines, surgery, and nontraditional treatment approaches.

Exercise

Research shows that exercise is one of the best treatments for osteoarthritis. Exercise can improve mood and outlook, decrease pain, increase flexibility, improve the heart and blood flow, maintain weight, and promote general physical fitness. Exercise is also inexpensive and, if done correctly, has few negative side effects. The amount and form of exercise will depend on which joints are involved, how stable the joints are, and whether a joint replacement has already been done.

You can use exercises to keep strong and limber, extend your range of movement, and reduce your weight. Some different types of exercise include the following:

- Strength exercises: These can be performed with exercise bands, inexpensive devices that add resistance.

- Aerobic activities: These keep your lungs and circulation systems in shape.

- Range of motion activities: These keep your joints limber.

- Agility exercises: These can help you maintain daily living skills.

- Neck and back strength exercises: These can help you keep your spine strong and limber.

Ask your doctor or physical therapist what exercises are best for you. Ask for guidelines on exercising when a joint is sore or if swelling is present. Also, check if you should (1) use pain-relieving drugs, such as analgesics or anti-inflammatories (also called NSAIDs), to make exercising easier, or (2) use ice afterward.

Rest and Joint Care

Treatment plans include regularly scheduled rest. Patients must learn to recognize the body's signals, and know when to stop or slow down, which prevents pain caused by overexertion. Some patients find that relaxation techniques, stress reduction, and biofeedback help. Some use canes and splints to protect joints and take pressure off them. Splints or braces provide extra support for weakened joints. They also keep the joint in proper position during sleep or activity. Splints should be used only for limited periods because joints and muscles need to be exercised to prevent stiffness and weakness. An occupational therapist or a doctor can help the patient get a properly fitting splint.

Nondrug Pain Relief

People with osteoarthritis may find nondrug ways to relieve pain. Warm towels, hot packs, or a warm bath or shower to apply moist heat to the joint can relieve pain and stiffness. In some cases, cold packs (a bag of ice or frozen vegetables wrapped in a towel) can relieve pain or numb the sore area. (Check with a doctor or physical therapist to find out if heat or cold is the best treatment.) Water therapy in a heated pool or whirlpool also may relieve pain and stiffness. For osteoarthritis in the knee, patients may wear insoles or cushioned shoes to redistribute weight and reduce joint stress.

Weight Control

Osteoarthritis patients who are overweight or obese need to lose weight. Weight loss can reduce stress on weight-bearing joints and limit further injury. A dietitian can help patients develop healthy eating habits. A healthy diet and regular exercise help reduce weight.

Medicines

Doctors prescribe medicines to eliminate or reduce pain and to improve functioning. Doctors consider a number of factors when choosing medicines for their patients with osteoarthritis. Two important factors are the intensity of the pain and the potential side effects of the medicine. Patients must use medicines carefully and tell their doctors about any changes that occur.

The following types of medicines are commonly used in treating osteoarthritis:

- Acetaminophen: Acetaminophen is a pain reliever (for example, Tylenol) that does not reduce swelling. Acetaminophen does not irritate the stomach and is less likely than nonsteroidal anti-inflammatory drugs (NSAIDs) to cause long-term side effects. Research has shown that acetaminophen relieves pain as effectively as NSAIDs for many patients with osteoarthritis. [Warning: People with liver disease, people who drink alcohol heavily, and those taking blood-thinning medicines or NSAIDs should use acetaminophen with caution.]

- NSAIDs (nonsteroidal anti-inflammatory drugs): Many NSAIDs are used to treat osteoarthritis. Patients can buy some over the counter (for example, aspirin, Advil, Motrin IB, Aleve, ketoprofen). Others require a prescription. All NSAIDs work similarly: they fight inflammation and relieve pain. However, each NSAID is a different chemical, and each has a slightly different effect on the body. Side effects: NSAIDs can cause stomach irritation or, less often, they can affect kidney function. The longer a person uses NSAIDs, the more likely he or she is to have side effects, ranging from mild to serious. Many other drugs cannot be taken when a patient is being treated with NSAIDs because NSAIDs alter the way the body uses or eliminates these other drugs. Check with your health care provider or pharmacist before you take NSAIDs in addition to another medication. Also, NSAIDs sometimes are associated with serious gastrointestinal problems, including ulcers, bleeding, and perforation of the stomach or intestine. People over age 65 and those with any history of ulcers or gastrointestinal bleeding should use NSAIDs with caution.

- COX-2 inhibitors: Several new NSAIDs—valdecoxib (Bextra), celecoxib (Celebrex), and rofecoxib (Vioxx)—form a class of drugs known as COX-2 inhibitors. These medicines reduce inflammation similarly to traditional NSAIDs, but they cause fewer gastrointestinal side effects. [Editor's Note: In September 2004, Vioxx was withdrawn from the market due to concerns regarding an increased risk of cardiovascular events (including heart attack and stroke). Visit http://www.fda.gov/cder/drug/infopage/vioxx/default.htm for more information.]

- Other medications: Doctors may prescribe several other medicines for osteoarthritis, including the following: topical pain-relieving creams, rubs, and sprays (for example, capsaicin cream), which are applied directly to the skin; mild narcotic painkillers, which—although very effective—may be addictive and are not commonly used; and corticosteroids, powerful anti-inflammatory hormones made naturally in the body or manmade for use as medicine. Corticosteroids may be injected into the affected joints to temporarily relieve pain. This is a short-term measure, generally not recommended for more than two or three treatments per year. Oral corticosteroids should not be used to treat osteoarthritis. Doctors may also prescribe hyaluronic acid, a medicine for joint injection, used to treat osteoarthritis of the knee. This substance is a normal component of the joint, involved in joint lubrication and nutrition.

Most medicines used to treat osteoarthritis have side effects, so it is important for people to learn about the medicines they take. Even nonprescription drugs should be checked. Several groups of patients are at high risk for side effects from NSAIDs, such as people with a history of peptic ulcers or digestive tract bleeding, people taking oral corticosteroids or anticoagulants (blood thinners), smokers, and people who consume alcohol. Some patients may be able to help reduce side effects by taking some medicines with food. Others should avoid stomach irritants such as alcohol, tobacco, and caffeine. Some patients try to protect their stomachs by taking other medicines that coat the stomach or block stomach acids. These measures help, but they are not always completely effective.

Surgery

For many people, surgery helps relieve the pain and disability of osteoarthritis. Surgery may be performed to:

- Remove loose pieces of bone and cartilage from the joint if they are causing mechanical symptoms of buckling or locking

- Resurface (smooth out) bones

- Reposition bones

- Replace joints

Surgeons may replace affected joints with artificial joints called prostheses. These joints can be made from metal alloys, high-density plastic, and ceramic material. They can be joined to bone surfaces by special cements. Artificial joints can last 10 to 15 years or longer. About 10 percent of artificial joints may need revision. Surgeons choose the design and components of prostheses according to their patient's weight, sex, age, activity level, and other medical conditions.

The decision to use surgery depends on several things. Both the surgeon and the patient consider the patient's level of disability, the intensity of pain, the interference with the patient's lifestyle, the patient's age, and occupation. Currently, more than 80 percent of osteoarthritis surgery cases involve replacing the hip or knee joint. After surgery and rehabilitation, the patient usually feels less pain and swelling, and can move more easily.

Nontraditional Approaches

Among the alternative therapies used to treat osteoarthritis are the following:

- Acupuncture: Some people have found pain relief using acupuncture (the use of fine needles inserted at specific points on the skin). Preliminary research shows that acupuncture may be a useful component in an osteoarthritis treatment plan for some patients.

- Folk remedies: Some patients seek alternative therapies for their pain and disability. Some of these alternative therapies have included wearing copper bracelets, drinking herbal teas, and taking mud baths. Although these practices are not harmful, some can be expensive. They also cause delays in seeking medical treatment. To date, no scientific research shows these approaches to be helpful in treating osteoarthritis.

- Nutritional supplements: Nutrients such as glucosamine and chondroitin sulfate have been reported to improve the symptoms of people with osteoarthritis, as have certain vitamins. Additional studies are being carried out to further evaluate these claims.

Self-Care for People with Arthritis

People with osteoarthritis can enjoy good health despite having the disease. How? By learning self-care skills and developing a good-health attitude. Self-care is central to successfully managing the pain and disability of osteoarthritis. People have a much better chance of having a rewarding lifestyle when they educate themselves about the disease and take part in their own care. Working actively with a team of health care providers enables people with the disease to minimize pain, share in decision making about treatment, and feel a sense of control over their lives. Research shows that people with osteoarthritis who take part in their own care report less pain and make fewer doctor visits. They also enjoy a better quality of life.

Self-Help and Education Programs

Three kinds of programs help people learn about osteoarthritis, learn self-care, and improve their good-health attitude. These programs include:

- Patient education programs

- Arthritis self-management programs

- Arthritis support groups

These programs teach people about osteoarthritis, its treatments, exercise and relaxation, patient and health care provider communication, and problem solving. Research has shown that these programs have clear and long-lasting benefits.

Exercise

Regular physical activity plays a key role in self-care and wellness. Two types of exercise are important in osteoarthritis management. The first type, therapeutic exercises, keeps joints working as well as possible. The other type, aerobic conditioning exercises, improves strength and fitness and controls weight. Patients should be realistic when they start exercising. They should learn how to exercise correctly because exercising incorrectly can cause problems.

Most people with osteoarthritis exercise best when their pain is least severe. Start with an adequate warmup and begin exercising slowly. Resting frequently ensures a good workout. It also reduces the risk of injury. A physical therapist can evaluate how a patient's muscles are working. This information helps the therapist develop a safe, personalized exercise program to increase strength and flexibility.

Many people enjoy sports or other activities in their exercise program. Good activities include swimming and aquatic exercise, walking, running, biking, cross-country skiing, and using exercise machines and exercise videotapes.

People with osteoarthritis should check with their doctor or physical therapist before starting an exercise program. Health care providers will suggest what exercises are best for you, how to warm up safely, and when to avoid exercising a joint affected by arthritis. Pain medications and applying ice after exercising may make exercising easier.

Body, Mind, Spirit

Making the most of good health requires careful attention to the body, mind, and spirit. People with osteoarthritis must plan and develop daily routines that maximize their quality of life and minimize disability. They also need to evaluate these routines periodically to make sure they are working well.

Good health also requires a positive attitude. People must decide to make the most of things when faced with the challenges of osteoarthritis. This attitude—a good-health mindset—doesn't just happen. It takes work, every day. And with the right attitude, you will achieve it.

Current Research

The leading role in osteoarthritis research is played by the National Institute of Arthritis and Musculoskeletal and Skin Diseases (NIAMS), within the National Institutes of Health (NIH). The NIAMS funds many researchers across the United States to study osteoarthritis. It has established a Specialized Center of Research devoted to osteoarthritis. Also, many researchers study arthritis at NIAMS Multipurpose Arthritis and Musculoskeletal Diseases Centers and Multidisciplinary Clinical Research Centers. These centers conduct basic, laboratory, and clinical research aimed at understanding the causes, treatment options, and prevention of arthritis and musculoskeletal

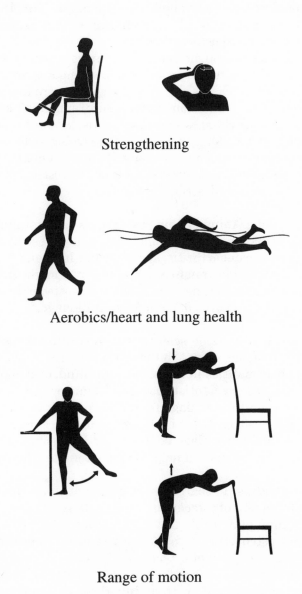

Strengthening

Aerobics/heart and lung health

Range of motion

Figure 37.2. People with osteoarthritis should do different kinds of exercise for different benefits to the body.

diseases. Center researchers also study epidemiology, health services, and professional, patient, and public education. The NIAMS also supports multidisciplinary clinical research centers that expand clinical studies for diseases like osteoarthritis.

For years, scientists thought that osteoarthritis was simply a disease of wear and tear that occurred in joints as people got older. In the last decade, however, research has shown that there is more to the disorder than aging alone. The production, maintenance, and breakdown of cartilage, as well as bone changes in osteoarthritis, are now seen as a series or cascade of events. Many researchers are trying to discover where in that cascade of events things go wrong. By understanding what goes wrong, they hope to find new ways to prevent or treat osteoarthritis. Some key areas of research are described below.

Animal Models: Animals help researchers understand how diseases work and why they occur. Animal models help researchers learn many things about osteoarthritis, such as what happens to cartilage, how treatment strategies might work, and what might prevent the disease. Animal models also help scientists study osteoarthritis in very early stages before it causes detectable joint damage.

Diagnostic Tools: Some scientists want to find ways to detect osteoarthritis at earlier stages so that they can treat it earlier. They seek specific abnormalities in the blood, joint fluid, or urine of people with the disease. Other scientists use new technologies to analyze the differences between the cartilage from different joints. For example, many people have osteoarthritis in the knees or hips, but few have it in the ankles. Can ankle cartilage be different? Does it age differently? Answering these questions will help us understand the disease better.

Genetics Studies: Researchers suspect that inheritance plays a role in 25 to 30 percent of osteoarthritis cases. Researchers have found that genetics may play a role in approximately 40 to 65 percent of hand and knee osteoarthritis cases. They suspect inheritance might play a role in other types of osteoarthritis, as well. Scientists have identified a mutation (a gene defect) affecting collagen, an important part of cartilage, in patients with an inherited kind of osteoarthritis that starts at an early age. The mutation weakens collagen protein, which may break or tear more easily under stress. Scientists are looking for other gene mutations in osteoarthritis. Recently, researchers found that the daughters of women who have knee osteoarthritis have a significant increase in cartilage breakdown, thus making them more susceptible to disease. In the future, a test to determine who carries the genetic defect (or defects) could help people reduce their risk for osteoarthritis with lifestyle adjustments.

Tissue Engineering: This technology involves removing cells from a healthy part of the body and placing them in an area of diseased or damaged tissue in order to improve certain body functions. Currently, it is used to treat small traumatic injuries or defects in cartilage, and, if successful, could eventually help treat osteoarthritis. Researchers at the NIAMS are exploring three types of tissue engineering. The two most common methods being studied today include cartilage cell replacement and stem cell transplantation. The third method is gene therapy.

- *Cartilage cell replacement:* In this procedure, researchers remove cartilage cells from the patient's own joint and then clone or grow new cells using tissue culture and other laboratory techniques. They then inject the newly grown cells into the patient's joint. Patients with cartilage cell replacement have fewer symptoms of osteoarthritis. Actual cartilage repair is limited, however.

- *Stem cell transplantation:* Stem cells are primitive cells that can transform into other kinds of cells, such as muscle or bone cells. They usually are taken from bone marrow. In the future, researchers hope to insert stem cells into cartilage, where the cells will make new cartilage. If successful, this process could be used to repair damaged cartilage and avoid the need for surgical joint replacements with metal or plastics.

- *Gene therapy:* Scientists are working to genetically engineer cells that would inhibit the body chemicals, called enzymes, that may help break down cartilage and cause joint damage. In gene therapy, cells are removed from the body, genetically changed, and then injected back into the affected joint. They live in the joint and protect it from damaging enzymes.

Comprehensive Treatment Strategies: Effective treatment for osteoarthritis takes more than medicine or surgery. Getting help from a variety of care professionals often can improve patient treatment and self-care. Research shows that adding patient education and social support is a low-cost, effective way to decrease pain and reduce the amount of medicine used.

Exercise plays a key part in comprehensive treatment. Researchers are studying exercise in greater detail and finding out just how to use it in treating or preventing osteoarthritis. For example, several scientists have studied knee osteoarthritis and exercise. Their results included the following:

- Strengthening the thigh muscle (quadriceps) can relieve symptoms of knee osteoarthritis and prevent more damage.

- Walking can result in better functioning, and the more you walk, the farther you will be able to walk.

- People with knee osteoarthritis who were active in an exercise program feel less pain. They also function better.

Research has shown that losing extra weight can help people who already have osteoarthritis. Moreover, overweight or obese people who do not have osteoarthritis may reduce their risk of developing the disease by losing weight.

Using NSAIDs: Many people who have osteoarthritis have persistent pain despite taking simple pain relievers such as acetaminophen. Some of these patients take NSAIDs instead. Health care providers are concerned about long-term NSAID use because it can lead to an upset stomach, heartburn, nausea, and more dangerous side effects, such as ulcers.

Scientists are working to design and test new, safer NSAIDs. One example currently available is a class of selective NSAIDs called COX-2 inhibitors. Traditional NSAIDs prevent inflammation by blocking two related enzymes in the body called COX-1 and COX-2. The gastrointestinal side effects associated with traditional NSAIDs seems to be associated mainly with blocking the COX-1 enzyme, which helps protect the stomach lining. The new selective COX-2 inhibitors, however, primarily block the COX-2 enzyme, which helps control inflammation in the body. As a result, COX-2 inhibitors reduce pain and inflammation but are less likely than traditional NSAIDs to cause gastrointestinal ulcers and bleeding. However, research shows that some COX-2 inhibitors may not protect against heart disease as well as traditional NSAIDs, so check with your doctor if you have concerns.

Drugs to Prevent Joint Damage: No treatment actually prevents osteoarthritis or reverses or blocks the disease process once it begins. Present treatments just relieve the symptoms. Researchers are looking for drugs that would prevent, slow down, or reverse joint damage. One experimental antibiotic drug, doxycycline, may stop certain enzymes from damaging cartilage. The drug has shown some promise in clinical studies, but more studies are needed. Researchers also are studying growth factors and other natural chemical messengers. These potential medicines may be able to stimulate cartilage growth or repair.

Acupuncture: During an acupuncture treatment, a licensed acupuncture therapist inserts very fine needles into the skin at various points on the body. Scientists think the needles stimulate the release of natural, pain-relieving chemicals produced by the brain or the nervous system. Researchers are studying acupuncture treatment of patients who have knee osteoarthritis. Early findings suggest that traditional Chinese acupuncture is effective for some patients as an additional therapy for osteoarthritis, reducing pain and improving function.

Nutritional Supplements: Nutritional supplements are often reported as helpful in treating osteoarthritis. Such reports should be viewed with caution, however, since very few studies have carefully evaluated the role of nutritional supplements in osteoarthritis.

- *Glucosamine and chondroitin sulfate*: Both of these nutrients are found in small quantities in food and are components of normal cartilage. Scientific studies on these two nutritional supplements have not yet shown that they affect the disease. They may relieve symptoms and reduce joint damage in some patients, however. The National Center for Complementary and Alternative Medicine at the NIH is supporting a clinical trial to test whether glucosamine, chondroitin sulfate, or the two nutrients in combination reduce pain and improve function. Patients using this therapy should do so only under the supervision of their doctor, as part of an overall treatment program with exercise, relaxation, and pain relief.

- *Vitamins D, C, E, and beta carotene:* The progression of osteoarthritis may be slower in people who take higher levels of vitamin D, C, E, or beta carotene. More studies are needed to confirm these reports.

- *Hyaluronic acid:* Injecting this substance into the knee joint provides long-term pain relief for some people with osteoarthritis. Hyaluronic acid is a natural component of cartilage and joint fluid. It lubricates and absorbs shock in the joint. The Food and Drug Administration (FDA) approved this therapy for patients with osteoarthritis of the knee who do not get relief from exercise, physical therapy, or simple analgesics. Researchers are presently studying the benefits of using hyaluronic acid to treat osteoarthritis.

- *Estrogen:* In studies of older women, scientists found a lower risk of osteoarthritis in women who had used oral estrogens for hormone replacement therapy. The researchers suspect having low levels of estrogen could increase the risk of developing osteoarthritis. Additional studies are needed to answer this question.

Hope for the Future

Research is opening up new avenues of treatment for people with osteoarthritis. A balanced, comprehensive approach is still the key to staying active and healthy with the disease. People with osteoarthritis should combine exercise, relaxation education, social support, and medicines in their treatment strategies. Meanwhile, as scientists unravel the complexities of the disease, new treatments and prevention methods should appear. They will improve the quality of life for people with osteoarthritis and their families.

Chapter 38

Sacroiliac Joint Syndrome

In the first part of the 20th century, sacroiliac (SI) joint syndrome was the most common diagnosis for lumbago (low back pain). Any pain in the low back, buttock, or adjacent leg was usually referred to as SI joint syndrome. Before 1932, SI joint syndrome was a particularly popular diagnosis. There was actually a period referred to as the "Era of the SI Joint."

In the late 1980s, many physicians rediscovered the SI joints as a possible source of back pain. Yet even today, SI joint pain is often overlooked. Many physicians have not been trained to consider it. Many are still reluctant to believe a joint that has so little movement can cause back pain.

Anatomy

In order to understand your symptoms and treatment options, it helps to begin with a basic understanding of the anatomy of your low back. This includes becoming familiar with the various parts that make up the lumbar spine and how these parts work together.

There are two sacroiliac (SI) joints in your pelvis that connect the sacrum (tailbone) and the ilium (large pelvic bone). The SI joints connect your spine to the pelvis, and thus, to the entire lower half of the skeleton.

Like any other joints, there is articular cartilage on both sides of the SI joint surfaces. But unlike most other joints, the SI joints are covered by two different kinds of cartilage. The articular surfaces have both hyaline (glassy, slick) and fibrocartilage (spongy) surfaces that rub against each other. The joints also have many large ridges (bumps) and depressions (dips in the surface that fit together like a puzzle).

The SI joints are also unique in that they are not designed for much motion. It is common for the SI joint to become stiff and actually lock as people age. The SI joint only moves about two to four millimeters during weight bearing and forward flexion. This small amount of motion occurring in the joint is described as a gliding type of motion. Due to the small amount of movement and the complexity, finding out about the SI joint's motion is very difficult during a physical exam.

The SI joints are viscoelastic joints, meaning that the major movement comes from giving or stretching. This motion is quite different than the hinge motion of the knee or the ball and socket motion of the hip. The main function of the SI joints is to provide shock absorption for the spine through stretching in various directions. The SI joints may also provide a self-locking mechanism that helps you to walk. The joints lock on one side as weight is transferred from one leg to the other.

Causes

Many problems can lead to degenerative arthritis of the SI joints. It is often hard to determine exactly what caused the wear and tear to the joints. One of the most common causes of problems at the SI joint is an injury. The injury can come from a direct fall on the buttocks, a motor vehicle accident, or even a blow to the side of your pelvis. The force from these injuries can strain the ligaments around the joint. Ligaments are the tough bands of connective tissue that hold joints together. Tearing of these ligaments can lead to too much motion in the joint. The excessive motion can eventually lead to wear and tear of the joint and pain from degenerative arthritis. Injuries can also cause direct injury of the articular cartilage lining the joint. Over time this will lead to degenerative arthritis in the joint.

Pain can also be caused by an abnormality of the sacrum bone. The sacrum bone is actually a very specialized set of vertebrae. When your body is undergoing development in the womb, several vertebrae fuse together to form the sacrum. In some people the bones that make up the sacrum never fuse together. In these cases, two or more of the vertebra that should fuse together remain separated. This creates an odd situation where the SI joint is malformed and a false joint occurs (sometimes called a transitional syndrome). This abnormality can be seen on x-rays. People who have this syndrome seem to have more problems with their SI joints, as well as back pain that appears to come from that area.

Women are at risk for developing SI joint problems later in life due to childbirth. Female hormones are released during pregnancy that allow the connective tissues in the body to relax. The relaxation is necessary so that during delivery, the female pelvis can stretch enough to allow birth. This stretching results in changes to the SI joints, making them hypermobile (extra or overly mobile). Over a period of years these changes can eventually lead to wear-and-tear arthritis. During pregnancy, the SI joints can cause discomfort both from the effects of the hormones that loosen them and from the stress of carrying a growing baby in the pelvis. The more pregnancies a woman has, the higher her chances of SI joint problems.

Symptoms

Symptoms of SI joint syndrome are often difficult to distinguish from other types of low back pain. In most cases, there is a confusing pattern of back and pelvic pain that mimic each other, making diagnosis of SI joint syndrome very difficult. The most common symptoms include:

- low back pain

- buttock pain

- thigh pain

- difficulty sitting in one place for too long due to pain

Diagnosis

The diagnosis usually begins with a complete history and physical exam. Your clinical exam may include the following orthopedic tests used to determine if the SI joints are involved. Pain during these tests is generally an indicator that the SI joints are indeed a problem.

- Distraction Test—The doctor stresses the SI joints by attempting to pull them apart a bit.

- Compression Test—The two sides of a joint are forced together. Pain may indicate that this SI joint is involved.

- Gaenslen's Test—The examiner will have you lie on a table with both legs brought up to the chest. You will then shift to the side of the table, so that one buttock is over the edge. The unsupported leg drops over the edge and the supported leg is flexed. In this position, SI joint problems will cause pain due to stress to the joint.

- Patrick's Test—The heel of one leg is crossed on top of the opposite knee, and the top knee is pressed down to test for hip mobility and pain.

- X-rays may also be recommended by your provider to determine if there are abnormalities of the joint.

- A CT scan can sometimes show more detail about the joint surfaces and the surrounding bone. If the X-rays suggest something may be affecting the SI joints, the provider may recommend a CT scan to get a better look.

- A bone scan can be useful in determining if the joint is inflamed. An inflamed SI joint usually shows up as a hot spot on a bone scan of the pelvis.

SI Joint Injection

Your doctor may also recommend that you undergo a fluoroscopic injection into the joint. During this test, a local anesthetic is injected into the joint. The doctor uses the fluoroscope to make sure the needle is actually in the joint before injecting the medication. The SI joints are located fairly deep in the upper buttocks and are covered by thick muscle. It is difficult to put a needle into the joint without some guidance. A fluoroscope is a special TV camera that uses x-rays to allow the doctor to see on the screen the exact placement of the needle and to make sure it is positioned accurately.

Once the needle is in the right place, anesthetic is injected to numb the joint. If the pain goes away, your doctor can be relatively sure that the problem is coming from the SI joint and not somewhere else in the spine. The doctor may also add a dose of cortisone to the injection to help ease the pain. Cortisone is a powerful anti-inflammatory medication that calms the arthritis inside the joint and reduces pain. The effect is usually temporary, but may last up to several months.

Treatment Options

Physical Therapy

Patients commonly receive physical therapy treatment for SI joint problems. A well-rounded rehabilitation program assists in calming pain and inflammation, improving your mobility and strength, and helping you do your daily activities with greater ease and ability.

Treatment choices depend on whether the SI joint is stiff or loose. A stiff or locked joint responds best to mobilization, a form of stretching used to improve joint movement. Along with hands-on techniques used by the therapist, mobilization includes specific exercises to improve SI joint mobility. For conditions where the joint is too loose, such as arthritis or SI ligament injuries, stabilization treatments are chosen to hold the joint in correct alignment. Stabilization exercises involve posture and muscle training.

Therapy sessions may be scheduled two to three times each week for up to six weeks.

The goals of physical therapy are to help you:

- learn ways to control symptoms and manage your condition

- learn correct posture and body movements to reduce SI joint strain

- obtain optimal movement and alignment of the SI joint

Sacroiliac Belt

A sacroiliac belt may be issued to help stabilize a loose and painful SI joint. The belt wraps around the hips to squeeze and hold the SI joints together. This supports and stabilizes the pelvis and the SI joints.

SI Joint Injection

An injection into the SI joint using cortisone is helpful for calming pain and inflammation. The injection usually gives temporary relief for several weeks or months.

Surgical Treatment

Surgery may become an option if all conservative methods of treatment fail. Surgery on the SI joint usually consists of a fusion of the joint (also called an arthrodesis). Fusing the two sides of a joint together to reduce pain has been used for many years as a treatment for arthritic joints.

An incision is made over the SI joint in the lower back. The joints are opened so the surgeon can see each joint surface. The articular cartilage lining the joints is removed from both surfaces. This leaves a fresh surface of bone instead of the normal cartilage. The bone surfaces are then held together until they heal or fuse. Without the articular cartilage of the joint, the body treats the two raw bone surfaces just like a fracture, and tries to heal them like any broken bone.

To hold the bones together, the surgeon will usually insert several metal screws across the joint. Bone graft may also be placed around the joint to help fuse it. The bone graft is usually removed from the pelvic bone right beside the SI joint.

Chapter 39

Sciatica

If you suddenly start feeling pain in your lower back or hip that radiates down from your buttock to the back of one thigh and into your leg, your problem may be a protruding disk in your lower spinal column pressing on the roots to your sciatic nerve. Sciatica (lumbar radiculopathy) may feel like a bad leg cramp that lasts for weeks before it goes away. You may have pain, especially when you sit, sneeze, or cough. You may also feel weakness, "pins and needles" numbness, or a burning or tingling sensation down your leg. See a doctor to have your condition diagnosed and start a course of treatment.

You're most likely to get sciatica when you're 30 to 50 years old. It may happen due to the effects of general wear and tear, plus any sudden pressure on the disks that cushion the vertebrae of your lower (lumbar) spine. The gel-like inside (nucleus) of a disk may protrude into or through the disk's outer lining (annulus). This herniated disk may press directly on nerve roots that become the sciatic nerve. The nerve may also get inflamed and irritated by chemicals from the disk's nucleus. About one in every 50 people experiences a herniated disk. Of these, 10 to 25 percent have symptoms lasting more than six weeks. About 80 to 90 percent of people with sciatica get better, over time, without surgery.

Treatment

The condition usually heals itself if you give it enough time and rest. Tell your doctor how your pain started, where it travels, and exactly what it feels like. A physical exam may help pinpoint the irritated nerve root. Your doctor may ask you to squat and rise, walk on your heels and toes, or perform a straight leg-raising test or other tests. Most cases of sciatica affect the L5 or S1 nerve roots. Later, x-rays and other specialized imaging tools such as MRI (magnetic resonance imaging) may confirm your doctor's diagnosis of which nerve roots are affected.

Treatment is aimed at helping you manage your pain without long-term use of medications. First, you'll probably need at least a few days of bed rest while the inflammation goes away. Nonsteroidal anti-inflammatory medications (NSAIDs) such as ibuprofen, aspirin, or muscle relaxants may also help. You may find it soothing to put gentle heat or cold on your painful muscles. Find positions that are comfortable, but be as active as possible. Motion helps to reduce inflammation. Most of the time, your condition will get better within a few weeks. Sometimes, your doctor may inject your spine area with a cortisone-like drug. As soon as possible, start physical therapy with stretching exercises to help you resume your physical activities without sciatica pain. To start, your doctor may want you to take short walks.

You might need surgery only if after 3 months or more of treatment you still have disabling leg pain. A part of the herniated disk may be removed to stop it from pressing on your nerve. The surgery (laminotomy) may be done under local, spinal, or general anesthesia. You have a 90 percent chance of successful surgery if most of your pain is in your leg. Avoid driving, excessive sitting, lifting, or bending forward for at least a month after surgery. Your doctor may give you exercises to strengthen your back.

Following treatment for sciatica, you will probably be able to resume your normal lifestyle and keep your pain under control. However, it's always possible for your disk to rupture again. This happens to about 5 percent of people with sciatica.

Emergency Situation

In rare cases, a herniated disk may press on nerves that cause you to lose control of your bladder or bowel. If this happens, you may also have numbness or tingling in your groin or genital area. This is an emergency situation that requires surgery. Phone your doctor immediately.

Chapter 40

Scoliosis

Chapter Contents

Section 40.1

What Is Scoliosis?

Introduction

A normal, healthy spine curves both to the back and front of the body. Each curve provides unique support to the back, allowing back muscles to work efficiently and nerves to function unimpeded. From the back view, however, the normal spine is straight, providing a balanced and stable structure for the body.

What Is Scoliosis?

Scoliosis results from an abnormal curvature of the spine when seen from the back.

When the curvature is more than 10 degrees, scoliosis is present. This side-to-side curvature might only be seen on x-ray, but may also be obvious simply by looking at or feeling the back. This curvature develops slowly and may not have any symptoms at first.

Adult scoliosis generally is one of two types: those with beginning stages of scoliosis during childhood and those who develop abnormal curvature with age. Symptoms are generally in the lower area of the spine and are due to degeneration (wear and tear) of the supporting structures, such as the intervertebral disks—the cushions between the vertebrae. Spinal curvature, along with arthritic changes, put pressure on the nerves by reducing the space available for the nerves. Besides back pain and stooped posture, problems with the legs may occur such as numbness, pain, weakness, heaviness, and tingling, which limit activity and make walking difficult.

What Causes Scoliosis?

Primary (idiopathic) scoliosis occurs most frequently in young females, but may occur in any child. Idiopathic means its cause is unknown, but usually develops during the growth years of ages 12 to 16. Secondary scoliosis may result from the spine compensating for a nonstructural spine problem such as muscle spasms, inflammatory conditions, poor posture, injury, disease, or difference in leg lengths. It may also be caused by birth defects, tumors, or other diseases such as muscular dystrophy or cerebral palsy.

Can Scoliosis Be Prevented?

Good spinal care includes good nutrition, especially during the growth years, but continuing as an adult. Calcium intake needs to be maintained throughout adulthood. Sensible exercise programs that maintain the strength of leg and back muscles helps reduce injury and deformity. Good posture is vitally important to maintain the supporting structures. Early treatment and intervention of beginning scoliosis through the use of physical therapy, chiropractic, and exercise can reduce the degree of curvature.

What Treatment Options Are There for Scoliosis?

Depending on the cause of the scoliosis, a variety of treatment options are now available.

Endoscopic Thoracic Release

An endoscope is a small instrument that permits a doctor to peer into the body through a small opening, minimizing the size of skin and muscle incisions. Endoscopic thoracic release involves the removal of disks, the separation of ligaments, and in some cases the removal of a portion of several ribs to facilitate correction of a deformed spinal column.

The thoracoscopic release technique involves general anesthesia with the patient lying on the side. The endoscope and other specialized instruments are introduced through skin incisions approximately 1 inch long in the side of the chest. The lung in the surgical area is deflated. A camera attachment on the endoscope allows the doctor to see the chest cavity and spinal column on a TV monitor.

The disks, ligaments, and rib segments are resected to gain motion across the deformed spine. Once this has been achieved, the lung is reinflated, the small skin incisions are closed, and the procedure is completed.

Endoscopic Correction of Scoliosis

Traditional open spine surgery for scoliosis leaves a large scar. Endoscopes, fiberoptic video cameras, and other specially designed surgical tools have made it possible for surgery to be performed through small holes instead of large incisions. Endoscopic surgery has potentially less blood loss and scarring, reduced disruption to the rib cage and other surrounding areas, less post-operative pain, and faster rehabilitation and recovery.

Endoscopic correction is not possible with all types of scoliosis, but single right thoracic curve is ideal for this method.

Spinal Fusion

Fusion is a surgically created solid bone bridge between two or more adjacent (usually freely mobile) bones. In the spine, this procedure is used to create stability between vertebrae. In order to achieve a fusion, bone must grow across the desired area in a gradual and solid fashion. A number of techniques can increase the chance of this to occur. The basis principle is to place bone tissue (bone graft) into the area of desired fusion, ensure sufficient immobility across that area (brace, cast, spinal instrumentation), and then wait for the fusion to take place (6 to 9 months or more).

Instrumentation

To straighten the spine in scoliosis patients, the doctor attaches hooks to the vertebral bodies. Then two titanium rods are inserted to either side of the spine. A piece of bone from the patient's hip (a bone graft) is applied to portions of the spine to assist fusion by growing into the spaces between the vertebrae and acting like a cement to hold them straight. This is called a spinal fusion. Until these bones heal together, they need to be supported and kept from curving again. The rods accomplish this purpose by holding the spine straight until the bones are fused together. Many types of instrumentation (rods) are now available.

Section 40.2

Scoliosis in Children and Adolescents

"Questions and Answers about Scoliosis in Children and Adolescents" from the National Institute of Arthritis and Musculoskeletal and Skin Diseases (NIAMS), July 2001. Available online at http://www.niams.nih.gov; accessed May 2004.

What Is Scoliosis?

Scoliosis is a musculoskeletal disorder in which there is a sideways curvature of the spine, or backbone. The bones that make up the spine are called vertebrae. Some people who have scoliosis require treatment. Other people, who have milder curves, may only need to visit their doctor for periodic observation. The section, "Does Scoliosis Have To Be Treated? What Are the Treatments?" describes how doctors decide whether to treat scoliosis.

Who Gets Scoliosis?

People of all ages can have scoliosis, but this material focuses on children and adolescents. Of every 1,000 children, 3 to 5 develop spinal curves that are considered large enough to need treatment. Adolescent idiopathic scoliosis (scoliosis of unknown cause) is the most common type and occurs after the age of 10. Girls are more likely than boys to have this type of scoliosis. Since scoliosis can run in families, a child who has a parent, brother, or sister with idiopathic scoliosis should be checked regularly for scoliosis by the family physician.

Idiopathic scoliosis can also occur in children younger than 10 years of age, but is very rare. Early onset or infantile idiopathic scoliosis occurs in children less than 3 years old. It is more common in Europe than in the United States. Juvenile idiopathic scoliosis occurs in children between the ages of 3 and 10.

What Causes Scoliosis?

In 80 to 85 percent of people, the cause of scoliosis is unknown; this is called idiopathic scoliosis. Before concluding that a person has

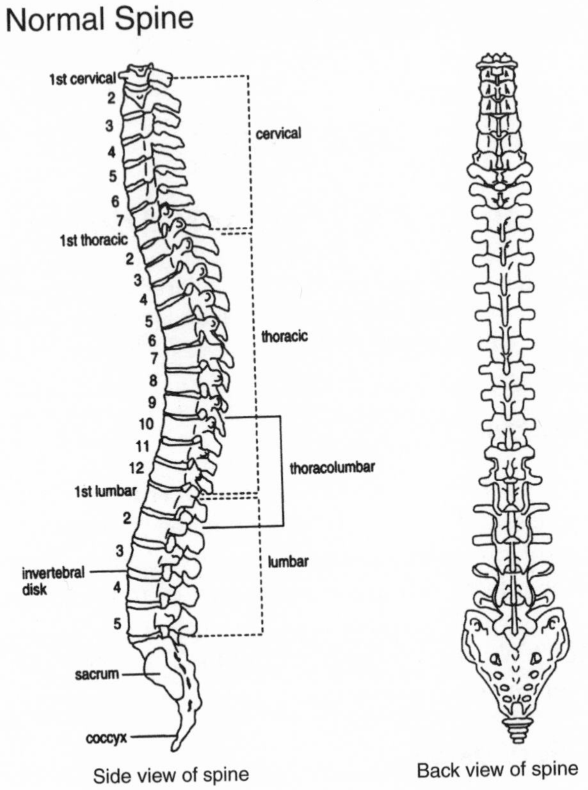

Normal Spine
1st cervical
2
3
4
5
6
7
1st thoracic
2
3
4
5
6
7
8
9
10
11
12
1st lumbar
2
3
4
5
invertebral disk
sacrum
coccyx
cervical
thoracic
thoracolumbar
lumbar
Side view of spine
Back view of spine

Figure 40.1. A side and back view of the spine.

Curve Patterns
•46°
Thoracic
Lumbar
Thoracolumbar
Double

Figure 40.2. Scoliosis curve patterns.

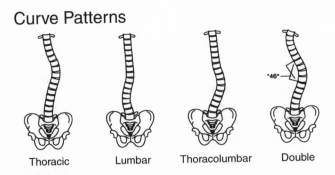

idiopathic scoliosis, the doctor looks for other possible causes, such as injury or infection. Causes of curves are classified as either nonstructural or structural.

- **Nonstructural (functional) scoliosis**—A structurally normal spine that appears curved. This is a temporary, changing curve. It is caused by an underlying condition such as a difference in leg length, muscle spasms, or inflammatory conditions such as appendicitis. Doctors treat this type of scoliosis by correcting the underlying problem.

- **Structural scoliosis**—A fixed curve that doctors treat case by case. Sometimes structural scoliosis is one part of a syndrome or disease, such as Marfan syndrome, an inherited connective tissue disorder. In other cases, it occurs by itself. Structural scoliosis can be caused by neuromuscular diseases (such as cerebral palsy, poliomyelitis, or muscular dystrophy), birth defects (such as hemivertebra, in which one side of a vertebra fails to form normally before birth), injury, certain infections, tumors (such as those caused by neurofibromatosis, a birth defect sometimes associated with benign tumors on the spinal column), metabolic diseases, connective tissue disorders, rheumatic diseases, or unknown factors (idiopathic scoliosis).

How Does the Doctor Diagnose Scoliosis?

The doctor takes the following steps to evaluate a patient for scoliosis:

- Medical history—The doctor talks to the patient and the patient's parent or parents and reviews the patient's records to look for medical problems that might be causing the spine to curve, for example, birth defects, trauma, or other disorders that can be associated with scoliosis.

- Physical examination—The doctor looks at the patient's back, chest, pelvis, legs, feet, and skin. The doctor checks if the patient's shoulders are level, whether the head is centered, and whether opposite sides of the body look level. The doctor also examines the back muscles while the patient is bending forward to see if one side of the rib cage is higher than the other. If there is a significant asymmetry (difference between opposite sides of the body), the doctor will refer the patient to an orthopaedic spine specialist (a doctor who has experience treating people with scoliosis). Certain changes in the skin, such as so-called café au lait (coffee-with-milk-colored) spots, can suggest that the scoliosis is caused by a birth defect.

- X-ray evaluation—Patients with significant spinal curves, unusual back pain, or signs of involvement of the central nervous system (brain and spinal cord) such as bowel and bladder control problems need to have an x-ray. The x-ray should be done with the patient standing with his or her back to the x-ray machine. The view is of the entire spine on one long (36-inch) film. Occasionally, doctors ask for more tests to see if there are other problems.

- Curve measurement—The doctor measures the curve on the x-ray image. He or she finds the vertebrae at the beginning and end of the curve and measures the angle of the curve. Curves that are greater than 20 degrees require treatment.

Doctors group curves of the spine by their location, shape, pattern, and cause. They use this information to decide how best to treat the scoliosis.

- Location—To identify a curve's location, doctors find the apex of the curve (the vertebra within the curve that is the most off-center); the location of the apex is the location of the curve. A thoracic curve has its apex in the thoracic area (the part of the spine to which the ribs attach). A lumbar curve has its apex in the lower back. A thoracolumbar curve has its apex where the thoracic and lumbar vertebrae join.

- Shape—The curve usually is S- or C-shaped.

- Pattern—Curves frequently follow patterns that have been studied in previous patients. The larger the curve is, the more likely it will progress (depending on the amount of growth remaining).

Does Scoliosis Have to Be Treated? What Are the Treatments?

Many children who are sent to the doctor by a school scoliosis screening program have very mild spinal curves that do not need treatment. When a child does need treatment, the doctor may send him or her to an orthopaedic spine specialist.

The doctor will suggest the best treatment for each patient based on the patient's age, how much more he or she is likely to grow, the degree and pattern of the curve, and the type of scoliosis. The doctor may recommend observation, bracing, or surgery.

- Observation—Doctors follow patients without treatment and re-examine them every 4 to 6 months when the patient is still growing (is skeletally immature) and has an idiopathic curve of less than 25 degrees.

- Bracing—Doctors advise patients to wear a brace to stop a curve from getting any worse when the patient: is still growing and has an idiopathic curve that is more than 25 to 30 degrees; has at least 2 years of growth remaining, has an idiopathic curve that is between 20 and 29 degrees, and, if a girl, has not had her first menstrual period; or is still growing and has an idiopathic curve between 20 and 29 degrees that is getting worse. As a child nears the end of growth, the indications for bracing will depend on how the curve affects the child's appearance, whether the curve is getting worse, and the size of the curve.

- Surgery—Doctors advise patients to have surgery to correct a curve or stop it from worsening when the patient is still growing, has a curve that is more than 45 degrees, and has a curve that is getting worse.

Are There Other Ways to Treat Scoliosis?

Some people have tried other ways to treat scoliosis, including manipulation by a chiropractor, electrical stimulation, dietary supplements, and corrective exercises. So far, studies of the following treatments have not been shown to prevent curve progression or worsening:

- Chiropractic manipulation

- Electrical stimulation

- Nutritional supplementation

- Exercise—Studies have shown that exercise alone will not stop progressive curves. However, patients may wish to exercise for the effects on their general health and well being.

Which Brace Is Best?

The decision about which brace to wear depends on the type of curve and whether the patient will follow the doctor's directions about how many hours a day to wear the brace.

There are two main types of braces. Braces can be custom-made or can be made from a prefabricated mold. All must be selected for the specific curve problem and fitted to each patient. To have their intended effect (to keep a curve from getting worse), braces must be worn every day for the full number of hours prescribed by the doctor until the child stops growing.

- Milwaukee brace—Patients can wear this brace to correct any curve in the spine. This brace has a neck ring.

- Thoracolumbosacral orthosis (TLSO)—Patients can wear this brace to correct curves whose apex is at or below the eighth thoracic vertebra. The TLSO is an underarm brace, which means that it fits under the arm and around the rib cage, lower back, and hips.

If the Doctor Recommends Surgery, Which Procedure Is Best?

Many surgical techniques can be used to correct the curves of scoliosis. The main surgical procedure is correction, stabilization, and fusion of the curve. Fusion is the joining of two or more vertebrae. Surgeons can choose different ways to straighten the spine and also different implants to keep the spine stable after surgery. (Implants are devices that remain in the patient after surgery to keep the spine aligned.) The decision about the type of implant will depend on the cost; the size of the implant, which depends on the size of the patient; the shape of the implant; its safety; and the experience of the surgeon. Each patient should discuss his or her options with at least two experienced surgeons.

Patients and parents who are thinking about surgery may want to ask the following questions:

- What are the benefits from surgery for scoliosis?

- What are the risks from surgery for scoliosis?

- What techniques will be used for the surgery?

- What devices will be used to keep the spine stable after surgery?

- Where will the incisions be made?
- How straight will the patient's spine be after surgery?
- How long will the hospital stay be?
- How long will it take to recover from surgery?
- Is there chronic back pain after surgery for scoliosis?
- Will the patient's growth be limited?
- How flexible will the spine remain?
- Can the curve worsen or progress after surgery?
- Will additional surgery be likely?
- Will the patient be able to do all the things he or she wants to do following surgery?

Can People with Scoliosis Exercise?

Although exercise programs have not been shown to affect the natural history of scoliosis, exercise is encouraged in patients with scoliosis to minimize any potential decrease in functional ability over time. It is very important for all people, including those with scoliosis, to exercise and remain physically fit. Girls have a higher risk than boys of developing osteoporosis (a disorder that results in weak bones that can break easily) later in life. The risk of osteoporosis is reduced in women who exercise regularly all their lives; and weight-bearing exercise, such as walking, running, soccer, and gymnastics, increases bone density and helps prevent osteoporosis. For both boys and girls, exercising and participating in sports also improves their general sense of well-being.

What Are Researchers Trying to Find out about Scoliosis?

Researchers are looking for the cause of idiopathic scoliosis. They have studied genetics, growth, structural and biochemical alterations in the disks and muscles, and central nervous system changes. The changes in the disks and muscles seem to be a result of scoliosis and not the cause. Scientists are still hopeful that studying changes in the central nervous system in people with idiopathic scoliosis may reveal a cause of this disorder.

Researchers continue to examine how a variety of braces, surgical procedures, and surgical instruments can be used to straighten the spine or to prevent further curvature. They are also studying the long-term effects of a scoliosis fusion and the long-term effects of untreated scoliosis.

Where Can People Get More Information about Scoliosis?

National Scoliosis Foundation
5 Cabot Place
Stoughton, MA 02072
Toll-Free: (800) 673-6922
Fax: (781) 341-8333
Website: http://www.scoliosis.org
E-mail: NSF@scoliosis.org

This is a nonprofit voluntary organization that provides pamphlets, a newsletter, and other information materials on childhood and adult scoliosis. The foundation also provides support group information and lists of physicians in each state who specialize in scoliosis.

Scoliosis Association, Inc.
P.O. Box 811705
Boca Raton, FL 33481-1705
Toll-Free: (800) 800-0669
Phone: (561) 991-4435
Fax: (561) 994-2455
Website: http://www.scoliosis-assoc.org

This association publishes a quarterly newsletter and pamphlets. A single copy of their fact sheet is available free by sending a self-addressed, stamped envelope. The association also provides information about local chapters and support groups.

Scoliosis Research Society
611 East Wells Street
Milwaukee, WI 53202-3892
Phone: (414) 289-9107
Fax: (414) 276-3349
Website: http://www.srs.org

This is a professional organization for orthopaedic surgeons interested in scoliosis. It provides pamphlets about the diagnosis and treatment of scoliosis. Their free pamphlet is offered on their website as well as through the mail. The society also can provide referrals to physicians.

Chapter 41

Slipped (Herniated) Disk

Chapter Contents

Section 41.1

Facts about Slipped Disk

What adult has not complained of an aching back at one time or another? How many people have experienced the sudden pain of "throwing one's back out?"

In most instances, back pain is simply the result of unusual exertion, fatigue, or a twist or sharp movement, but in some cases, there has been an injury to the spine and medical attention is required. One of the most common injuries to the spine is a slipped, or herniated, disk. This condition can be extremely painful, and may damage surrounding muscle and nerve systems. If pain is very severe, if it persists or worsens when you lie down, if it travels down your leg or if numbness sets in, then a physician must be consulted.

What Is a Disk?

A disk is a small mass of elastic, gristle-like tissue. Located between each vertebra in the spinal column, disks act as shock absorbers for the spinal bones. Thick ligaments attached to the vertebrae hold the pulpy disk material in place.

What Is a Slipped Disk?

When some of the disk material pops out of place and bulges into the spinal canal, this is also known as a herniated or ruptured disk.

Why Do Disks Herniate?

Occasionally, a single excessive strain may cause a slipped disk. However, disk material degenerates naturally as we age, and the ligaments that hold it in place begin to weaken. As this degeneration progresses, a relatively minor strain or twisting movement can cause a disk to pop out of place.

Certain individuals may be more vulnerable to disk problems, and as a consequence may suffer herniations at several places along the spine. Research has shown that a predisposition for slipped disks may exist in families, with several members affected.

What Are the Symptoms of a Slipped Disk?

Extreme, sudden pain is usually the first symptom. Since most herniations involve the bottom two disks in the spinal column, the pain usually begins in the lower back. The bulging disk in this location exerts pressure on the sciatic nerve, and sharp pain may follow that nerve all the way down the leg and into the foot. Pressure on this nerve may eventually cause numbness or a pins and needles sensation. Over time, the surrounding muscles can weaken and shrink in size.

Disks can also rupture at higher levels in the spine causing pain and weakness in the neck, shoulders, and arms.

Even if the initial pain subsides, it is important that the condition be diagnosed and treated in order to prevent further damage.

How Is a Slipped Disk Diagnosed?

A number of tests are used to make a precise diagnosis and to pinpoint the site of the herniation, such as x-rays, myelography, computed tomography (CT) scans, and magnetic resonance imaging (MRI).

What Is the Treatment for a Slipped Disk?

The first goal of treatment is to relieve pain by decreasing the muscle spasm. Physicians may prescribe pain relievers, muscle relaxants, and bed rest. As the muscle spasm subsides, the pressure in the nerve root at the disk protrusion eases.

When the herniation is higher on the spinal column, special collars or even traction may relieve the pressure.

Most slipped disks respond well to this kind of treatment, and a carefully designed exercise program to strengthen the surrounding muscles can be very helpful in preventing future ruptures.

In some cases, however, the pain is severe and intractable; there may even be nerve damage. In these instances, a neurological surgeon may have to remove the disk material. When the disk is removed, the pressure on the nerve is released, and this may rapidly relieve pain and permit restoration of lost muscle function.

Role of the Neurosurgeon

Neurological surgery is the medical specialty concerned with the diagnosis and treatment of disorders affecting the nervous system, the brain, or the spinal cord. Neurosurgeons may treat injuries to the head, spinal cord, or nerves; strokes (or patients in danger of a stroke due to clogged arteries in the neck); brain or spinal cord tumors or malformations; or the back and neck pain associated with a slipped disk. Depending on the nature of the surgery or illness, neurosurgeons may provide surgical or non-surgical treatment. Neurological surgeons undergo six to eight years of rigorous training following medical school. After completing this training, two years of practice, and an examination, neurological surgeons can become board certified.

Section 41.2

Cervical Disk Herniation

Reprinted with permission from John Regan, M.D., Co-Director, Cedars-Sinai Institute for Spinal Disorders, Los Angeles, California. For additional information about spinal disorders and treatments, visit Dr. Regan's website at http://www.spinesource.com. © 2004 John Regan. All rights reserved.

Introduction to Cervical Disk Herniation

The seven cervical (neck) vertebrae support the head, allowing rotation and movement and providing pathways for the spinal cord and the cervical nerves. Besides the vertebral foramen (the spinal canal through which the spinal cord passes), the cervical vertebra have smaller foramina (canals) through which a large artery and the cervical nerves pass.

The cervical nerves are responsible for controlling the neck, arms, and upper body. The portion of the cervical nerve as it exits the spinal column is called the nerve root. The functions of the cervical vertebrae—spinal cord and artery pathways, support, and movement—make them especially significant for spinal health.

What Is a Cervical Disk Herniation?

The disks between the cervical vertebrae are much smaller than the other disks in the back. They can become weakened, causing some of the disk material to protrude. This generally occurs at the lower level of the neck, at the fifth or sixth vertebra (C-5 or C-6 or C-7). In a cervical disk herniation, the herniated disk generally pushes outward rather than inward on the spinal nerve. This outward protrusion places pressure on the cervical nerve roots, resulting in dysfunction and pain in the neck, arms, and upper body.

What Causes Cervical Disk Herniation?

Accidents, especially those with an abrupt change in speed, are one cause of cervical disk herniation. The weight of the head, when whipped rapidly or violently, exerts tremendous force on the neck muscles and structures. This force can weaken the wall (annulus fibrosus) of the disk, causing the disk material to bulge outward. Disk degeneration related to repetitive minor trauma can also lead to disk herniation.

Because the disks between the cervical vertebrae are much smaller and generally bear a lesser load than disks in the lumbar region, herniations occur less often than in other areas of the spine. Posture or position problems, when chronic, may also weaken the muscles and structures of the spinal column.

Can Cervical Disk Herniation Be Prevented?

The best way to prevent cervical disk herniation is to prevent accidents and reduce the severity of injuries. Seat belts and air bags in cars are designed especially for this purpose. Ergonomic working positions and appropriate exercise and rest all help to prevent injuries and achieve good neck health.

What Treatment Options Are There for Cervical Disk Herniation?

Surgical Treatment

If conservative treatment fails to relieve the pain after 2 or 3 months, surgery may be necessary to relieve the pressure on the cervical nerves. After using an MRI or CT scan to determine the exact presence of the herniation, the herniated disk may be surgically removed either from the front (anterior) or the back (posterior) of the neck. Surgery may also be urgently recommended for progressive weakness, numbness, or severe neck and arm pain.

Most cervical herniated disks are removed from the front as this procedure allows the surgeon to more easily place bone graft in the disk space. This results in a wider opening for the nerve root. The posterior route may be more appropriate if the disk is large and soft and protrudes to the side of the canal. In either case, most patients are able to return home after one night in the hospital.

The use of advanced microscopic imaging, computers, software, and tracking technology allow the surgeon to clearly visualize structures, make decisions based upon precise measurements and information, and maneuver in exacting detail.

Types of Surgery

Microscopic Posterior Cervical Foraminotomy

The foramen, the small canal within or between the vertebra, provides the passageway for a nerve. If the disk has ruptured or the body of a vertebra has collapsed, the foramen is distorted or made smaller, which presses on the nerve. Using advanced microscopic imaging, computers, software, and tracking technology, the surgeon is able to clearly see and maneuver at the same time within a very limited area, reducing injury to surrounding tissues. Tiny portions of the bone surrounding the foramen are removed, leaving a larger canal for the nerve to occupy without pressure. The new technologies help the surgeon avoid injury to the nerve during the procedure.

Anterior Cervical Discectomy and Fusion

Removal of a cervical herniated disk (cervical discectomy) is necessary when the disk has ruptured and lost its ability to retain its form, thereby placing pressure on the nerves. From an incision on the back of the neck, the disk is carefully and precisely removed and the two bordering vertebrae are joined to create stability. Very small sections of bone may be used from another part of the body to bridge the gap left from the removed herniated disk (fusion).

Cervical Laminaplasty

The lamina is a flat portion of bone that is the back portion of the vertebra. When the spinal canal has become too small due to injury or disease, it may be made larger by use of laminaplasty. An incision is made down the back of the neck to expose the cervical vertebrae. On one side of the vertebral column, the lamina are cut through just far enough to create a hinge-like movement, much like a door. Then the lamina on the other side are cut all the way through to, in effect, open the door. The back portion of the vertebrae, the spinous processes (bumps you feel on the back) are removed to make more room for the door to open. After gently opening the door of each vertebra to create more room for the spinal cord and nerve roots behind it, bone wedges are inserted to keep the door from totally closing. Then the door is closed securely onto the wedges, resulting in an expanded doorway for the nerves.

By increasing the space for the spinal cord and nerve roots, laminaplasty reduces the cause of pain and may help prevent progression of spinal deformity. It preserves the stability of the neck, but may result in loss of the ability to extend the neck backward and may reduce other cervical motion. A relapse of pain may occur if excessive bone growth occurs as the bone heals.

Cervical Instrumentation

Advanced imaging equipment also provides the surgeon with the ability to precisely determine what the final position of the vertebrae, and subsequently the nerve canals, should be. Thorough and accurate measurements of positions of the vertebral structures assure the surgeon that both bone and manufactured implants precisely align the spine and the nerve canals. The correct sizing of the implant, using interactive templating, is critical in obtaining an ideal outcome. This precision is possible using microscopic imaging, computers, software, and tracking technology.

Artificial Cervical Disk Replacement

The Cedars Sinai Institute for Spinal Disorders is currently participating in a randomized 12-center FDA clinical trial for cervical disk replacement using the Bryan cervical disk prosthesis. This technique involves removing the disk and replacing it with an artificial prosthetic disk. The benefits of using an artificial disk include maintaining motion of the cervical spine.

Section 41.3

Thoracic Disk Herniation

Introduction

The spine is composed of 33 vertebrae, uniquely aligned to support the body and provide a passageway for the spinal cord and nerves. At the top of the spine are seven cervical (neck) vertebrae, followed by 12 thoracic vertebrae from which the 12 pairs of ribs originate. Next are 5 lumbar vertebrae, followed by the 5 fused sacral bones (the back of the pelvis) and 4 fused bones of the coccyx (tailbone).

What Is Thoracic Disk Herniation?

The cervical, thoracic, and lumbar vertebrae are separated from each other by intervertebral disks that cushion and separate the vertebra, providing space for the nerves roots to exit the spinal canal. Disks are composed of cartilage that lies between the bony vertebral bodies of the spine. The disk and vertebral bodies are considered joints since there is motion. The disks are composed of an outer wall of tough fibrous tissue called the annulus fibrosus, and a softer, inner substance called the nucleus pulposus. The nucleus pulposus contains water, which like a water-filled balloon, gives cushioning to the disk. If a disk degenerates (a herniated disk), it flattens and puts pressure on the spinal cord. Because the space between the vertebrae is shorter, the bones may put pressure on the nerves also.

What Causes Thoracic Disk Herniation?

The natural curvature of the spine provides the skeleton with strength and stability. The curves act like a coiled spring to distribute the mechanical stress as the body moves. As disks age, they lose their water content and begin to degenerate. The annulus fibrosis (outer ring), may also be damaged through general wear and tear or by injury in which the nucleus, under extreme pressure, bulges out through the annulus fibrosis ring.

Can Thoracic Disk Herniation Be Prevented?

Like other disks in the spine, the thoracic disks are vulnerable to injury when the person practices poor posture. Sensible exercises, designed to strengthen the upper back, help to improve posture and prevent injury. Maintaining a healthy lifestyle with good nutrition is key, as well as preventing accidents. The spine, designed for flexibility, will perform best if cared for properly.

What Treatment Options Are There for Thoracic Disk Herniation?

VATS—Video Assisted Thoracic Surgery

The standard open surgical approaches to the thoracic spine usually involve creating a large opening in the chest wall. Video Assisted Thoracic Surgery (VATS) is a minimally invasive (keyhole) surgical procedure. It allows the surgeon to directly examine the chest cavity without a big incision. Three or four small incisions will be made to allow the surgeon to use the special instruments (video camera and endoscope) needed for this operation. A very small video camera is used to project pictures of the chest cavity onto a screen during the procedure.

VATS avoids the extensive damage to the chest wall. Specific tools and implant systems permit the spine surgeon to remove thoracic disks, biopsy vertebral masses/tumors, release scoliotic curves, perform bone grafts on the disk spaces, and even to instrument the spine working through these small (1- to 2-inch) puncture incisions.

Discectomy

A discectomy is a surgical procedure in which part or all of an intervertebral disk is removed from the spine. This is commonly done when a disk is herniated (slipped disk) and is causing symptoms of pain and nerve irritation or injury. In the thoracic area, discectomies are usually done through an incision on the side of the ribcage. A small window is created in the bone overlying the disk herniation. The nerve root is gently retracted to expose the disk herniation. The disk material is then removed using special instruments.

Fusion

Fusion is a surgically created solid bone bridge between two or more adjacent (usually freely mobile) bones. In the spine, this procedure is used to create a stability between vertebrae. In order to achieve a fusion, bone must grow across the desired area in a gradual and solid fashion. A number of techniques can increase the chance of this occurring. The basis principle is to place bone tissue (bone graft) into the area of desired fusion, ensure sufficient immobility across that area (brace, cast, and spinal instrumentation), and then wait for the fusion to take place (6 to 9 months or more).

Spinal Instrumentation

For spine operations to be successful, solid healing of bone across the spine must be achieved. The use of metal devices, also called instrumentation (screws, rods, plates, cables, wires) can help correct a deformed spine and will also increase the probability of obtaining a solid spinal fusion.

Spinal instrumentation can be placed in the front or in the back portion of the spine. The devices are usually made of metal, commonly stainless steel or titanium. In order to place this instrumentation into the spine, the spine is at first exposed by making a skin incision, and then gently clearing the muscles, ligaments, and other soft tissues from the levels of the vertebrae to be fused. Specific tools are used to carefully prepare the bone in such a way to obtain good seating of the implants (screw, rod, wire, cable, or other). When these devices are in the proper position, a rod or plate is positioned to link the implants together. Screws are inserted into the pedicles, which are part of the arch of the vertebra. This essentially forms a rigid scaffolding to hold the spine in the desired position. The bone graft which has been placed into the area of fusion gradually solidifies over several months. The spinal instrumentation is gradually covered by scar tissue and sometimes bone which the body lays down.

Chapter 42

Spina Bifida and Tethered Spinal Cord Syndrome

Chapter Contents

Section 42.1

What Is Spina Bifida?

What are neural tube defects?

Neural tube defects (NTDs) are serious birth defects that involve incomplete development of the brain, spinal cord, and/or protective coverings for these organs. There are three types of NTDs: anencephaly, encephalocele, and spina bifida.

Babies born with anencephaly have underdeveloped brains and incomplete skulls. Most infants born with anencephaly do not survive more than a few hours after birth. Encephalocele results in a hole in the skull through which brain tissue protrudes. Although most babies with encephalocele do not live or are severely retarded, early surgery has been able to save a few children.

What is spina bifida?

Spina bifida is the most frequently occurring permanently disabling birth defect. It affects approximately one out of every 1,000 newborns in the United States.

Spina bifida, the most common NTD, is one of the most devastating of all birth defects. It results from the failure of the spine to close properly during the first month of pregnancy. In severe cases, the spinal cord protrudes through the back and may be covered by skin or a thin membrane. Surgery to close a newborn's back is generally performed within 24 hours after birth to minimize the risk of infection and to preserve existing function in the spinal cord.

Because of the paralysis resulting from the damage to the spinal cord, people born with spina bifida may need surgeries and other extensive medical care. The condition can also cause bowel and bladder complications. A large percentage of children born with spina bifida also have hydrocephalus, the accumulation of fluid in the brain.

Hydrocephalus is controlled by a surgical procedure called shunting, which relieves the fluid build up in the brain by redirecting it into the abdominal area. Most children born with spina bifida live well into adulthood as a result of today's sophisticated medical techniques.

Who is at higher risk?

Women who:

- have a child with spina bifida
- have spina bifida themselves
- have already had a pregnancy affected by any neural defect

are at greater risk of having a child affected by spina bifida or another neural tube defect.

These women may need to get a prescription for folic acid before trying to become pregnant, so it's important to plan any future pregnancy. Please speak with your health care provider about folic acid.

I've heard that children with spina bifida have learning problems. Is this true?

Some children with spina bifida do experience learning problems. They may have difficulty with paying attention, expressing or understanding language, organizing, sequencing, and grasping reading and math.

How can we help those with learning problems?

Early intervention can help considerably to prepare these children for school. Students should be in the least restrictive environment and their day to day activities should be as normal as possible. It often helps to have a psychological evaluation, which tests the child's intelligence, academic levels (reading, spelling, math, etc.), and basic learning abilities (visual perception, receptive and expressive language skills).

What about the physical limitations?

Children with spina bifida need to learn mobility skills and often with the use of crutches, braces, or wheelchairs can achieve more independence. Also, with new techniques children can become independent in managing their bowel and bladder problems. Physical disabilities like spina bifida can have profound effects on the child's emotional and social development. It is important that health care professionals, teachers, and parents understand the child's physical capabilities and limitations. To promote personal growth, they should encourage children (within the limits of safety and health) to be independent, to participate in activities with their non-disabled peers and to assume responsibility for their own care.

What are secondary conditions associated with spina bifida?

Special attention is needed to identify and treat secondary disabilities. Due to the wide range of neurological damage and mobility impairment it can be difficult to identify some secondary disabilities. Attention should be focused on the psychological and social development of children and young adults with spina bifida. Many recent studies, including the Spina Bifida Association of America (SBAA)'s Adult Network Survey, clearly indicate the presence of emotional problems that result from factors such as low self-esteem and lack of social skills training.

Examples of secondary conditions associated with spina bifida are latex allergy, tendinitis, obesity, skin breakdown, gastrointestinal disorders, learning disabilities, attaining and retaining mobility, depression, and social and sexual issues.

What is latex allergy?

Allergic responses to latex (rubber) products. Typical symptoms include watery eyes, wheezing, hives, rash, swelling, and in severe cases, anaphylaxis (a life threatening reaction). These responses can occur when items containing latex touch the skin, the mucous membranes (like the mouth, genitals, bladder or rectum), open areas, or bloodstream (especially during surgery).

Who is allergic to latex?

While it is not known exactly how this allergy develops, anybody can develop a latex allergy. However, certain groups of individuals have been identified as having a greater risk of becoming latex allergic. Those at higher risk include people who are frequently exposed to latex, such as children and adults with spina bifida and health professionals. Research has shown that spina bifida patients have the potential to become allergic (to some degree) to latex. Anyone with a latex allergy should avoid exposure to all products that contain latex.

What are some common products that contain latex?

Catheters, elastic bandages, baby bottle nipples, pacifiers, and balloons are just a few common products that contain latex. For a more extensive list of items containing latex often found at home, in your community, and in hospitals, contact the SBAA. If you are in doubt about a specific product, check with its distributor or manufacturer.

Can anything be done to prevent spina bifida?

Birth defects can happen in any family. Many things can affect a pregnancy, including family genes and things women may come in contact with during pregnancy. Recent studies have shown that folic acid is one factor that may reduce the risk of having an NTD baby.

Taking folic acid cannot guarantee having a healthy baby, but it can help. Taking folic acid before and during early pregnancy reduces the risk of spina bifida and other neural tube defects. Here's what you can do:

- Take a vitamin with 400 micrograms (mcg) folic acid every day. This amount is also written as 0.4 milligrams (mg). All women should take this amount every day while not planning to become pregnant.

- If you have a child with spina bifida, have spina bifida yourself, or have had a history of pregnancy affected by a neural tube defect, and you are thinking about becoming pregnant, you need a higher dose of folic acid. You should take 4000 micrograms (mcg) of folic acid by prescription for 1 to 3 months before becoming pregnant. This amount is also written as 4.0 milligrams (mg). Taking this amount of folic acid by prescription may reduce the chance of a neural tube defect like spina bifida in future pregnancies. Please see your doctor. Do not take this extra folic acid by taking more multivitamins because too much of some of the other vitamins could harm you and your future baby.

- Plan your next pregnancy. Speak with your health care provider about your personal risk of having a baby with a neural tube defect. You may need to get a prescription for folic acid before you try to become pregnant.

What is folic acid?

Folic acid, a common water-soluble B vitamin, is essential for the functioning of the human body. During periods of rapid growth, such as pregnancy and fetal development, the body's requirement for this vitamin increases. Folic acid can be found in multivitamins, fortified breakfast cereals, dark green leafy vegetables such as broccoli and spinach, egg yolks, and some fruits and fruit juices. However, the average American diet does not supply the recommended level of folic acid.

Section 42.2

What Is Tethered Spinal Cord Syndrome?

"Tethered Spinal Cord Information Page" is from the National Institute of Neurological Disorders and Stroke (NINDS), July 1, 2001. Available online at http://www.ninds.nih.gov; accessed May 2004.

What is tethered spinal cord syndrome?

Tethered spinal cord syndrome is a neurological disorder caused by an abnormal stretching of the spinal cord. The course of the disorder is progressive. In children, symptoms may include lesions, hairy patches, dimples, or fatty tumors on the lower back; foot and spinal deformities; weakness in the legs; low back pain; scoliosis; and incontinence. Tethered spinal cord syndrome may go undiagnosed until adulthood, when symptoms such as sensory and motor problems and loss of bowel and bladder control emerge. This delayed presentation of symptoms is related to the degree of strain placed on the spinal cord over time. Tethered spinal cord syndrome appears to be the result of improper development of the neural tube, and is closely linked with spina bifida.

Is there any treatment?

In children, early surgery is recommended to prevent further neurological deterioration. If surgery is not advisable, spinal cord nerve roots may be cut to relieve pain. Other treatment is symptomatic and supportive.

What is the prognosis?

With treatment, patients with tethered spinal cord syndrome have a normal life expectancy. However, some neurological and motor impairments may not be fully correctable.

What research is being done?

The National Institute of Neurological Disorders and Stroke (NINDS) conducts and supports research on disorders of the spinal cord. The goals of this research are to find ways to prevent, treat, and cure these disorders.

Chapter 43

Spinal Stenosis

This chapter contains general information about spinal stenosis. It describes the condition's causes, symptoms, diagnosis, and treatments. At the end is a list of additional resources. If you have further questions after reading this chapter, you may wish to discuss them with your doctor.

What Is Spinal Stenosis?

Spinal stenosis is a narrowing of spaces in the spine (backbone) that results in pressure on the spinal cord and/or nerve roots. This disorder usually involves the narrowing of one or more of three areas of the spine: (1) the canal in the center of the column of bones (vertebral or spinal column) through which the spinal cord and nerve roots run, (2) the canals at the base or roots of nerves branching out from the spinal cord, or (3) the openings between vertebrae (bones of the spine) through which nerves leave the spine and go to other parts of the body. The narrowing may involve a small or large area of the spine. Pressure on the lower part of the spinal cord or on nerve roots branching out from that area may give rise to pain or numbness in the legs. Pressure on the upper part of the spinal cord (that is, the neck area) may produce similar symptoms in the shoulders, or even the legs.

"Questions and Answers About Spinal Stenosis," National Institute of Arthritis and Musculoskeletal and Skin Diseases, October 1999. Available online at http://www.niams.nih.gov; accessed April 2004. Reviewed by David A. Cooke, M.D., on April 11, 2004.

Who Gets Spinal Stenosis?

This disorder is most common in people over 50 years of age. However, it may occur in younger people who are born with a narrowing of the spinal canal or who suffer an injury to the spine.

What Structures of the Spine Are Involved?

The spine is a column of 26 bones that extend in a line from the base of the skull to the pelvis. Twenty-four of the bones are called vertebrae. The bones of the spine include 7 cervical vertebrae in the neck; 12 thoracic vertebrae at the back wall of the chest; 5 lumbar vertebrae at the inward curve (small) of the lower back; the sacrum, composed of 5 fused vertebrae between the hip bones; and the coccyx, composed of 3 to 5 fused bones at the lower tip of the vertebral column. The vertebrae link to each other and are cushioned by shock-absorbing disks that lie between them.

The vertebral column provides the main support for the upper body, allowing humans to stand upright or bend and twist, and it protects the spinal cord from injury. Following are structures of the spine most involved in spinal stenosis.

- Intervertebral disks—pads of cartilage between vertebrae that act as shock absorbers.

- Facet joints—joints located on both sides and on the top and bottom of each vertebra. They connect the vertebrae to each other and permit back motion.

- Intervertebral foramen (also called neural foramen)—an opening between vertebrae through which nerves leave the spine and extend to other parts of the body.

- Lamina—part of the vertebra at the upper portion of the vertebral arch that forms the roof of the canal through which the spinal cord and nerve roots pass.

- Ligaments—elastic bands of tissue that support the spine by preventing the vertebrae from slipping out of line as the spine moves. A large ligament often involved in spinal stenosis is the ligamentum flavum, which runs as a continuous band from lamina to lamina in the spine.

- Pedicles—narrow stem-like structures on the vertebrae that form the walls of the bottom part of the vertebral arch.

- Spinal cord/nerve roots—a major part of the central nervous system that extends from the base of the brain down to the lower back and that is encased by the vertebral column. It consists of nerve cells and bundles of nerves. The cord connects the brain to all parts of the body via 31 pairs of nerves that branch out from the cord and leave the spine between vertebrae.

- Synovium—a thin membrane that produces fluid to lubricate the facet joints, allowing them to move easily.

- Vertebral arch—a circle of bone around the canal through which the spinal cord passes. It is composed of a floor at the back of the vertebra, walls (the pedicles), and a ceiling where two laminae join.

What Causes Spinal Stenosis?

The normal vertebral canal provides adequate room for the spinal cord. Narrowing of the canal, which occurs in spinal stenosis, may be inherited or acquired. Some people inherit a small spinal canal or have a curvature of the spine (scoliosis) that produces pressure on nerves and soft tissue and compresses or stretches ligaments. In an inherited condition called achondroplasia, defective bone formation results in abnormally short and thickened pedicles that reduce the diameter of (distance across) the spinal canal.

Acquired conditions that can cause spinal stenosis are explained in more detail in the sections that follow.

Degenerative (Aging) Conditions, Including Osteoarthritis

Spinal stenosis most often results from a gradual, degenerative aging process. Either structural changes or inflammation can begin the process. As people age, the ligaments of the spine may thicken and calcify (harden from deposits of calcium salts). Bones and joints may also enlarge, and osteophytes (bone spurs) may form. When the health of one part of the spine fails, it usually places increased stress on other parts of the spine. For example, a degenerative condition affecting the facet joints may eventually cause secondary changes, such as a herniated (bulging) disk that places pressure on the spinal cord or nerve root. When a segment of the spine becomes too mobile, the capsules (enclosing membranes) of the facet joints thicken in an effort to stabilize the segment, and bone spurs may occur. This decreases the space (neural foramen) available for nerve roots leaving the spinal cord.

Aging with secondary changes is the most common cause of spinal stenosis. Two forms of arthritis that may affect the spine are osteoarthritis and rheumatoid arthritis. Osteoarthritis is the most common form of arthritis and is more likely to occur in middle-aged and older people. It is a chronic, degenerative process that may involve multiple joints of the body. It wears away the surface cartilage layer of joints, and is often accompanied by overgrowth of bone, formation of bone spurs, and impaired function. If the degenerative change affects the facet joint(s) and the disk, the condition is sometimes referred to as spondylosis. This condition may be accompanied by disk degeneration, and an enlargement or overgrowth of bone that narrows the central and root canals.

Spondylolisthesis, a condition in which one vertebra slips forward on another, may result from a degenerative condition or an accident, or may be acquired at birth. Poor alignment of the spinal column when a vertebra slips forward onto the one below it can place pressure on the spinal cord or nerve roots at that place.

Rheumatoid Arthritis

Rheumatoid arthritis usually affects people at an earlier age than osteoarthritis does and is associated with inflammation and enlargement of the soft tissues of the joints. Although not a common cause of spinal stenosis, damage to ligaments, bones, and joints that begins as synovitis (inflammation of the synovial membrane) has a severe and disrupting effect on joint function. The portions of the vertebral column with the greatest mobility (for example, the neck area) are often the ones most affected in people with rheumatoid arthritis.

Nonarthritic Acquired Spinal Stenosis

The following conditions that are not related to arthritis or degenerative disease are causes of acquired spinal stenosis:

- *Tumors of the spine* are abnormal growths of soft tissue that may affect the spinal canal directly by inflammation or by growth of tissue into the canal. Tissue growth may lead to bone resorption (bone loss due to overactivity of certain bone cells) or displacement of bone and the eventual collapse of the supporting framework of the vertebral column.

- *Trauma* (accidents) may either dislocate the spine and the spinal canal or cause burst fractures that produce fragments of bone that penetrate the canal.

- Although surgery that involves fusion (union) of vertebrae may be skillfully performed, *tissue swelling after surgery* may place pressure on the spinal cord.

- *Paget's disease of bone* is a chronic (long-term) disorder that typically results in enlarged and deformed bones. Excessive bone breakdown and formation cause thick and fragile bone. As a result, bone pain, arthritis, noticeable deformities, and fractures can occur. The disease can affect any bone of the body, but is often found in the spine. The blood supply that feeds healthy nerve tissue may be diverted to the area of involved bone. Also, structural deformities of the involved vertebrae can cause narrowing of the spinal canal, producing a variety of neurological symptoms.

- *Fluorosis* is an excessive level of fluoride in the body. It may result from chronic inhalation of industrial dusts or gases contaminated with fluorides, prolonged ingestion of water containing large amounts of fluorides, or accidental ingestion of fluoride-containing insecticides. The condition may lead to calcified spinal ligaments or softened bones and to degenerative conditions like spinal stenosis.

What Are the Symptoms of Spinal Stenosis?

Spaces within the spine can narrow without producing any symptoms. However, if narrowing places pressure on the spinal cord or nerve roots, there may be a slow onset and progression of symptoms. The back itself may or may not hurt. More often, people experience numbness, weakness, cramping, or general pain in the legs that occurs during flexing the lower back while sitting. (The flex position opens up the spinal column, enlarging the spaces between vertebrae at the back of the spine.) If a disk between vertebrae is compressed, people may feel pain radiating down the leg (sciatica).

People with more severe stenosis may experience abnormal bowel and bladder function and foot disorders. For example, cauda equina syndrome is a partial or complete loss of control of the bowel or bladder and sometimes sexual function; it is due to compression of the collection of spinal roots that descend from the lower part of the spinal cord and occupy the vertebral canal below the cord. In very rare instances, compression above the area where the lumbar vertebrae and sacrum meet results in partial or complete paralysis of the legs.

How Is Spinal Stenosis Diagnosed?

The doctor may use a variety of approaches to diagnose spinal stenosis and rule out other conditions.

- Medical history—the patient tells the doctor details about symptoms and about any injury, condition, or general health problem that might be causing the symptoms.

- Physical examination—the doctor (1) examines the patient to determine the extent of limitation of movement; (2) checks for pain or symptoms when the patient hyperextends the spine (bends backwards); and (3) looks for the loss of extremity reflexes, which may be related to numbness or weakness in the arms or legs.

- X ray—an x-ray beam is passed through the back to produce a two-dimensional picture. An x ray may be done before other tests to look for signs of an injury, tumor, or inherited abnormality. This test can show the structure of the vertebrae and the outlines of joints, and can detect calcification.

- MRI (magnetic resonance imaging)—energy from a powerful magnet (rather than x-rays) produces signals that are detected by a scanner and analyzed by computer. This produces a series of cross-sectional images (slices) and/or a three-dimensional view of parts of the back. An MRI is particularly sensitive for detecting damage or disease of soft tissues, such as the disks between vertebrae or ligaments. It shows the spinal cord, nerve roots, and surrounding spaces, as well as enlargement, degeneration, or tumors.

- Computerized axial tomography (CAT)—x-rays are passed through the back at different angles, detected by a scanner, and analyzed by a computer. This produces a series of cross-sectional images and/or three-dimensional views of the parts of the back. The scan shows the shape and size of the spinal canal, its contents, and structures surrounding it.

- Myelogram—a liquid dye that x-rays cannot penetrate is injected into the spinal column. The dye circulates around the spinal cord and spinal nerves, which appear as white objects against bone on an x-ray film. A myelogram can show pressure on the spinal cord or nerves from herniated disks, bone spurs, or tumors.

- Bone scan—an injected radioactive material attaches itself to bone, especially in areas where bone is actively breaking down or being formed. The test can detect fractures, tumors, infections, and arthritis, but may not tell one disorder from another. Therefore, a bone scan is usually performed along with other tests.

Who Treats Spinal Stenosis?

Nonsurgical treatment of spinal stenosis may be provided by internists or general practitioners. The disorder is also treated by specialists such as rheumatologists, who treat arthritis and related disorders; and neurologists, who treat nerve diseases. Orthopaedic surgeons and neurosurgeons also provide nonsurgical treatment and perform spinal surgery if it is required. Allied health professionals such as physical therapists may also help treat patients.

What Are Some Nonsurgical Treatments for Spinal Stenosis?

In the absence of severe or progressive nerve involvement, a doctor may prescribe one or more of the following conservative treatments:

- Nonsteroidal anti-inflammatory drugs, such as aspirin, naproxen (Naprosyn), ibuprofen (Motrin, Nuprin, Advil), or indomethacin (Indocin), to reduce inflammation and relieve pain.

- Analgesics, such as acetaminophen (Tylenol), to relieve pain.

- Corticosteroid injections into the outermost of the membranes covering the spinal cord and nerve roots to reduce inflammation and treat acute pain that radiates to the hips or down a leg.

- Restricted activity (varies depending on extent of nerve involvement).

- Physical therapy and/or prescribed exercises to maintain motion of the spine and build endurance, which help stabilize the spine.

- A lumbar brace or corset to provide some support and help the patient regain mobility. This approach is sometimes used for patients with weak abdominal muscles or older patients with degeneration at several levels of the spine.

When Should Surgery Be Considered and What Is Involved?

In many cases, the conditions causing spinal stenosis cannot be permanently altered by nonsurgical treatment, even though these measures may relieve pain for a time. To determine the extent to which nonsurgical treatment will help, a doctor seldom recommends surgery during the first 3 months of treatment. However, surgery might be considered within the 3-month period if a patient experiences numbness or weakness that interferes with walking, impaired bowel or bladder function, or other neurological involvement.

The purpose of surgery is to relieve pressure on the spinal cord or nerves and restore and maintain alignment and strength of the spine. This can be done by removing, trimming, or adjusting diseased parts that are causing the pressure or loss of alignment. The most common surgery is called decompressive laminectomy: removal of the lamina (roof) of one or more vertebrae to create more space for the nerves. A surgeon may perform a laminectomy with or without fusing vertebrae or removing part of a disk. Various devices may be used to enhance fusion and strengthen unstable segments of the spine following decompression surgery.

Patients with spinal stenosis caused by spinal trauma or achondroplasia may need surgery at a young age. When surgery is required in patients with achondroplasia, laminectomy (removal of the roof) without fusion is usually sufficient.

What Are the Major Risks of Surgery?

All surgery, particularly that involving general anesthesia and older patients, carries risks. The most common complications of surgery for spinal stenosis are a tear in the membrane covering the spinal cord at the site of the operation, infection, or a blood clot that forms in the veins. These conditions can be treated but may prolong recovery.

What Are the Long-Term Outcomes of Surgical Treatment for Spinal Stenosis?

Removal of the obstruction that has caused the symptoms usually gives patients some relief; most patients have less leg pain and are able to walk better following surgery. However, if nerves were badly damaged prior to surgery, there may be some remaining pain or numbness or no improvement. Also, the degenerative process will likely continue, and pain or limitation of activity may reappear 5 or more years after surgery.

What Research on Spinal Stenosis Is Being Supported by the NIAMS?

The National Institute of Arthritis and Musculoskeletal and Skin Diseases (NIAMS) is supporting several research projects on spinal stenosis. For example, at the Multipurpose Arthritis and Musculoskeletal Disease Center at the Hospital for Special Surgery in New York City, doctors are comparing the effectiveness of injecting a steroid (cortisone-like) medicine with that of injecting an analgesic medicine into the epidura (outermost membrane covering the spinal cord) for relief of pain and disability due to spinal stenosis. In another NIAMS-funded study involving 11 different medical centers, researchers are comparing surgical versus nonsurgical treatment of spinal stenosis and two other conditions that cause back pain.

Other researchers are exploring why spinal cord changes lead to a decreased pain threshold or an increased sensitivity to pain, and how fractures of the spine and their repair affect the spinal canal and intervertebral foramen.

What Are Other Sources of Information on Spinal Stenosis?

American Academy of Orthopaedic Surgeons (AAOS)
6300 North River Road
Rosemont, IL 60018-4262
Toll-Free: (800) 824-BONE (2663)
Phone: (847) 823-7186
Fax: (847) 823-8125
Website: http://www.aaos.org
E-mail: custserv@aaos.org

North American Spine Society
22 Calendar Ct., 2nd Floor
LaGrange, IL 60525
Toll-Free Phone: (877) 774-6337
Phone: (708) 588-8080
Fax: (708) 588-1080
Website: http://www.spine.org

American College of Rheumatology
1800 Century Place, Suite 250
Atlanta, GA 30345-4300
Phone: (404) 633-3777
Fax: (404) 633-1870
Website: http://www.rheumatology.org

Arthritis Foundation
1330 West Peachtree Street
Atlanta, GA 30309
Toll-Free: (800) 283-7800
Phone: (404) 872-7100
Website: http://www.arthritis.org
E-mail: arthritis@finelinesolutions.com

Spondylitis Association of America
P.O. Box 5872
Sherman Oaks, CA 91413
Toll-Free: (800) 777-8189
Website: http://www.spondylitis.org
E-mail: info@spondylitis.org

National Institute of Arthritis and Musculoskeletal and Skin Diseases
1 AMS Circle
Bethesda, MD 20892-3675
Toll-Free: (877) 22-NIAMS (226-4267)
Phone: (301) 495-4484
TTY: (301) 565-2966
Fax: (301) 718-6366
Website: http://www.niams.nih.gov
E-mail: niamsinfo@mail.nih.gov

Chapter 44

Spinal Tumors and Cysts

Chapter Contents

Section 44.1

Facts about Spinal Tumors

"Brain and Spinal Cord Tumors—Hope Through Research" is from the National Institute of Neurological Disorders and Stroke (NINDS), July 1, 2001. Available online at http://www.ninds.nih.gov; accessed May 2004.

Introduction

The diagnosis of a brain or spinal cord tumor often comes as a shock, leaving confusion, uncertainty, fear, or even anger in its wake. After the diagnosis, a physician's explanation can fall on ears deafened by this blow. Although it cannot substitute for the advice and expertise of a physician, this information is designed to convey the latest research information on the diagnosis, course, and possible treatment of various brain and spinal cord tumors, so that patients and their families have the information they need to become active participants in their treatment.

What Are Brain and Spinal Cord Tumors?

Brain and spinal cord tumors are abnormal growths of tissue found inside the skull or the bony spinal column. The word tumor is used to describe both abnormal growths that are new (neoplasms) and those present at birth (congenital tumors). This section will focus primarily on neoplasms.

No matter where they are located in the body, tumors are usually classed as benign (or non-cancerous) if the cells that make up the growth are similar to other normal cells, grow relatively slowly, and are confined to one location. Tumors are called malignant (or cancerous) when the cells are very different from normal cells, grow relatively quickly, and can spread easily to other locations.

In most parts of the body, benign tumors are not particularly harmful. This is not necessarily true in the brain and spinal cord, which are the primary components of the central nervous system (CNS). Because the CNS is housed within rigid, bony quarters (that is, the skull and spinal column), any abnormal growth can place pressure on sensitive tissues and impair function. Also, any tumor located near vital brain structures or sensitive spinal cord nerves can seriously threaten health. If a benign tumor is found deep inside the brain, surgery to remove it may be very risky because of the chances of damaging vital brain centers. On the other hand, a benign tumor located near the brain's surface can often be removed surgically.

An important difference between malignant tumors in the CNS and those elsewhere in the body lies with their potential to spread. While malignant cells elsewhere in the body can easily seed tumors inside the brain and spinal cord, malignant CNS tumors rarely spread out to other body parts. Laboratory and clinical investigators are exploring the basis of these unusual characteristics of CNS tumors, because these unique properties may suggest new strategies to prevent or treat them.

What Causes These Tumors?

When newly formed tumors begin within the brain or spinal cord, they are called primary tumors. Primary CNS tumors rarely grow from neurons—nerve cells that perform the nervous system's important functions—because once neurons are mature they no longer divide and multiply. Instead, most tumors are caused by out-of-control growth among cells that surround and support neurons. Primary CNS tumors—such as gliomas and meningiomas—are named by the types of cells comprising them, their location, or both.

In a small number of individuals, primary tumors may result from specific genetic diseases—such as neurofibromatosis and tuberous sclerosis—or exposure to radiation or cancer-causing chemicals. Although smoking, alcohol consumption, and certain dietary habits are associated with some types of cancers, they have not been linked to primary brain and spinal cord tumors.

In fact, the cause of most primary brain and spinal cord tumors—and most cancers—remains a mystery. Scientists do not know exactly why and how cells in the nervous system or elsewhere in the body lose their normal identity as nerve, blood, skin, or other cell types and grow uncontrollably. Research scientists are looking for clues to this process with the goals of learning why and how cancer begins and developing new tools to stop it. Some of the possible causes under investigation include viruses, defective genes, and chemicals.

Metastatic tumors are caused by cancerous cells that shed from tumors in other parts of the body, travel through the bloodstream, burrow through the blood vessel walls, latch onto tissue, and spawn new tumors inside the brain or spinal cord.

For every four people who have cancer that has spread within the body, one develops metastasis within the CNS. The top two culprits that lead to these secondary CNS tumors are lung and breast cancer. Other, less frequent causes of CNS metastases include kidney (renal) cancer, lymphoma (a cancer affecting immune cells), prostate cancer, and melanoma, a form of skin cancer.

Brain and spinal cord tumors are not contagious or, at this time, preventable.

How Many People Have These Tumors?

Research studies suggest that new brain tumors arise in more than 40,000 Americans each year. About half of these tumors are primary, and the remainder are metastatic.

Individuals of any age can develop a brain tumor. In fact, they are the second most common cause of cancer-related death in people up to the age of 35, with a slight peak in occurrence among children between the ages of 6 and 9. However, brain tumors are most common among middle-aged and older adults. People in their 60s face the highest risk—each year 1 of every 5,000 people in this age group develops a brain tumor.

Spinal cord tumors are less common than brain tumors. About 10,000 Americans develop primary or metastatic spinal cord tumors each year. Although spinal cord tumors affect people of all ages, they are most common in young and middle-aged adults.

By studying the epidemiology of CNS tumors, scientists can learn if different tumors are more common at certain ages or in certain people. This information, in turn, may reveal environmental factors that are linked to tumors, connections between tumors and other disorders, or patterns of tumor occurrence, all of which offer clues about why tumors develop.

What Are the Symptoms?

Brain and spinal cord tumors cause many diverse symptoms, which can make detection tricky. Whatever specific symptoms a patient has, the symptoms generally develop slowly and worsen over time.

Brain Tumors

A 3.5-pound wrinkled mass of tissue, the brain orchestrates behavior, movement, feeling, and sensation. It controls automatic functions like breathing and heartbeat. Many of these important functions are controlled by specialized brain areas. For example, the brain's left and right hemispheres jointly control hearing and vision; the front part of each hemisphere controls voluntary movements, like writing, for the opposite side of the body; and the brain stem is responsible for basic life-sustaining functions, including blood pressure, heartbeat, and breathing.

As a result, brain tumors can cause a bewildering array of symptoms depending on their size, type, and location. Certain symptoms are quite specific because they result from damage to particular brain areas. Other, more general symptoms are triggered by increased pressure within the skull as the growing tumor encroaches on the brain's limited space or blocks the flow of cerebrospinal fluid (fluid that bathes the brain and spinal cord). Some of the more common symptoms of a brain tumor include:

- **Headaches.** More than half of people with brain tumors experience headaches. Because the skull cannot expand, the growing mass places pressure on pain-sensitive areas. The headaches recur, often at irregular periods, and can last several minutes or hours. They may worsen when coughing, changing posture, or straining. As the tumor grows, headaches often last longer, become more frequent, and grow more severe.

- **Seizures.** The abnormal tissue found in a brain tumor can disrupt the normal flow of electricity through which brain cells communicate. The resulting bursts of electrical activity cause seizures with a variety of symptoms, such as convulsions, loss of consciousness, or loss of bladder control. Seizures that first start in adulthood (in a patient who has not been in an accident or had an illness that causes seizures) are a key warning sign of brain tumors. Sometimes, seizures are the only sign of a slowly growing brain tumor.

- **Nausea and vomiting.** Increased pressure within the skull can cause nausea and vomiting. These symptoms sometimes accompany headaches.

- **Vision or hearing problems.** Increased intracranial pressure can also decrease blood flow in the eye and trigger swelling of the optic nerve, which in turn causes blurred vision, double vision, or partial visual loss. Tumors growing on or near sensory nerves often trigger visual or hearing disturbances, such as ringing or buzzing sounds, abnormal eye movements or crossed eyes, and partial or total loss of vision or hearing. Tumors that grow in the brain's occipital lobe, which interprets visual images, may also cause partial vision loss.

- **Behavioral and cognitive symptoms.** Because they strike at the core of the individual's identity, changes in behavior and personality can be the most frightening and devastating symptoms of a brain tumor. These symptoms usually occur when the tumor is located in the brain's cerebral hemispheres, which are responsible, in part, for personality, communication, thinking, behavior, and other vital functions. Examples include problems with speech, language, thinking, and memory, or psychotic episodes and changes in personality.

- **Motor problems.** When tumors affect brain areas responsible for command of body movement, they can cause motor symptoms, including weakness or paralysis, lack of coordination, or trouble with walking. Often, muscle weakness or paralysis affects only one side of the body.

- **Balance problems.** Brain tumors that disrupt the normal control of equilibrium can cause dizziness or difficulty with balance.

Spinal Cord Tumors

The spinal cord is, in part, like a living telephone cable. Lying protected inside the bony spine, it contains bundles of nerves that carry messages between the brain and the body's nerves, such as instructions from the brain to move an arm or information from the skin that signals pain.

A tumor that forms on or near the spinal cord can disrupt this communication. Often, these tumors exert pressure on the spinal cord or the nerves that exit from it; sometimes, they restrict the cord's supply of blood. Common symptoms that result from this include:

- **Pain.** Normally, the spinal cord carries important warnings about pain from the body's nerves to the brain. By putting pressure on the spinal cord, a tumor can trigger these circuits and cause pain that feels as if it is coming from various parts of the body. This pain is often constant, sometimes severe, and can have a burning or aching quality.

- **Sensory changes.** Many people with spinal cord tumors suffer a loss of sensation. This usually takes the form of numbness and decreased skin sensitivity to temperature.

- **Motor problems.** Since the nerves control the muscles, tumors that affect nerve communication can trigger a number of muscle-related symptoms. Early symptoms include muscle weakness; spasticity in which the muscles stay stiffly contracted; and impaired bladder and/or bowel control. If untreated, symptoms may worsen to include muscle wasting and paralysis. In addition, some people develop an abnormal walking rhythm known as ataxia.

The parts of the body affected by these symptoms vary with tumor location along the spinal cord. In general, symptoms strike body areas at the same level or at a level below that of the tumor. For example, a tumor midway along the spinal cord (in the thoracic spine) can cause pain that spreads over the chest in a girdle-shaped pattern and gets worse when the individual coughs, sneezes, or lies down. A tumor that grows in the top fourth of the spinal column (or cervical spine) can cause pain that seems to come from the neck or arms. And a tumor that grows in the lower spine (or lumbar spine) can trigger back or leg pain.

In some cases, one or more tumors extend over several sections of the spinal cord. This results in symptoms that are spread over various parts of the body. Sometimes sensory symptoms occur in a patchy, confusing pattern in which some parts of the body are unaffected even though they lie between affected areas.

Doctors divide spinal cord tumors into three major groups based on where they are found. Extradural tumors grow between the bony spinal canal and the tough membrane called dura mater that protects the spinal cord. Tumors inside the dura (intradural tumors) are further divided into those outside the spinal cord (extramedullary tumors) and those inside the spinal cord (intramedullary tumors).

How Are CNS Tumors Diagnosed?

Research has made major strides in the ability to detect and diagnose CNS tumors. When a doctor suspects a brain or spinal cord tumor because of a patient's medical history and symptoms, he or she can turn to a number of specialized tests and techniques to confirm the diagnosis. However, the first test is often a traditional neurological exam. A neurological exam checks:

Eye movement, eye reflexes, and pupil reaction. For example, the doctor can shine a pen light into the eye to see if the pupil contracts normally or ask the patient to follow a moving object, such as a finger.

- **Reflexes.** Tests like tapping below the knee with a rubber hammer can identify changes in reflexes.

- **Hearing.** Using a tuning fork, the physician can check for changes in hearing.

- **Sensation.** The doctor can use something sharp like a pin to test the sense of touch.

- **Movement.** Problems with movement are often tested by asking the patient to move his or her tongue, head, or facial muscles—as in smiling—and to perform tasks with the arms and legs.

- **Balance and coordination.** Typical tests include maintaining balance with the eyes closed, walking heel-to-toe in a straight line, or touching the nose with the eyes closed.

The next step in diagnosing brain tumors often involves x-rays or special imaging techniques and laboratory tests that can detect the presence of a tumor and provide clues about its location and type.

Imaging and X-rays

Special imaging techniques developed through recent research, especially computed tomography (CT) and magnetic resonance imaging (MRI), have dramatically improved the diagnosis of CNS tumors in recent years. In many cases, these scans can detect the presence of a tumor even if it is less than half an inch across.

CT uses a sophisticated x-ray machine and a computer to create a detailed picture of the body's tissues and structures. Often, doctors will inject a special dye into the patient before performing a CT scan. The dye, also called contrast material, makes it easier to see abnormal tissue. A CT scan often gives doctors a good idea of where the tumor is located in the brain or spinal cord and can sometimes help them determine the tumor's type. It can also help doctors detect swelling, bleeding, and other associated conditions. In addition, CT scans can help doctors check the results of treatment and watch for tumor recurrence.

MRI uses a magnetic field and radio waves, rather than x-rays, and can often distinguish accurately between healthy and diseased tissue. MRI gives better pictures of tumors located near bone than CT, does not use radiation as CT does, and provides pictures from various angles that can enable doctors to construct a three-dimensional image of the tumor.

A third imaging technique called positron emission tomography (PET) provides a picture of brain activity rather than structure by measuring levels of injected glucose (sugar) that has been labeled with a radioactive tracer. Glucose is used by the brain for energy. Detectors placed around the head can spot the labeled glucose, and a computer uses the pattern of glucose distribution to form an image of the brain. Since malignant tissue uses more glucose than normal, it usually shows up on the scan as brighter or lighter than surrounding tissue. Currently, PET is not widely used in tumor diagnosis, in part because the technique requires very elaborate, expensive equipment, including a cyclotron to create the radioactive glucose.

Although it is not widely used for diagnosis now that CT and MRI scans are possible, angiography continues to help doctors distinguish certain types of brain tumors and make decisions about surgery. In angiography, doctors inject dye into a major blood vessel, usually one of the large arteries in the neck. This dye deflects x-rays and makes it possible for doctors to see the network of blood vessels by taking a series of x-ray pictures as the dye flows through the brain. Since some tumors have a characteristic pattern of blood vessels and blood flow, the pictures can provide clues about the tumor's type. Information from angiography can also tell physicians if a tumor is located close to important, normal blood vessels that must be avoided during surgery.

Widespread use of CT and MRI has largely displaced use of traditional x-rays for diagnosis of brain and spinal cord tumors, since x-rays do not provide very useful images of brain tissue. They are occasionally helpful when tumors cause changes in the skull or spinal cord or when they contain tiny deposits of bone-like material made of calcium.

Physicians may also use a specialized x-ray technique, called a myelogram, when diagnosing spinal cord tumors. In myelography, a special dye that absorbs x-rays is injected into the spinal cord. This dye outlines the spinal cord but will not pass through a tumor. The resulting x-ray picture shows a dark area or narrowing that reveals the tumor's location.

Laboratory Tests

Laboratory tests commonly used include the electroencephalogram (or EEG) in patients whose tumors cause epilepsy and lumbar puncture, also known as the spinal tap. The EEG uses special patches placed on the scalp or fine needles placed in the brain to record abnormal electrical currents inside the brain.

In lumbar puncture, doctors obtain a small sample of cerebrospinal fluid. This fluid can be examined for abnormal cells or unusual levels of various compounds that suggest a brain or spinal cord tumor.

In the future, diagnosis of brain tumors should grow more accurate as additional techniques—including new ways to image the CNS and advanced laboratory tests—are developed through basic laboratory studies and clinical research.

What Is a Biopsy and How Is It Used?

A biopsy is a surgical procedure in which a small sample of tissue is taken from the suspected tumor, often during surgery aimed at removing as much tumor as possible.

A biopsy gives doctors the clues they need to specifically diagnose the type of tumor. By examining the sample under a microscope, the pathologist—a physician who specializes in understanding how disease affects the body's tissues—can tell what kinds of cells are in a tumor. Pathologists also look carefully for certain changes that signal cancer. These signs include abnormal growths or changes in the cell membranes and telltale problems in the cell nuclei, which normally control cell characteristics and growth. For example, cancerous cells may grow small finger-like projections on their normally smooth surface or have extra nuclei.

Using this information, the pathologist provides a diagnosis of the tumor type. The tumor may also be classified as benign or malignant and given a numbered score that reflects how malignant it is. This score can help doctors determine how to treat a tumor and predict the likely outcome, or prognosis, for the patient.

Although biopsy has long been a mainstay of brain tumor diagnosis, it is still an important research area. Scientists continue to look for better ways to identify and classify types of abnormal cells in order to improve the accuracy of prognosis and provide the best possible information for treatment decisions.

How Are Brain and Spinal Cord Tumors Treated?

The three most commonly used treatments—surgery, radiation, and chemotherapy—are largely the result of recent research. For some patients, doctors may suggest a new treatment still being tested. In any case, the doctor will recommend a treatment or a combination of treatments based on the tumor's location and type, any previous treatment the patient may have received, and the patient's medical history and general health.

Surgery

Surgery to remove as much tumor as possible is usually the first step in treating an accessible tumor—that is, a tumor that can be removed without unacceptable risk of neurological damage. Fortunately, research has led to advances in neurosurgery that make it possible for doctors to reach many tumors that were previously considered inaccessible. These new techniques and tools equip neurosurgeons to operate in the tight, vulnerable confines of the CNS. Some recently developed approaches in use in the operating room include:

- **Microsurgery.** In this widely used technique, the surgeon looks through a high-powered microscope to get a magnified view of the operating area. This makes it easier to see—and remove—tumor tissue while sparing surrounding healthy tissue.

- **Stereotaxic procedures.** In these procedures, a computer uses information from CT or MRI to create a three-dimensional map of the operation site. The computer uses the map to help the surgeon guide special, computer-assisted tools. This makes it possible for surgeons to approach certain difficult-to-reach tumors with greater precision. Many procedures can be performed using this approach, including biopsy, certain types of surgery, and planting radiation pellets in a tumor.

- **Ultrasonic aspirators.** Ultrasonic aspirators use sound waves to vibrate tumors and break them up. Like a vacuum, the aspirator then sucks up the tumor fragments.

- **Evoked potentials.** Doctors use this test during surgery to determine the role of specific nerves and thus avoid damage. In this technique, small electrodes are used to stimulate a nerve so its electrical response, or evoked potential, can be measured.

• **Shunts.** Shunts are flexible tubes used to reroute and drain fluid. Doctors sometimes insert a shunt into the brain when a tumor blocks the flow of cerebrospinal fluid and causes hydrocephalus. Shunting of the fluid can relieve headaches, nausea, and other symptoms caused by too much pressure inside the skull.

Surgery may be the beginning and end of treatment if the biopsy shows a benign tumor. If the tumor is malignant, however, doctors often recommend additional treatment following surgery, including radiation, chemotherapy, or experimental treatments.

An inaccessible or inoperable tumor is one that cannot be removed surgically because of the risk of severe nervous system damage. These tumors are frequently located deep within the brain or near vital structures such as the brain stem—the part of the brain that controls many crucial functions including breathing and heart rate. Malignant, multiple tumors may also be inoperable. Doctors treat most malignant, inaccessible, or inoperable CNS tumors with radiation and/or chemotherapy.

Among patients who have metastatic CNS tumors, doctors usually focus on treating the original cancer first. However, when a metastatic tumor causes serious disability or pain, doctors may recommend surgery or other treatments to reduce symptoms even if the original cancer has not been controlled.

Radiation Therapy

In radiation therapy, the tumor is bombarded with beams of energy that kill tumor cells. Traditional radiation therapy delivers radiation from outside the patient's body, usually begins a week or two after surgery, and continues for about 6 weeks. The dosage is fairly uniform throughout the treated areas, making it especially useful for tumors that are large or have infiltrated into surrounding tissue.

However, when traditional radiation therapy is given to the brain, it may also cause damage to healthy tissue. Depending on the type of tumor, doctors may be able to choose a modified form of radiation therapy to help prevent this and to improve the effectiveness of treatment. Modifying therapy can be as simple as changing the dosage schedule and amount of radiation that a patient receives. For example, an approach called hyperfractionation uses smaller, more frequent doses. Neurological investigators are also testing several other, more complex techniques to improve radiation therapy.

Chemotherapy

Chemotherapy uses tumor-killing drugs that are given orally or injected into the bloodstream. Because not all tumors are vulnerable to the same anticancer drugs, doctors often use a combination of drugs for chemotherapy.

Chemotherapeutic drugs generally kill cells that are growing or dividing. This property makes them more deadly to malignant tissue, which contains a high proportion of growing and dividing cells, than to most normal cells. It also causes some of the side effects that can accompany chemotherapy—such as skin reactions, hair loss, or digestive problems—because a high proportion of these normal cell types are also growing and dividing at any given time. The drugs most commonly used for CNS tumors are known by the initials BCNU (sometimes called carmustine) and CCNU (or lomustine). Research scientists are also testing many promising drugs to learn if they can improve treatment for brain and spinal cord tumors and reduce side effects.

Other Drugs

Tumors, surgery, and radiation therapy can all result in swelling inside the CNS. Doctors may prescribe steroids for short or long periods to reduce this swelling. Examples of such drugs include dexamethasone, methylprednisolone, and prednisone.

Whether new treatment approaches involve surgery, radiation therapy, chemotherapy, or completely new avenues to treating CNS tumors, carefully planned clinical trials of new and experimental therapies are vital for identifying promising treatments and learning the best applications of current therapies. Experimental treatments, in turn, would not be possible without research by basic and clinical scientists who identify new approaches.

Where Should Patients Go for Treatment?

Brain and spinal cord tumors are often difficult to diagnose, and surgery to remove them demands great skill. Experience, therefore, is probably the most important factor in choosing among physicians. Brain and spinal cord tumors are also relatively rare. Many physicians see only a few patients with CNS tumors each year. Others, however, have made treating brain and spinal cord tumors their specialty. Patients should consider how many patients a physician treats each year. Because many patients are understandably perplexed or frightened by a CNS tumor diagnosis, it is also important that they choose a physician who will answer questions and describe treatment options clearly and fully.

Patients should also learn what techniques and tools are available at the physician's hospital. Teaching hospitals affiliated with a medical college or university are more likely to be involved in research and, thus, have the equipment and specialists necessary to offer experimental treatments. Finally, if a patient is dissatisfied with a physician or a physician's recommendations, he or she may wish to seek another opinion.

What Research Is Being Done?

Scientists are attacking CNS tumors through biomedical research to improve medical understanding and treatment. CNS tumor research ranges from bench-side studies on the origins and characteristics of tumors to bedside studies that test new tumor-killing drugs and other innovative treatments. Much of this work is supported by the National Institute of Neurological Disorders and Stroke (NINDS) and by the National Cancer Institute (NCI), as well as other agencies within the Federal Government, non-profit groups, and private institutions.

Some key areas of brain tumor research include:

- **Radiosurgery.** In radiosurgery, computerized localization techniques permit delivery of a very large dose of radiation to a well-defined, precisely targeted region. This technique can deliver a large dose of radiation to the tumor while minimizing radiation of normal tissue. Through research, scientists thus far have found that radiosurgery is most useful for small tumors that do not invade the brain and that are difficult to remove surgically. Research scientists continue to examine whether this technique can help patients with other tumor types as well.

- **Drugs and techniques for chemotherapy.** Dozens of new chemotherapeutic drugs are in various stages of development. Scientists are testing these drugs in animals and patients to determine what side effects they cause, what doses are appropriate, and whether they can improve survival and recovery. Patients interested in up-to-date information on current trials are encouraged to contact the resources listed on the pocket card at the end of the brochure.

Scientists are also working to overcome an obstacle to effective chemotherapy for brain and spinal cord tumors—the blood-brain barrier. The blood-brain barrier—an elaborate meshwork of fine blood vessels and cells that filters blood reaching the CNS—normally helps protect the sensitive tissues of the CNS from potentially dangerous compounds in the bloodstream and changes in its environment. But the blood-brain barrier also stymies many efforts to deliver anticancer drugs that may help patients with CNS tumors. Investigators are testing drugs that may help open the barrier. If these drugs prove useful and safe in animal models and humans, then physicians would be equipped to test promising anticancer drugs that normally cannot cross the blood-brain barrier.

Another experimental path aimed at improving drug delivery into the CNS is called interstitial chemotherapy. With this technique a slow infusion into the interstitial spaces of the tumor permits delivery of large molecules to the tumor. In another technique, doctors place disc-shaped specially designed polymers, wafers soaked with chemotherapeutic drugs, directly into tumor tissue. These techniques may help physicians increase the dose of life-prolonging drugs while limiting side effects—since less of the drug spreads elsewhere in the body. Most trials of these techniques currently involve patients with recurrent gliomas.

- **Drugs to improve radiation therapy.** Many scientists are testing the usefulness of drugs known as radiosensitizers that make tumor tissue more vulnerable to radiation. Early results with the two most commonly studied radiosensitizers, metronidazole and misonidazole, have been mixed; some trials suggest these drugs may improve survival in certain patients, while other trials have shown little benefit.

- **Gamma knife.** The gamma knife, used for a procedure known technically as stereotactic gamma knife radiosurgery, combines precise stereotactic guidance and a sharply focused beam of radiation energy to deliver a single, precise dose of radiation. Despite its name, the gamma knife does not require a surgical incision. Investigators using this tool have found it can help

383

them reach and treat some small tumors that are not accessible through surgery.

- **Gene therapy.** Gene therapy, an innovative approach to treating CNS cancer, is in the early stages of research in laboratories around the country. Genes are the blueprints the body's cells use to make proteins and other vital substances. In gene therapy, scientists insert a new gene into specific cells. In the case of gene therapy for brain tumors, this inserted gene could make the tumor cells sensitive to certain drugs, program the cancerous cells to self-destruct, or instruct them to manufacture substances that would slow their growth. Scientists are using tumor cells and animal models to learn how various genes, once introduced, hinder cancer growth and to identify the best methods for inserting new genes into tumor cells.

- **Hyperthermia.** Tumors are more sensitive to heat than normal tissue, partly because they have less blood flow to cool them. Research scientists testing hyperthermia take advantage of this sensitivity by placing special heat-producing antennae into the tumor region after surgery. Most often, these antennae send out microwaves that raise the temperature in nearby tissues. Hyperthermia is a new treatment for tumors in the brain, and scientists are still testing its effectiveness. They are also looking at heat sources that may be more effective than microwaves, including electromagnetic energy and radiofrequencies.

- **Immunotherapy.** The body's immune system normally seeks out and destroys foreign tissue such as cancerous cells by detecting antigens, telltale proteins found on foreign cells that alert the body to the foreign cells' presence. Stimulated by the antigens, the body manufactures a variety of immune cells and special proteins called antibodies. These antibodies then latch onto the antigens, working as tiny flags that alert immune cells to attack and destroy the foreign cells. In immunotherapy—an exciting and very new field of CNS tumor research—scientists are looking for ways to duplicate or enhance the body's immune response to fight against brain and spinal cord cancer.

Some scientists are testing the effectiveness of giving the body's immune system a general boost. Much like the way coffee can stimulate the nervous system, certain naturally occurring body chemicals trigger immune cells to grow and divide. In numerous studies, researchers have supplied patients with extra amounts of immune stimulants, such as interleukin-2, in the hope that they will improve the body's ability to fight CNS cancer. However, this technique has produced mixed results. A second type of general immunotherapy involves removing immune cells from a patient, growing and activating these cells and then returning them to the patient where they can work against the cancer. This approach has also yielded mixed results.

Another, still more recent approach in immunotherapy research specifically targets tumor cells using monoclonal antibodies. Like duplicate keys for the same lock, monoclonal antibodies are multiple copies of a single antibody; they fit one—and only one—antigen. Scientists are now producing monoclonal antibodies against tumor cell antigens and testing their usefulness. For example, scientists at the NINDS and elsewhere are linking these antibodies to toxins that can kill tumor cells. The armed monoclonal antibodies then function like guided missiles; they seek out the tumor cells with a matching antigen, bind to these tumor cells, and deliver their toxin. Early experiments with this therapy suggest it has more promise for treating widespread cancer cells than solid tumors. Studies are underway to corroborate these early results and to learn if this therapy has promise for other types of CNS tumors. Monoclonal antibodies may also prove helpful in improving brain tumor diagnosis, because they can be attached to special tracers to make tumor cells more visible.

- **Intraoperative ultrasound.** This technique, which uses sound waves, provides the surgeon with an image of brain tissues during the operation. Ultrasound is less expensive and complex than other imaging techniques. Some scientists conducting research on intraoperative ultrasound have found the technique makes it easier for the surgeon to locate the outer edges of tumor tissue, which can be hard to find. Thus, this technique may help improve tumor surgery by increasing the amount of tumor that can be safely removed.

- **Oncogenes.** The body contains a number of genes that are important in normal cell growth and development. Changes in some of these genes—which might be triggered by such events as exposure to chemicals or radiation—can transform them into dangerous, cancer-causing oncogenes. A number of oncogenes have already been found, and scientists continue to look for more. They are also working to identify specific events that can create oncogenes and to learn if there may be ways to prevent oncogenes from forming or to impair oncogene function in cancerous cells.

- **PET.** Based on recent research, some scientists believe that PET scans offer important clues for diagnosis of brain tumors. For example, physicians sometimes have trouble detecting recurrent tumors with CT or MRI scans. Recent studies have shown that PET may make it easier to detect recurrent brain tumors. Scientists are also examining whether PET can help physicians tell the difference between benign and malignant tumors before performing a biopsy or surgery.

- **Physiological mapping.** Mapping brain functions has promise for improving the safety and effectiveness of brain tumor surgery, particularly when the tumor lies in or next to in critical brain regions. In physiological mapping, the physician locates brain areas responsible for key functions, such as language or sensation. The surgeon then has a map to help avoid these critical areas, thus reducing the chance of serious complications.

- **Photodynamic therapy.** Photodynamic therapy uses drugs that collect in tumor cells and can be turned on or activated by special light. The drugs may be given by injection or placed directly into the tumor during an initial surgery. In order to activate the tumor-killing drug, the physician must expose the tumor tissue to light during surgery. Thus far, this technique has been found useful only for small amounts of tumor tissue, although researchers continue the search for new light-sensitive drugs and better light sources that can penetrate tumors.

- **Tumor growth factors.** Cancerous tumors are often rich in an array of substances, called growth factors, that enable them to grow and spread rapidly. In recent years, scientists have identified a number of these factors, including one that triggers growth of nerve tissue and another that stimulates blood vessels to grow. Many investigators continue the search for more such factors. Meanwhile, other researchers have begun testing antibodies that can block these factors. Early results in animals have shown that blocking growth factors with antibodies may help slow tumor growth, suggesting this research arena could lead to new therapies for brain tumors.

Although many new approaches to treatment thus appear promising, it is important to remember that all potential therapies must stand the tests of well-designed, carefully controlled clinical trials and long-term follow-up of treated patients before any conclusions can be drawn about their safety or effectiveness. Past research has led to improved tumor treatments and techniques, providing longer survival and richer lives for many CNS tumor patients.

Current research promises to generate further improvements. In the years ahead, physicians and patients can look forward to new forms of therapy developed through an understanding of the unique traits of CNS tumors.

Where Can I Find More Information?

The National Institute of Neurological Disorders and Stroke, a component of the National Institutes of Health, is the leading federal supporter of research on brain and nervous system disorders. The Institute also sponsors an active public information program that offers information about diagnosis, treatment, and research on painful neurological disorders.

For information on other neurological disorders or research programs funded by the National Institute of Neurological Disorders and Stroke, contact the Institute's Brain Resources and Information Network (BRAIN) at:

BRAIN
P.O. Box 5801
Bethesda, MD 20824
Toll-Free: (800) 352-9424
Phone: (301) 496-5751
Website: http://www.ninds.nih.gov

Section 44.2

Syringomyelia

"Syringomyelia Fact Sheet" is from the National Institute of Neurological Disorders and Stroke (NINDS), July 1, 2001. Available online at http://www.ninds.nih.gov; accessed May 2004.

What Is Syringomyelia?

Syringomyelia is a disorder in which a cyst forms within the spinal cord. This cyst, called a syrinx, expands and elongates over time, destroying the center of the spinal cord. Since the spinal cord connects the brain to nerves in the extremities, this damage results in pain, weakness, and stiffness in the back, shoulders, arms, or legs. Other symptoms may include headaches and a loss of the ability to feel extremes of hot or cold, especially in the hands. Each patient experiences a different combination of symptoms.

Other, more common disorders share the early symptoms of syringomyelia. In the past, this has made diagnosis difficult. The advent of one outpatient test, however, called magnetic resonance imaging (MRI), has significantly increased the number of syringomyelia cases diagnosed in the beginning stages of the disorder.

About 21,000 American men and women have syringomyelia, with symptoms usually beginning in young adulthood. Signs of the disorder tend to develop slowly, although sudden onset may occur with coughing or straining. If not treated surgically, syringomyelia often leads to progressive weakness in the arms and legs, loss of hand sensation, and chronic, severe pain.

What Causes Syringomyelia?

A watery, protective substance known as cerebrospinal fluid normally flows around the spinal cord and brain, transporting nutrients and waste products. It also serves to cushion the brain.

A number of medical conditions can cause an obstruction in the normal flow of cerebrospinal fluid, redirecting it into the spinal cord itself. For reasons that are only now becoming clear, this results in syrinx formation. Cerebrospinal fluid fills the syrinx. Pressure differences along the spine cause the fluid to move within the cyst. Physicians believe that it is this continual movement of fluid that results in cyst growth and further damage to the spinal cord.

What Are the Different Forms of Syringomyelia?

Generally, there are two forms of syringomyelia. In most cases, the disorder is related to an abnormality of the brain called a Chiari I malformation, named after the physician who first characterized it. This anatomic abnormality causes the lower part of the cerebellum to protrude from its normal location in the back of the head into the cervical or neck portion of the spinal canal. A syrinx may then develop in the cervical region of the spinal cord. Because of the relationship that was once thought to exist between the brain and spinal cord in this type of syringomyelia, physicians sometimes refer to it as communicating syringomyelia. Here, symptoms usually begin between the ages of 25 and 40 and may worsen with straining or any activity that causes cerebrospinal fluid pressure to fluctuate suddenly. Some patients, however, may have long periods of stability. Some patients with this form of the disorder also have hydrocephalus, in which cerebrospinal fluid accumulates in the skull, or a condition called arachnoiditis, in which a covering of the spinal cord—the arachnoid membrane—is inflamed.

The second major form of syringomyelia occurs as a complication of trauma, meningitis, hemorrhage, a tumor, or arachnoiditis. Here, the syrinx or cyst develops in a segment of the spinal cord damaged by one of these conditions. The syrinx then starts to expand. This is sometimes referred to as noncommunicating syringomyelia. Symptoms may appear months or even years after the initial injury, starting with pain, weakness, and sensory impairment originating at the site of trauma.

The primary symptom of post-traumatic syringomyelia is pain, which may spread upward from the site of injury. Symptoms, such as pain, numbness, weakness, and disruption in temperature sensation, may be limited to one side of the body. Syringomyelia can also adversely affect sweating, sexual function, and, later, bladder and bowel control.

Some cases of syringomyelia are familial, although this is rare. In addition, one form of the disorder involves a part of the brain called the brainstem. The brainstem controls many of our vital functions, such as respiration and heartbeat. When syrinxes affect the brainstem, the condition is called syringobulbia.

How Is Syringomyelia Diagnosed?

Physicians now use magnetic resonance imaging (MRI) to diagnose syringomyelia. The MR imager takes pictures of body structures, such as the brain and spinal cord, in vivid detail. This test will show the syrinx in the spine or any other conditions, such as the presence of a tumor. MRI is safe, painless, and informative and has greatly improved the diagnosis of syringomyelia.

The physician may order additional tests to help confirm the diagnosis. One of these is called electromyography (EMG), which measures muscle weakness. The doctor may also wish to test cerebrospinal fluid pressure levels and to analyze the cerebrospinal fluid by performing a lumbar puncture. In addition, computed tomography (CT) scans of a patient's head may reveal the presence of tumors and other abnormalities such as hydrocephalus.

Like MRI and CT scans, another test, called a myelogram, takes x-ray-like pictures and requires a contrast medium or dye to do so. Since the introduction of MRI this test is rarely necessary to diagnose syringomyelia.

How Is Syringomyelia Treated?

Surgery is usually recommended for syringomyelia patients. The main goal of surgery is to provide more space for the cerebellum (Chiari malformation) at the base of the skull and upper neck, without entering the brain or spinal cord. This results in flattening or disappearance of the primary cavity. If a tumor is causing syringomyelia, removal of the tumor is the treatment of choice and almost always eliminates the syrinx.

Surgery results in stabilization or modest improvement in symptoms for most patients. Delay in treatment may result in irreversible spinal cord injury. Recurrence of syringomyelia after surgery may make additional operations necessary; these may not be completely successful over the long term.

In some patients it may be necessary to drain the syrinx, which can be accomplished using a catheter, drainage tubes, and valves. This system is also known as a shunt. Shunts are used in both the communicating and noncommunicating forms of the disorder. First, the surgeon must locate the syrinx. Then, the shunt is placed into it with the other end draining cerebrospinal fluid into a cavity, usually the abdomen. This type of shunt is called a ventriculoperitoneal shunt and is used in cases involving hydrocephalus. By draining syrinx fluid, a shunt can arrest the progression of symptoms and relieve pain, headache, and tightness. Without correction, symptoms generally continue.

The decision to use a shunt requires extensive discussion between doctor and patient, as this procedure carries with it the risk of injury to the spinal cord, infection, blockage, or hemorrhage and may not necessarily work for all patients.

In the case of trauma-related syringomyelia, the surgeon operates at the level of the initial injury. The cyst collapses at surgery but a tube or shunt is usually necessary to prevent re-expansion.

Drugs have no curative value as a treatment for syringomyelia. Radiation is used rarely and is of little benefit except in the presence of a tumor. In these cases, it can halt the extension of a cavity and may help to alleviate pain.

In the absence of symptoms, syringomyelia is usually not treated. In addition, a physician may recommend not treating the condition in patients of advanced age or in cases where there is no progression of symptoms. Whether treated or not, many patients will be told to avoid activities that involve straining.

What Research Is Being Done?

The precise causes of syringomyelia are still unknown. Scientists at the National Institute of Neurological Disorders and Stroke in Bethesda, Maryland, and at grantee institutions across the country continue to explore the mechanisms that lead to the formation of syrinxes in the spinal cord. For instance, Institute investigators have found that as the heart beats, the syrinx fluid is abruptly forced downward. They have also demonstrated the presence of a block to the free flow of cerebrospinal fluid that normally occurs in and out of the head during each heartbeat.

Surgical techniques are also being refined by the neurosurgical research community. In one treatment approach currently being evaluated, neurosurgeons perform a decompressive procedure where the dura mater, a tough membrane covering the cerebellum and spinal cord, is enlarged with a graft. Like altering a suit of clothing, this procedure expands the area around the cerebellum and spinal cord, thus improving the flow of cerebrospinal fluid and eliminating the syrinx.

It is also important to understand the role of birth defects in the development of hindbrain malformations that can lead to syringomyelia.

Learning when these defects occur during the development of the fetus can help us understand this and similar disorders, and may lead to preventive treatment that can stop the formation of many birth abnormalities. Dietary supplements of folic acid during pregnancy have already been found to reduce the number of cases of certain birth defects.

Diagnostic technology is another area for continued research. Already, MRI has enabled scientists to see conditions in the spine, including syringomyelia, even before symptoms appear. A new technology, known as dynamic MRI, allows investigators to view spinal fluid pulsating within the syrinx. CT scans allow physicians to see abnormalities in the brain, and other diagnostic tests have also improved greatly with the availability of new, non-toxic, contrast dyes. Patients can expect even better techniques to become available in the future from the research efforts of scientists today.

Where Can I Go for More Information?

For information on other neurological disorders or research programs funded by the National Institute of Neurological Disorders and Stroke, contact the Institute's Brain Resources and Information Network (BRAIN) at:

BRAIN
P.O. Box 5801
Bethesda, MD 20824
Toll-Free: (800) 352-9424
Phone: (301) 496-5751
Website: http://www.ninds.nih.gov

The organization listed below provides printed information and assistance to syringomyelia patients and other interested individuals.

American Syringomyelia Alliance Project
P.O. Box 1586
Longview, TX 75606-1586
Phone: (903) 236-7079
Fax: (903) 757-7456
Toll-Free: (800) 272-7282
Website: http://www.asap.org
E-mail: info@asap.org

Several lay organizations are directly concerned with chronic pain. They are excellent sources of additional information, research updates, and specific help and referrals:

National Chronic Pain Outreach Association, Inc.
7979 Old Georgetown Road, Suite 100
Bethesda, MD 20814-2429
Phone: (301) 652-4948
Fax: (301) 907-0745
Website: http://neurosurgery.mgh.harvard.edu/ncpainoa.htm

American Chronic Pain Association
P.O. Box 850
Rocklin, CA 95677
Toll-Free: (800) 533-3231
Phone: (916) 632-0922
Fax: (916) 632-3208
Website: http://www.theacpa.org
E-mail: ACPA@pacbell.net

The following national organizations are concerned with research, care, and treatment of spinal cord injury and other paralyzing or disabling conditions, and are sources of information, publications, and advice:

Christopher Reeve Paralysis Foundation/ Paralysis Resource Center
500 Morris Avenue
Springfield, NJ 07081
Toll-Free: (800) 539-7309
Phone: (973) 379-2690
Fax: (973) 912-9433
Website: http://www.christopherreeve.org
E-mail: info@crpf.org

National Spinal Cord Injury Association
6701 Democracy Blvd. #300-9
Bethesda, MD 20817
Toll-Free: (800) 962-9629
Phone: (301) 214-4006
Fax: (301) 881-9817
Website: http://www.spinalcord.org
E-mail: info@spinalcord.org

Paralyzed Veterans of America (PVA)
801 18th Street, NW
Washington, DC 20006-3517
Toll-Free: (800) 424-8200
Phone: (202) 872-1300; Fax: (202) 785-4452
Website: http://www.pva.org
E-mail: info@pva.org

Spinal Cord Society
19051 County Highway 1
Fergus Falls, MN 56537
Phone: (218) 739-5252 or (218) 739-5261
Fax: (218) 739-5262
Website: http://members.aol.com/scsweb

Additional information about Arnold-Chiari malformation may be available from:

Spina Bifida Association of America
4590 MacArthur Blvd., NW, Suite 250
Washington, DC 20007-4226
Toll-Free: (800) 621-3141
Phone: (202) 944-3285; Fax:(202) 944-3295
Website: http://www.sbaa.org
E-mail: sbaa@sbaa.org

March of Dimes Birth Defects Foundation
1275 Mamaroneck Avenue
White Plains, NY 10605
Toll-Free: (888) 663-4637
Phone: (914) 428-7100; Fax: (914) 428-8203
Website: http://www.marchofdimes.com
E-mail: askus@marchofdimes.com

National Organization for Rare Disorders
P.O. Box 1968
55 Kenosia Avenue
Danbury, CT 06813-1968
Toll-Free: (800) 999-6673
Phone: (203) 744-0100; Fax: (203) 798-2291
Website: http://www.rarediseases.org
E-mail: orphan@rarediseases.org

Section 44.3

Tarlov Cysts

"Tarlov Cysts Information Page" is from the National Institute of Neurological Disorders and Stroke (NINDS), July 10, 2003. Available online at http://www.ninds.nih.gov; accessed May 2004.

What Are Tarlov Cysts?

Tarlov cysts are fluid-filled sacs that most often affect nerve roots in the sacrum, the group of bones at the base of the spine. These cysts can compress nerve roots, causing lower back pain, sciatica (shock-like or burning pain in the lower back, buttocks, and down one leg to below the knee), urinary incontinence, sexual dysfunction, and some loss of feeling or control of movement in the leg and/or foot. Pressure on the nerves next to the cysts can also cause pain. Tarlov cysts may become symptomatic following shock, trauma, or exertion that causes the buildup of cerebrospinal fluid. Women are at much higher risk of developing these cysts than are men.

Is There Any Treatment?

Tarlov cysts may be drained to relieve pressure and pain, but relief is often only temporary and fluid buildup in the cysts will recur. Corticosteroid injections may also temporarily relieve pain. Other drugs may be prescribed to treat chronic pain and depression. Filling the cysts with fat has not been shown to work. Injecting the cysts with fibrin glue (a combination of naturally occurring substances based on the clotting factor in blood) may provide temporary relief of pain. Some scientists believe the herpes simplex virus, which thrives in an alkaline environment, can cause Tarlov cysts to become symptomatic; making the body less alkaline, through diet or supplements, may lesson symptoms. Surgical resection may be needed when the cysts cause continued pain or progressive neurological damage.

What Is the Prognosis?

Most Tarlov cysts do not cause pain, weakness, or nerve root compression. The cysts do not appear to recur following complete resection by an experienced neurosurgeon. Acute and chronic pain may require changes in lifestyle. If left untreated, nerve root compression can cause permanent neurological damage.

What Research Is Being Done?

The National Institute of Neurological Disorders and Stroke (NINDS), a component of the National Institutes of Health within the U.S. Department of Health and Human Services, vigorously pursues a research program seeking new treatments to reduce and prevent pain and nerve damage.

Chapter 45

Spondylolisthesis

Introduction

There are 33 vertebrae in the human spine: 7 in the neck area (cervical), 12 in the chest area (thoracic), 5 in the lumbar (lower back), 5 fused vertebrae in the pelvic area (sacrum), and 4 fused vertebrae forming the tailbone (coccyx).

The cervical, thoracic, and lumbar vertebrae are held in place, one above the next, by projections on each vertebra called superior and inferior processes. The inferior (lower) process of the top vertebra fit into the superior (upper) process of the lower vertebra, forming a joint that holds the vertebrae in place. Between each vertebra (except in the sacrum and coccyx) intervertebral (between the vertebrae) disks cushion and separate the vertebrae.

What Is Spondylolisthesis?

Spondylolisthesis is a Latin term meaning improper forward movement of a vertebra over the vertebra below it. Most often, this forward slip of the vertebra occurs in the lumbar area of the spine. This slippage and herniation (deformity) of the disk places pressure on the nerve roots associated with the affected vertebrae, causing pain and dysfunction. While the herniation of the disk causes pain, discectomy alone is unable to provide relief. The reduction in disk space height and abnormal amount of movement allowed by the joint also causes pressure on the nerves. This intervertebral space must be restored in order to provide adequate space for the nerves.

What Causes Spondylolisthesis?

Spondylolisthesis occurs only in people who are able to stand upright and walk, so is virtually nonexistent among newborns. The upright position of human walking seems to have a direct effect on the development. It is more common in persons who participate is sports such as diving, weight lifting, wrestling, and gymnastics. All of these activities require repetitive hyperextension, which can contribute to instability of the spine.

Can Spondylolisthesis Be Prevented?

Good spinal care, both in developing good musculature and in preventing overuse or injuries, is key into reducing the chance of developing spondylolisthesis. Athletes, especially, need to be knowledgeable about body mechanics and the importance of both strengthening and resting the muscles of the back.

What Treatment Options Are There for Spondylolisthesis?

Anterior or Posterior Decompression with Fusion Cages

The goals of surgery are to remove pressure on spinal nerves (decompression), and to provide stability to the lumbar spine. Decompression involves removing the damaged structures that are causing the spondylolisthesis. In most cases of spondylolisthesis, lumbar decompression is accompanied by the uniting of one spinal vertebra to the next (spinal fusion) with spinal instrumentation (implants that are used to assist the healing process). Surgery can be performed from the back of the spine (posterior) or from the front of the spine (anterior). A structural graft is inserted into the place previously occupied by the removed structure. The purpose of this graft is to hold the disk space open until the fusion is complete. The graft is often held in place by a cage device, such as the BAK cage.

Laminectomy Decompression with Graft

In the laminectomy procedure, the spine is approached through a two-inch to five-inch incision in the midline of the back, and the left and right back muscles are detached from the lamina on both sides. The lamina are flat bone projections on each side of the vertebra. After this is accomplished, the lamina is removed (laminectomy), allowing the doctor to see the nerve roots. The facet joints, which are directly over the nerve roots, may then be trimmed to give the nerve roots more room. Once the nerve roots have adequate space made by the removed lamina and facet joint trimmings, pressure is eliminated, thereby alleviating pain. Bone graft chips may be placed between the vertebrae to create a solid section of bone, preventing motion that may detract from healing.

Posterolateral Fusion

The posterolateral fusion involves placing bone graft in the posterolateral portion of the spine (behind and to one side of the spine).The surgical approach to the spine is from the back through a midline incision that is approximately three inches to six inches long. First, bone graft is obtained from the pelvis (the iliac crest). Most surgeons work through the same incision to obtain the bone graft and perform the spinal fusion.

Next, the harvested bone graft applied to the posterolateral portion of the spine. This region lies on the outside of the spine and is rich in blood to supply the nutrients for it to grow. A small extension of the vertebral body in this area (transverse process) is a bone that serves as a muscle attachment site. The large back muscles that attach to the transverse processes are elevated to create a bed to lay the bone graft on. The back muscles are then laid back over the bone graft, creating tension to hold the bone graft in place.

After surgery, the body uses a natural process to repair itself, which usually means growing bone. As the harvested bone graft grows and adheres to the transverse processes, the spinal fusion is achieved and motion at that segment is stopped. Spine surgery instrumentation (medical devices) is sometimes used as an adjunct to obtain a solid fusion.

Spinal Instrumentation with Pedicle Screws

For spine operations to be successful, solid healing of bone across the spine must be achieved. The use of metal devices, also called instrumentation (screws, rods, plates, cables, wires) can help correct a deformed spine and will also increase the probability of obtaining a solid spinal fusion.

Spinal instrumentation can be placed in the front or in the back portion of the spine. The devices are usually made of metal and commonly stainless steel or titanium. In order to place this instrumentation into the spine, the spine is at first exposed by making a skin incision, and then gently clearing the muscles, ligaments, and other soft tissues from the levels of the vertebrae to be fused. Specific tools are used to carefully prepare the bone in such a way to obtain good seating of the implants (screw, rod, wire, cable or other).

When these devices are in the proper position, a rod (or plate) is positioned to link the implants together. Screws are inserted into the pedicles, which are part of the arch of the vertebra. This essentially forms a rigid scaffolding to hold the spine in the desired position. The bone graft that has been placed into the area of fusion gradually solidifies over several months. The spinal instrumentation is gradually covered by scar tissue and sometimes bone that the body lays down.

Chapter 46

Torticollis

Chapter Contents

Section 46.1

Congenital Torticollis

Parents of a newborn are often fascinated by their child's every move. When a child doesn't move in a normal way, the parents are rightly concerned.

An infant who keeps his or her head tilted to one side may have a condition called congenital muscular torticollis. Congenital means that the condition is present at birth. Torticollis means twisted or bent neck. It is caused by a tight muscle on one side of the head that pulls the head (ear) down toward one shoulder as the chin tilts to the opposite side.

How It Develops

No one knows exactly what causes this condition, which is more common in first-born children. One theory is that the muscle was stretched or torn during the delivery. Bleeding and swelling create pressure on the muscle. Eventually, scar tissue forms and replaces some of the muscle. Another theory suggests that the condition develops while the infant is still in the womb.

Within the first month after birth, a lump or pseudotumor may be felt on the tight muscle, but this gradually disappears. About one in five babies born with congenital muscular torticollis also has developmental dysplasia of the hip. Early diagnosis and treatment is required to avoid permanent deformities.

Signs and Symptoms

- Head tilts to one side, and chin points to the opposite shoulder.

- Usually, the head tilts right and the chin points left, meaning the muscle on the right side is affected.

- Lump or swelling in the muscle that gradually disappears.

- Limited range of motion in neck muscles.

- One side of face may flatten and the skull may appear oblong instead of round.

Congenital muscular torticollis generally is painless and can be treated with a consistent program of exercises and stretching.

Diagnosis and Treatment

If you notice that your child consistently holds the head tilted to one side, consult your physician. Conditions other than congenital muscular torticollis may result in this head position, and the physician must eliminate them as possible causes. The physician will also want to check the child's hips to ensure that no dysplasia is present. He or she may request X-rays or an ultrasound of the hips.

The initial treatment consists of a series of exercises that must be done several times a day. The physician may refer you to a physical therapist, but most of the time, the parents will be doing the exercises with the child, turning and bending the child's head to stretch the muscle.

Placing toys and other objects in positions where the infant has to turn the head to see them encourages the infant to stretch the muscle. So does carrying the infant in a side-lying position, with the face away from you. Support the infant by putting one arm under the head on the side of the tight muscle, which will stretch the muscle. Place the other arm between the child's legs to hold the body.

Most of the time, this condition resolves by the time the child is a year old. If not, the physician may recommend surgical treatment to release and lengthen the tight muscle.

Section 46.2

Spasmodic Torticollis

What Is It?

Cervical dystonia, also known as spasmodic torticollis, is a focal dystonia characterized by neck muscles contracting involuntarily, causing abnormal movements and posture of the head and neck.

This term is used generally to describe spasms in any direction: forward (anterocollis), backward (retrocollis), and sideways (torticollis). The movements may be sustained or jerky. Spasms in the muscles or pinching nerves in the neck can result in considerable pain and discomfort.

Symptoms

In cervical dystonia, the neck muscles contract involuntarily in various combinations. Sustained contractions cause abnormal posture of the head and neck, while periodic spasms produce jerky head movements. The severity may vary from mild to severe. Movements are often partially relieved by a gentle touch on the chin or other parts of the face.

If cervical dystonia causes any type of impairment, it is because muscle contractions interfere with normal function. Features such as cognition, strength, and the senses, including vision and hearing, are normal. While dystonia is not fatal, it is a chronic disorder and prognosis is difficult to predict.

Cause

Cervical dystonia is believed to be due to abnormal functioning of the basal ganglia, which are deep brain structures involved with the control of movement. The basal ganglia assist in initiating and regulating movement. What goes wrong in the basal ganglia is still unknown.

An imbalance of dopamine, a neurotransmitter in the basal ganglia, may underlie several different forms of dystonia, but much more research needs to be done for a better understanding of the brain mechanisms involved with dystonia.

A history of head or neck injury may be obtained, but the relationship between trauma and dystonia is still unclear. Research to examine the role of trauma is being conducted, including whether there is evidence that trauma may precipitate dystonia in those who have genetic susceptibility. This remains a gray area. It is clear that the interval from trauma to the onset of dystonia can be years.

Cases of inherited cervical dystonia have been reported, usually in conjunction with early-onset generalized dystonia, which is associated with the DYT1 gene.

Diagnosis

Diagnosis of cervical dystonia is based on information from the affected individual and the physical and neurological examination. At this time, there is no test to confirm diagnosis of blepharospasm, and, in most cases, laboratory tests are normal.

Usually the torticollis reaches a plateau and remains stable within five years of onset. This form of focal dystonia is unlikely to spread or become generalized dystonia, though patients with generalized dystonia may also have cervical dystonia. Occasionally, there may be associated focal dystonia.

Cervical dystonia should not be confused with other conditions which cause a twisted neck such as local orthopedic, congenital problems of the neck, or ophthalmologic conditions where the head tilts to compensate for double vision. It is sometimes misdiagnosed as stiff neck, arthritis, or wry neck.

Treatment

Treatment for dystonia is designed to help lessen the symptoms of spasms, pain, and disturbed postures and functions. Most therapies are symptomatic, attempting to cover up or release the dystonic spasms. No single strategy will be appropriate for every case.

The goal of any treatment is to achieve the greatest benefits while incurring the fewest risks. It is to allow you to lead a fuller, more productive life by reducing the effects of dystonia. Establishing a satisfactory regimen requires patience on the part of both the affected individual and the physician.

The approach for treatment of dystonia is usually three-tiered: oral medications, botulinum toxin injections, and surgery. These therapies may be used in alone or in combination.

Complementary care, such as physical therapy and speech therapy, may also have a role in the treatment management depending on the form of dystonia. For many people, supportive therapy provides an important adjunct to medical treatment.

Although there is currently no known cure for dystonia, we are gaining a better understanding of dystonia through research and are developing new approaches to treatments.

Medications

A multitude of drugs have been studied to determine benefit for people with cervical dystonia, but none appear to be uniformly effective.

The categories of drugs reported to help relieve the symptoms associated with cervical dystonia include anticholinergic drugs [Artane (trihexyphenidyl), Cogentin (benztropine)]; dopaminergic drugs [Sinemet or Madopar (levodopa), Parlodel (bromocriptine), Symmetrel (amantadine)]; and GABAergic drugs [Valium (diazepam)].

Botulinum Toxin Injections

Botulinum toxin injections are the primary and most effective form of treatment for cervical dystonia. Injections are made directly into the affected neck muscles. A crucial element to successful botulinum toxin injections is that the appropriate muscles are injected.

For this reason it is important that the physician administering the injections be experienced with botulinum toxin injections and be very knowledgeable about the anatomy of the neck and surrounding areas. The muscular structure of the neck is very complicated and physicians must also be aware of anatomical variation.

It may be necessary to inject different muscles at some visits. Extensive EMG tests are helpful, as is listening to the affected person.

To avoid BOTOX® immunity, it's best to use the lowest possible dose. A typical, fairly low dose is 150 units. Doses that exceed 200 units seem to increase the risk of developing a resistance to the toxin, and too frequent injections (i.e., injections less than three to four months apart) are a real risk to antibody formation.

The term resistance means that the drug had no effect on the muscle injected. This is very different from an inadequate or inappropriate response. If the toxin is injected in the right dose and in the correct muscle, the patient should have a good result.

The side effects of botulinum toxin injections are usually exactly what the therapy is supposed to cause: muscle weakness. It's crucial to inject into the right place and with the appropriate dose. Sometimes the botulinum injections can cause difficulty swallowing, and, over the long term, immunity may occur (in less than 5% of people treated).

Surgery

Surgery may be considered when patients are no longer receptive to other treatments, including botulinum toxin injections and medications. Surgery may lose its effects over the years, but it can possibly provide some relief.

Surgery is undertaken to interrupt, at various levels of the nervous system, the pathways responsible for the abnormal neck movements. Some operations intentionally damage small regions of the thalamus (thalamotomy), globus pallidus (pallidotomy), or other deep centers in the brain in an attempt to rebalance movement and posture control. These surgeries have had widespread use in Parkinson's disease, and the results in dystonia have been promising.

Other surgical approaches include severing one or more of the contracting neck muscles (muscle resection), cutting nerves going to the nerve roots deep in the neck close to the spinal cord (anterior cervical rhizotomy), and removing the nerves at the point they enter the contracting muscles (selective peripheral denervation—The Bertrand Procedure).

Along with the type of torticollis a patient has, other factors influence the success of an operation. Every patient is unique and the muscles involved may vary from one patient to another. It is for this reason that the preoperative evaluation is important, so that the patient's head and neck movements and the muscular contractions causing it are identified and characterized. Also, surgery should only be considered when done by a neurosurgeon who has significant experience with these specific operations.

Complementary Therapy

Physical therapy may be helpful in the treatment of cervical dystonia. The goals of physical therapy for people with cervical dystonia are to help increase range of motion, to increase flexibility, to correct muscle imbalances, to improve posture, to increase balance, to enhance functional abilities in home and workplace, and to improve coordination. More is not better in physical therapy for people with dystonia, and "no pain, no gain" does not apply. Also, it is important to find a physical therapist who is experienced with dystonia.

The use and/or need for a soft cervical collar is sometimes helpful, especially if it is molded to provide the perfect fit.

The use of sensory tricks may also be effective in dealing with cervical dystonia, such as touching the chin or back of the head. Different sensory tricks work for different people, and if a person finds a sensory trick that works, it usually continues to work.

Support

By educating yourself with information, you have taken the first step in dealing with dystonia. Dystonia and its emotional offshoots affect every aspect of a person's life—how we think, the way we act, and how we cope.

Stress is an inevitable part of life, and although it clearly does not cause dystonia, it can aggravate dystonia symptoms. Stress reduction programs such as relaxation techniques, meditation, and journal writing may be beneficial.

Sometimes depression can be a by-product of dystonia. It, too, can aggravate symptoms and make them worse, but often, treating depression can result in an improvement of dystonia. It is important to remember that depression is a disease; it is treatable and not a reflection of one's self.

Thousands of people are experiencing similar symptoms, and you are not alone in coping with dystonia. Reassurance from family, friends, and others who have dystonia is beneficial. Support groups offer encouragement, camaraderie, and information about new treatments and medical advances. The Dystonia Medical Research Foundation maintains a network of support groups throughout North America along with many resources online.

Part Six

Medications and Rehabilitative Therapies for Spinal Problems

Chapter 47

Managing Chronic Pain

Helen Dearman, 52, of Houston, had a broken back for more than a decade and didn't know it. After falling from a ski lift in Mt. Hood, Oregon, when she was 23, Dearman was diagnosed with a broken left arm and thought that was her only injury. Her arm healed. But she developed excruciating back pain that made it hard to sleep and move around. "I worked as a teacher, so some doctors suggested that the problem was from standing on my feet all day," Dearman says. "Others told me it was all in my head. For years, I left doctors' offices feeling desperate for help."

The pain grew worse during her 30s. One morning, Dearman woke up with stabbing pains in her back and could barely walk. This time, her husband took her to an orthopedic surgeon who specialized in back problems. He took x-rays that revealed three old fractures in Dearman's spine.

"When the doctor showed me the x-rays, I cried," Dearman says. "Someone had finally given me the words and understanding for all the pain I had been suffering from for so long."

Pain That Persists

By definition, acute pain after surgery or trauma comes on suddenly and lasts for a limited time, whereas chronic pain persists.

"Managing Chronic Pain," by Michelle Meadows, U.S. Food and Drug Administration, *FDA Consumer,* March-April 2004. Available online at http://www.fda.gov/fdac; accessed April 2004.

"Acute pain is a direct response to disease or injury to tissue, and presumably it will subside when you treat the disease or injury," says Sharon Hertz, M.D., deputy director in the Food and Drug Administration's Division of Anti-Inflammatory, Analgesic, and Ophthalmologic Drug Products. "Chronic pain goes on and on—for months or even years."

Common types of chronic pain include back pain, headaches, arthritis, cancer pain, and neuropathic pain, which results from injury to nerves. In Dearman's case, her untreated back injury caused her spine to twist out of place, not only resulting in severe back pain, but also putting intense pressure on the nerves in her legs. "I often felt pain shooting down my legs," she says, "like a jolt of electricity."

Experts say the first step in treating chronic pain is to identify the source of the pain, if possible. Many people with chronic pain try to tough it out, according to research from the American Academy of Pain Medicine. But persistent pain should never be ignored because it could signal disease or injury that will worsen if left untreated. Sometimes, it turns out that the cause of pain is unknown. Fibromyalgia, for example, is characterized by fatigue and widespread pain in muscles and joints. Although scientists have theorized that the condition may be connected to injury, changes in muscle metabolism, or viruses, the exact cause is unclear.

Regardless of the type of chronic pain, the physical and emotional effects can be devastating. Dearman says, "My teaching career suffered, my children were confused about why I always felt bad, and our finances were ruined." Sometimes, she says, she even considered suicide.

Finding Relief

Dearman believes the first two surgeries she had to repair the fractures in her back and realign her spine were necessary. But she questions the four surgeries that followed. "I talked myself into the operating room more than once because I was desperate to feel better," Dearman says. "Even when doctors told me there was only a small chance another surgery would help, I wanted to take the chance." But after several surgeries, Dearman's pain only seemed to be getting worse.

The turning point occurred in 1995 when a physical therapist referred Dearman to a pain management specialist, a professional who takes a multidisciplinary approach to managing pain. She was treated by a team of pain experts. Doctors and nurses worked with her to manage pain medications. Psychologists addressed her depression and anger, and physical therapists helped improve her strength and mobility.

Dearman finally found effective drug treatment with a pump implanted into her abdomen that delivers morphine through a catheter into the fluid surrounding her spine. The pump, called an intrathecal drug infusion pump, is used for severe pain only after other oral and intravenous drug therapies have failed. The pump is programmed to deliver a controlled amount of medication continuously. Risks include surgical complications, such as infection, and complications with the catheter or pump. "It doesn't take away all the pain, but it's a drastic improvement and allows me to be in control of the pain," says Dearman, who also takes other pain medication as needed.

Seddon Savage, M.D., a pain specialist on the faculty of Dartmouth Medical School in Hanover, New Hampshire, says there are times when it's impossible to eliminate pain. "The goal of pain management is to provide as much pain relief as possible and improve functioning," Savage says.

Because pain varies from person to person, treatment is individualized. Someone with arthritis may do well with occasional use of an over-the-counter pain reliever, whereas someone else with arthritis may need a prescription pain reliever and regular aerobic exercise to feel good.

"Treatment for chronic pain is about much more than medication," Savage says. It can also involve stress relief and relaxation, physical therapy, improved sleep and nutrition habits, and exercise. Dearman says that through a multidisciplinary approach to pain management, she also learned to pace her activities so that she is realistic about how much she can do in a certain time period.

Savage recommends that people seek professional help for chronic pain when they feel that pain is interfering with their quality of life. "Start with your primary care physician, who may refer you to other specialists," she says.

"Consider asking your doctor about a pain management specialist if you feel that your pain is just not getting better over time." Another reason to seek advice from a specialist is if you are experiencing intolerable side effects from medications.

Concerns about Drug Abuse

One of Dearman's biggest fears was of becoming addicted to pain medications. "It's a common concern for both patients and health providers," says Savage, who specializes in addiction.

"Most forms of chronic pain respond to non-opioid drug treatments," she says. Examples of non-opioid pain relievers, which don't have addiction potential, include aspirin, acetaminophen, ibuprofen, naproxen, and other non-steroidal anti-inflammatory drugs. A combination of different types of analgesic medications at lower doses is often more effective than a single high-dose medication.

"But if opioids are prescribed for your pain, you are not abusing drugs if you are taking the medication as prescribed," Savage says. "Taking doses of drugs to relieve pain is not the same as taking drugs to get high."

Opioids are controlled substances that are potentially addictive. Pain medications containing opioids include Vicodin (hydrocodone), OxyContin and Percocet (oxycodone), MS-Contin (morphine), Tylenol #2, #3 and #4 (codeine), and the Duragesic Patch and Actiq (fentanyl).

June Dahl, Ph.D., director of the American Alliance of Cancer Pain Initiatives and professor of pharmacology at the University of Wisconsin-Madison Medical School, says she recently took a call from a man with cancer who said he stopped taking an opioid pain medication on his own for fear that he was becoming addicted. "But what he described were not signs of addiction, but signs of physical dependence," Dahl says.

Addiction is characterized by craving and compulsive use of drugs. Physical dependence occurs when a person's body adapts to the drug. If someone has become physically dependent on a drug and suddenly stops taking it, withdrawal may occur. These symptoms can include muscle aches, watery nose and eyes, irritability, sweating, and diarrhea. Physical dependence is a normal response to repeated use of opioids and is distinct from psychological addiction.

Savage says that in prescribing potentially addictive medications, doctors should consider patients' personal and family histories of addiction, as well as psychological and social stressors that may affect medication use. Also, some people who begin taking opioid medications for pain as prescribed may later discover that they are using the medication for its psychic brain effects. Physicians need to be aware of this potential adverse effect, and should educate patients and their families about appropriate use of addictive drugs.

To better guide physicians, the Federation of State Medical Boards adopted guidelines for the use of controlled substances for pain treatment in 1998. The guidelines advise physicians on patient evaluations, treatment plans, and medical records.

The use of opioids in pain treatment remains controversial for several reasons. The rate of addiction in the properly treated pain population is unknown. The media has highlighted problems of addiction to pain medicine among celebrities. And there has been considerable drug abuse involving OxyContin, which the FDA approved for moderate to severe pain in 1995. The FDA strengthened warnings for oxycodone in 2001, while continuing to recommend appropriate pain control for people living with severe pain.

But experts say that finding a balance between cracking down on drug abusers and protecting people in pain is an ongoing struggle. "Some doctors fear regulatory scrutiny for over-prescribing these drugs," Dahl says. "And concerns about the small segment of people who abuse drugs ends up interfering with effective pain management for others."

Sheryl Kaufman, 40, of Boston, who uses oxycodone and a fentanyl patch for severe pain associated with breast cancer, says she recently filed a grievance with a pharmacy over her struggles to get prescriptions filled. "They made me feel like a criminal," she says. "Sometimes I've had to go without pain medication for two to three days because of delays in filling prescriptions."

The Value of Support

Dearman's experiences with chronic pain led her to establish the National Chronic Pain Society in 2002. The organization provides peer support for people with chronic pain and their families.

"We give people support for dealing with all of the issues that can go along with chronic pain—not having your pain taken seriously, frustration over not finding relief, how to communicate your pain to your doctor, and how to maintain relations with your family," Dearman says.

Penney Cowan, executive director of the American Chronic Pain Association, another peer support organization in Rocklin, California, says support systems are important because they give people with pain the coping skills needed to take an active role in their recovery. "Sometimes doctors tell people they'll have to learn to live with the pain," Cowan says. "But too often they stop short of telling them how to accomplish that."

Dearman says finding effective treatment and gaining the skills to live with her pain made all the difference. "It's about being a person first and not letting pain define who you are," she says. "Our motto is: Pain may be unavoidable, but suffering is optional."

Chronic Headaches

More than 45 million Americans have chronic headaches, according to the National Headache Foundation. The most common types include tension headaches, which are associated with muscle tension.

These are sometimes described as feeling like a tight band squeezing the head. Cluster headaches are marked by severe pain around one eye. Migraines are characterized by throbbing pain on one side of the head. Most people with migraines also experience nausea and sensitivities to light and sound.

Andrew Fano, 38, of Lincolnshire, Illinois, who has had migraines since he was 12, says headaches used to wipe him out for days. But things improved in 1992 when the FDA approved Imitrex (sumatriptan), the first drug in a class known as triptans. This class of drugs marked a huge leap forward for headache sufferers.

Unlike some previous drugs that dulled the perception of pain, triptans stop the pain by narrowing blood vessels in the brain and reducing inflammation. Fano's migraine treatment now includes a newer triptan called Frova (frovatriptan). Side effects include nausea, dizziness, and dry mouth. He also takes the pain reliever Vicodin as needed, sticks to a regular sleep schedule, and avoids red wine and other migraine triggers.

Migraines, tension headaches, and cluster headaches are considered primary headaches because they are not caused by underlying illness. "But it's important to rule out disease, especially when headaches are resistant to treatment," says Seymour Diamond, M.D., founder and executive chairman of the National Headache Foundation.

Diamond performed an MRI (magnetic resonance imaging) on Fano a couple of years ago. "We assessed him for a possible brain aneurysm, but luckily, there wasn't a problem," he says.

Most headaches can be successfully treated with over-the-counter pain relievers. But you should seek professional help for headaches if they persist or get worse or if the headaches are keeping you from work and social activities. "You should also see a doctor if you've never had headaches before and you start having them, if you get headaches upon exertion, or if headaches are accompanied by a stiff neck, fever, or neurological symptoms like dizziness or blurred vision," Diamond says.

Pain Basics

People usually feel pain when receptors in skin, bones, joints, or other tissues are stimulated by an injury or threat to the body. Neuropathic pain is triggered by changes in the nerves themselves, or caused by changes in the brain or peripheral tissues.

Pain involves the interaction between several chemicals in the brain and spinal cord. These chemicals, called neurotransmitters, transmit nerve impulses from one nerve cell to another. Neurotransmitters stimulate receptors found on the surface of nerve and brain cells, which function like gates, allowing messages to pass from one nerve cell to the next. Many pain-relieving drugs work by acting on these receptors. For example, opioid drugs block pain by locking onto opioid receptors in the brain.

Other drugs control pain outside the brain, such as non-steroidal anti-inflammatory drugs (NSAIDs). These drugs, including aspirin, ibuprofen, and naproxen, inhibit hormones called prostaglandins, which stimulate nerves at the site of injury and cause inflammation and fever. Newer NSAIDs, including Celebrex (celecoxib) and Vioxx (rofecoxib) for rheumatoid arthritis, primarily block an enzyme called cyclooxygenase-2. Known as COX-2 inhibitors, these drugs may be less likely to cause the stomach problems associated with older NSAIDs.

[Editor's Note: In September 2004, Merck & Company, Inc. announced a voluntary withdrawal of Vioxx from the U.S. and worldwide market due to safety concerns regarding an increased risk of cardiovascular events (including heart attack and stroke). The U.S. Food and Drug Administration (FDA) announced it would monitor other drugs in this class for similar side effects. For more information from Merck, visit www.merck.com or www.vioxx.com or call 1-888-368-4699. For more information from FDA , visit www.fda.gov/cder/drug/infopage/vioxx/default.htm or call 1-888-INFO-FDA.]

For More Information

American Academy of Pain Management
13947 Mono Way #A
Sonora, CA 95370
Phone: (209) 533-9744
Fax: (209) 533-9750
Website: http://www.aapainmanage.org
E-mail: aapm@aapainmanage.org

American Pain Society
4700 West Lake Avenue
Glenview, IL 60025-1485
Phone: (847) 375-4715
Fax (Toll-Free): (877) 734-8758
http://www.ampainsoc.org
E-mail: info@ampainsoc.org

American Pain Foundation
201 N. Charles Street, Suite 710
Baltimore, MD 21201-4111
Toll-Free: (888) 615-PAIN (7246)
Website: http://www.painfoundation.org
E-mail: info@painfoundation.org

American Chronic Pain Association
P.O. Box 850
Rocklin, CA 95677
Toll-Free: (800) 533-3231
Phone: (916) 632-0922
Fax: (916) 632-3208
Website: http://www.theacpa.org
E-mail: ACPA@pacbell.net

National Chronic Pain Society
P.O. Box 903
Tomball, TX 77377
Phone: (281) 357-4673
Website: http://www.ncps-cpr.org

Chapter 48

All about Medications for Spinal Pain

Introduction

Mild pain medications can reduce inflammation and pain when taken properly. Pain medications cannot stop the effects of aging and wear and tear on the spine. But they can help control pain. If you are pregnant, you should not take any medication unless you have discussed it with your obstetrician.

General tips:

- Medications should be used wisely. Take them exactly as prescribed by your doctor and report any side effects.

- Some pain medications are highly addictive.

- Pain medication is less effective for controlling chronic pain if used over a long period.

- Medication will not cure pain of degenerative origin.

Medications for Back Pain

Medications prescribed for back pain include:

"Pain Medications" is reprinted with permission from www.allaboutback andneckpain.com, an informational website from DePuy Spine, Inc., a Johnson & Johnson company. © 2004 DePuy Spine, Inc. All rights reserved. Some illustrations on website by Marks Creative, © 2004 www.markscreative.com.

419

- aspirin
- NSAIDs (non-steroidal anti-inflammatory drugs)
- COX-2 (cyclooxygenase-2) inhibitors
- nonnarcotic prescription pain medications
- narcotic pain medications
- muscle relaxants
- antidepressants

Aspirin

Aspirin compounds are over-the-counter medications that can help relieve minor pain and back ache. The main potential side effect with aspirin is the development of stomach problems—particularly ulcers with or without bleeding.

NSAIDs

Non-steroidal anti-inflammatory drugs (NSAIDs) include over-the-counter pain relievers such as ibuprofen and naproxen. These medications were once only available by prescription. NSAIDs are very effective in relieving the pain associated with muscle strain and inflammation. Be aware that NSAIDs can decrease renal function if you are an older patient. Excessive use can lead to kidney problems.

COX-2 Inhibitors

A new class of NSAIDs is gaining wide acceptance in its ability to reduce inflammation. Commonly called COX-2 inhibitors, these newer NSAIDs work by selectively blocking the formation of pain-causing inflammatory chemicals. COX-2 inhibitors appear to be easier on the stomach, mainly because they don't interrupt stomach enzymes like traditional NSAIDs. Celecoxib (Celebrex) and rofecoxib (Vioxx) are two commonly prescribed COX-2 inhibitors. [See page 422 for information regarding the withdrawal of Vioxx from the market.]

Nonnarcotic Prescription Pain Medications

Nonnarcotic analgesics (pain relievers) are ideal in the treatment of mild to moderate chronic pain. Tylenol and aspirin are the most widely used over-the-counter analgesics. Medications that are analgesics and require a prescription from the doctor include NSAIDs, such as carprofen, fenoprofen, ketoprofen, and sulindac. To reduce side effects do not lie down for 15 to 30 minutes after taking the medication, avoid direct sunlight, and wear protective clothing and sunblock. Avoid using these medications if you have recurrent ulcers or liver problems.

Narcotic Pain Medications

If you experience severe pain, your doctor might prescribe a narcotic pain medication such as codeine or morphine. Narcotics relieve pain by acting as a numbing anesthetic to the central nervous system. The strength and length of pain relief differs for each drug.

Narcotics can have side effects such as nausea, vomiting, constipation, and sedation (drowsiness). These side effects are predictable and can often be prevented. Common preventive measures include not taking sleeping aids or antidepressants along with narcotics, avoiding alcohol, increasing fluid intake, eating a high fiber diet, and using a fiber laxative or stool softener to treat constipation. Remember that narcotics can be addictive if used excessively or improperly.

Muscle Relaxants

If you are having muscle spasms, muscle relaxants may help relieve pain. They have only been shown to be marginally effective. Muscle relaxants also have a significant risk of drowsiness and depression. Long-term use is not suggested; only three to four days is typically recommended.

Antidepressants

Back pain is a common symptom of depression and could be an indicator of its presence. Similarly back pain can lead to emotional distress and depression. It seems that the same chemical reactions in the nerve cells that trigger depression also control the pain pathways in the brain.

Antidepressants can relieve emotional stress associated with back pain. Some antidepressant medications seem to reduce pain-probably because they affect this chemical reaction in the nerve cells.

Some types of antidepressants make good sleeping medications. If you are having trouble sleeping due to your back pain, your doctor may prescribe an antidepressant to help you get back to a normal sleep routine. Antidepressants can have side effects such as drowsiness, loss of appetite, constipation, dry mouth, and fatigue.

Editor's Note Regarding Vioxx

The U.S. Food and Drug Administration (FDA) originally approved Vioxx (rofecoxib) in 1999. At that time, it was hoped that Vioxx and other COX-2 selective non-steroidal anti-inflammatory drugs (NSAIDs) would have a lower risk of gastrointestinal ulcers and bleeding than other NSAIDs (such as ibuprofen and naproxen).

In September 2004, Merck & Company, Inc. announced a voluntary withdrawal of Vioxx from the U.S. and worldwide market due to safety concerns regarding an increased risk of cardiovascular events (including heart attack and stroke). FDA announced it would monitor other drugs in the same class for similar side effects.

Additional information from Merck can be obtained from the websites at www.merck.com or www.vioxx.com or by calling 1-888-368-4699. For more information from FDA, visit www.fda.gov/cder/drug/infopage/vioxx/default.htm or call 1-888-INFO-FDA.

Chapter 49

What You Need to Know about Non-Steroidal Anti-Inflammatory Medications

What are non-steroidal anti-inflammatory medications?

Non-steroidal anti-inflammatory medications (NSAIDs) effectively reduce inflammation and relieve pain. Inflammation is the body's protective response to irritation or injury and is characterized by redness, warmth, swelling, and pain. NSAIDs are used to treat a variety of conditions that cause pain and swelling of joints such as rheumatoid arthritis and tendinitis. NSAIDs are also used to treat a variety of other conditions such as osteoarthritis, muscle sprains, back strains, and more.

How do NSAIDs work?

NSAIDs work by blocking the production of certain body chemicals that cause inflammation. NSAIDs are effective in treating pain caused by slow, prolonged tissue damage, such as the pain associated with an arthritic joint. NSAIDs are also effective in treating general or localized pain, such as back pain, menstrual cramps, and headaches.

NSAIDs work like corticosteroids (also called steroids) without many of the side effects associated with steroids. Steroids are manmade drugs that closely resemble cortisone, a naturally-occurring hormone. Like cortisone, NSAIDs are effective in reducing pain and inflammation often associated with joint and muscle diseases and injuries.

Are NSAIDs available without a prescription?

Yes. Over-the-counter NSAIDs are available without a prescription. Over-the-counter NSAIDs are available in much lower doses than comparable prescription NSAIDs. Current over-the-counter NSAIDs include:

- Aspirin compounds (such as Anacin, Ascriptin, Bayer, Bufferin, and Excedrin)

- Ketoprofen (such as Orudis KT)

- Ibuprofen (such as Motrin, Advil, Nuprin, and Medipren)

- Naproxen sodium (such as Aleve)

Over-the-counter NSAIDs are effective in treating mild osteoarthritis and some muscle injuries. Ibuprofen and naproxen are also used to treat fever. As with any medication, always follow the directions on the label and the instructions from your health care provider.

How long should I use an over-the-counter NSAID?

Never use an over-the-counter NSAID continuously for more than three days for fever and 10 days for pain without consulting your health care provider. Over-the-counter NSAIDs are effective pain relievers, but they are intended for short-term use. When taking NSAIDs for long periods of time, you should be carefully monitored by your health care provider so he or she can detect the development of harmful side effects and modify your treatment if necessary.

How long do NSAIDs take to work?

Some NSAIDs work within a few hours. Others may take a week or two before most benefits are achieved. Generally, for acute muscle injuries, we recommend NSAIDs that work quickly, but may need to be taken as often as every 4 to 6 hours because of their short action time.

For long-term treatment of osteoarthritis and rheumatoid arthritis, we generally recommend NSAIDs that need to be taken only once or twice a day. However, it generally takes longer for these drugs to have a therapeutic effect.

When are NSAIDs prescribed?

NSAIDs are often prescribed for rheumatologic diseases including rheumatoid arthritis and moderate to severe osteoarthritis. NSAIDs are also prescribed for moderately painful musculoskeletal conditions (such as back pain).

How are NSAIDs prescribed?

NSAIDs are prescribed in different doses, depending on your condition. Dosage may range from one to four doses per day.

Your health care provider may prescribe higher doses of NSAIDs if you have rheumatoid arthritis, for example, because there is frequently a significant degree of heat, swelling, redness, and stiffness in the joints. Lower doses may be prescribed for osteoarthritis and acute muscle injuries, since there is generally less swelling and frequently no warmth or redness to the joints.

No single NSAID is guaranteed to work. Your health care provider may prescribe several types of NSAIDs in order to find the one that works best for you.

Table 49.1. Generic and Brand Names for Non-Steroidal Anti-Inflammatory Drugs

Generic Name	Brand Name
celecoxib	Celebrex
diclofenac	Voltaren
diflunisal	Dolobid
etodolac	Lodine
fenoprofen	Nalfon
flurbiprofen	Ansaid
ibuprofen	Motrin
indomethacin	Indocin
ketoprofen	Orudis
ketorolac tromethamine	Toradol
meclofenamate sodium	Meclomen
nabumetone	Relafen
naproxen sodium	Anaprox
oxaprozin	Daypro
phenylbutazone	Butazolidin
piroxicam	Feldene
rofecoxib	Vioxx (withdrawn from the market Sept. 2004)
sulindac	Clinoril
tolmetin	Tolectin
salicylate	Trilisate, Disalcid
valdecoxib	Bextra

How will my health care provider choose a NSAID that is right for me?

The effectiveness and the risks of drugs are considered when your health care provider plans your treatment. Your health care provider will work with you to develop an appropriate treatment program. The drugs that will be prescribed will match the seriousness of your condition. Your health care provider will consider the results of your medical history, physical exam, x-rays, and blood tests to create your treatment plan. Your health care provider will also consider the presence of other medical conditions.

It is important to meet with your health care provider regularly so he or she can detect the development of any harmful side effects and modify your treatment if necessary. Your health care provider may periodically order blood tests or other tests (including a kidney function test) to determine the effectiveness of your treatment and the presence of any harmful side effects.

What are some common side effects of NSAIDs?

Side effects may occur if you are taking large doses of NSAIDs or if you are taking them for a long period of time. Some side effects are mild and go away, while others are more serious and need medical attention.

Please note: The side effects listed are the most common side effects. All possible side effects are not included. Always contact your health care provider if you have questions about your particular medication.

The most frequently reported side effects of NSAIDs are gastrointestinal symptoms, such as:

- Gas
- Feeling bloated
- Heartburn
- Stomach pain
- Nausea
- Vomiting
- Diarrhea and/or constipation

These side effects can generally be relieved by taking the drug with adequate amounts of food. NSAIDs may also be taken with milk or antacids (such as Maalox or Mylanta) to prevent gastrointestinal symptoms. If the symptoms continue, the NSAID may need to be stopped. You should contact your health care provider if the symptoms listed above do not stop after a few days of taking the NSAID with food, milk, or antacids.

Some other side effects of NSAIDs include:

- Dizziness

- Feeling lightheaded

- Problems with balance

- Difficulty concentrating

- Mild headaches

If these symptoms continue for more than a few days, stop taking the NSAID and contact your health care provider for more instructions.

What side effects should I tell my health care provider about right away?

If you experience any of the following side effects, it is important to call your health care provider right away.

- Fluid retention (recognized by swelling around the ankles, feet, lower legs, hands, and possibly around the eyes)

- Ringing in the ears

- Severe rash or hives or red, peeling skin

- Itching

- Unexplained bruising and bleeding

- Unusual weight gain

- Black stools—bloody or black, tarry stools

- Bloody or cloudy urine

- Severe stomach pain

- Bloody vomit

- Blurred vision

- Wheezing or trouble breathing

Can I take NSAIDs if I'm being treated for high blood pressure?

Nonsteroidal anti-inflammatory agents can raise blood pressure in some people. Some people with known high blood pressure (hypertension) may have to stop taking NSAIDs, if they notice their blood pressure increases in spite of taking their blood pressure medications and following their diet.

Is there anyone who should not take NSAIDs?

People who have the following conditions or circumstances should not use any type of NSAID until they are first evaluated by their health care provider:

- Children and teenagers with viral infections with or without fever should not receive aspirin or aspirin-containing products due to the risk of Reye syndrome

- Those who have an upcoming surgical procedure, including dental surgery

- Diabetes that is difficult to control

- Known kidney disease

- Known liver disease

- Known allergies to medications, especially aspirin

- Active peptic ulcer disease (stomach ulcers or previous history of stomach ulcer bleeding)

- Bleeding problems (people who have a history of prolonged bleeding time or who bruise easily)

- People who consume three or more alcoholic beverages per day

- High blood pressure that is difficult to control

- Active congestive heart failure

- Asthma that worsens when taking aspirin

- Pregnancy in the third trimester

- Simultaneous use with certain medications such as warfarin (Coumadin), phenytoin (Dilantin), cyclosporine (Neoral,

Sandimmune), probenecid (Benemid), lithium (Eskalith, Lithobid) and drugs used for arthritis, diabetes, high blood pressure, heart disease, and vitamins

Can NSAIDs cause allergic reactions?

Very rarely, a nonsteroidal anti-inflammatory agent can cause a generalized allergic reaction known as anaphylactic shock. If this happens, it generally occurs soon after the person starts taking the NSAID. The symptoms of this reaction include:

- Swollen eyes, lips, or tongue
- Difficulty swallowing
- Shortness of breath
- Rapid heart rate
- Chest pain
- Decrease in sedation

If any of these symptoms occur, call 911 or have someone drive you to the nearest emergency room immediately.

Before medication is prescribed, tell your health care provider:

- If you are allergic to any medications.
- If you are currently taking any other medications (including over-the-counter medications) and/or herbal dietary supplements.
- If you are pregnant or think you might be pregnant.
- If you have problems taking any medications.

Before you start taking any new medication, ask your health care provider:

- What is the name of the medication?
- Why do I need to take it?
- How often should I take it?
- What time of day should I take it?
- Should I take it on an empty stomach or with meals?
- Where should I store the medication?

- What should I do if I forget to take a dose?

- How long should I expect to take the medication?

- How will I know it is working?

- What side effects should I expect?

- Will the medication interfere with driving, working, or other activities?

- Does the medication interact with any foods, alcohol, or other medications (including over-the-counter medications, herbal, and/or dietary supplements)?

Chapter 50

A Patient's Guide to Spinal Injections

Introduction

In many cases of chronic back pain, spinal injections may be used both to find out what is causing your pain and to treat your pain. Doctors refer to these two separate uses of spinal injections as diagnostic and therapeutic. If an injection provides pain relief in the area that is injected, it is likely that this particular area is the source of the problem. Injections are also therapeutic in that they can provide temporary relief from pain.

Learn about spinal injections including:

- what medications are injected
- what types of injections are used
- why you might choose to have an injection
- why you might choose not to have an injection

Medications

With most spinal injections, a local anesthetic (numbing medication) called lidocaine (also known as Xylocaine) is injected into a ᵖecific area of the spine. Lidocaine is a fast-acting drug, but the effects wear off within about two hours. That is why lidocaine is used more often as a diagnostic tool rather than a long-lasting pain reliever. Bupivacaine (also known as Marcaine) is another type of anesthetic that can be used. It is slower to take effect, but it lasts longer, giving the patient more relief from pain.

Cortisone is a strong anti-inflammatory steroid medication. It is commonly injected along with a local anesthetic in order to reduce inflammation in the affected areas. Cortisone is long lasting and can be slow-releasing in order to give the best possible benefits of pain relief. Cortisone may not begin working for several days following the injection, but the effects can last for months. Sometimes a narcotic medication such as morphine or fentanyl is mixed with cortisone and the anesthetic to get increased pain relief.

Injections

Types of spinal injections include:

- epidural steroid injection (ESI)
- facet joint injections
- hardware injections
- sacroiliac (SI) joint injections
- differential lower extremity injections

Epidural Steroid Injection (ESI)

An ESI is a common type of injection that is given to provide relief from certain types of low back and neck pain. The epidural space is the space between the covering of the spinal cord (dura mater) and the inside of the bony spinal canal. It runs the entire length of your spine. When injected into this area the medication moves freely up and down the spine to coat the nerve roots and the outside lining of the facet joints near the area of injection. For example, if the injection is given in the lumbar spine, the medication will usually affect the entire lower portion of the spine.

The epidural needle is inserted into the back until the doctor feels sure it is in the epidural space. The doctor will then place a small amount of lidocaine into the epidural space and wait to see if you feel warmth and numbness in your legs. If so, the needle is most likely in the correct position. The remainder of the medication is injected and the needle is withdrawn.

There are three different ways to perform an epidural injection:

- caudal block
- translumbar
- transforaminal

Caudal Block

A caudal block is placed through the sacral gap (a space below the lumbar spine near the sacrum). The injection is placed into the epidural space. This type of block usually affects the spinal nerves at the end of the spinal canal near the sacrum. This collection of nerves is called the cauda equina. One of the benefits of this type of injection is less chance of puncturing the dura.

Translumbar

The translumbar approach is the most common way of performing an epidural injection. This type of injection is performed by placing a needle between two vertebrae from the back. The needle is inserted between the spinous processes of two vertebrae. You can actually feel the bumps that make up the spinous process by feeling along the back of your spine.

Transforaminal

The transforaminal approach is a very selective injection around a specific nerve root. The foramina are small openings between your vertebrae through which the nerve roots exit the spinal canal and enter the body. By injecting medication around a specific nerve root, the doctor can determine if this nerve root is causing the problem. This type of epidural injection is used most often for diagnostic purposes, and it is commonly used in the neck.

Facet Joint Injections

Facet joint injections are used to localize and treat low back pain caused by problems of the facet joints. These joints are located on each side of the vertebrae. They join the vertebrae together and allow the spine to move with flexibility. The facet joint injections form a pain block that allows the doctor to confirm that a facet joint is causing the pain. The medication used also decreases inflammation that occurs in the joint from arthritis and joint degeneration.

It is important to make sure that the injection goes directly into the facet joint. Fluoroscopy can be used to confirm that the needle is in the right position before any medication is injected. A fluoroscope uses X-rays to show a TV image. You doctor can watch on the screen as the needle is placed into the joint and magnify the image to increase accuracy.

There are two types of facet joint injections.

- Interarticular are injected directly into the joint to block the pain and reduce inflammation.

- Nerve blocks help determine whether the joint is indeed a source of pain by blocking the small nerves that connect with the joint.

A facet joint injection is perhaps the best way to diagnose facet joint syndrome. Joints that look abnormal on an x-ray may in fact be painless, while joints that look fine may actually be a source of pain. This is a rather simple procedure with little risk.

Hardware Injections

Your doctor may need to determine whether the metal hardware that has been used during surgery could be causing your discomfort. A hardware injection is performed by injecting lidocaine alongside the spinal hardware that was placed in the spine during surgery. If the pain is removed temporarily by the injection, it may indicate that the hardware is causing your pain.

These injections are used to determine whether a specific piece of hardware is causing the pain and needs to be removed surgically.

SI Joint Injections

Sacroiliac (SI) joint pain is easily confused with back pain from the spine. The SI joint is located between the sacrum and pelvic bones. Sometimes injecting the SI joint with lidocaine may help your doctor determine whether the SI joint is the source of your pain. If the joint is injected and your pain does not go away, it is probably coming from somewhere else. If the pain goes away immediately, your doctor may also inject cortisone into the joint before removing the needle. Cortisone is added to treat inflammation from SI joint arthritis. The injection usually gives temporary relief for several weeks or months.

SI joint injections can be used both to treat pain and to determine the source of the pain. This injection usually requires the use of fluoroscopic guidance or a CT scan in order to make sure the needle is placed correctly in the joint.

Differential Lower Extremity Injections

Various types of injections into certain areas of the lower extremities can help your doctor decide where the pain is starting. Pain that comes from problems with the back and the spinal nerves can mimic many other conditions. Sometimes it is impossible to tell if the pain you are experiencing is due to a back condition or a problem in your hip, knee, or foot.

To help determine whether a joint of your lower limb is causing you pain, your doctor may suggest injecting medication, such as lidocaine, into the joint to numb the area. Once the medication is injected, if the pain goes away immediately, that joint is more likely to be the source of the pain than your back. Your doctor can then focus on finding the problem in the joint.

General Contraindication

When certain medical conditions are present, doctors may determine it is unsafe to perform a spinal injection. Your doctor will discuss any concerns with you before making a final decision.

Bleeding Tendencies

If you have a tendency to heavy bleeding or are on anti-coagulant therapy (medication that prevents blood clotting), you are not a good candidate for spinal injections. The physician might ask you to stop all medications such as aspirin and ibuprofen five days before the injection. These medications can decrease the ability of the blood to clot and lead to problems. Make sure your provider has a list of your medications well ahead of your scheduled procedure.

Infections

If you have a local or systemic infection, a spinal injection may put you at greater risk for spreading the infection into the spine, causing meningitis (inflammation in the covering that surrounds the spinal cord). Make sure to tell your health care provider if you have any infected wounds, boils, or rashes anywhere on your body.

Unstable Medical Conditions

Injections are usually an elective procedure offered to patients without life-threatening conditions. A medically unstable patient should have his or her medical condition treated before any elective injections are given.

General Precautions

Consider these basic warnings before choosing to have a spinal injection.

- If you are chronically taking a platelet-inhibiting drug, such as aspirin or NSAIDs (non-steroidal anti-inflammatory drugs), you have an increased risk of bleeding and might not be a candidate for a spinal injection.

- If you are hypersensitive or have certain allergies to medications, you may have a negative reaction to the drugs used in the injection. Make sure to give your provider a list of your allergies.

- If you have an accompanying medical illness, you should discuss the risks of spinal injections with your physician. For instance, patients with diabetes mellitus might experience an increase in blood sugar after an injection with cortisone. Patients with congestive heart failure, renal failure, hypertension, or a significant cardiac disease may have problems due to the effects of fluid retention several days after an injection.

Chapter 51

Physical Therapy for Back and Neck Disorders

Chapter Contents

Section 51.1

Forms of Physical Therapy Used for Back and Neck Pain

After an episode of low back pain has lasted between two and six weeks, or if there are frequent recurrences of low back pain, it is reasonable to consider physical therapy for treatment. (Some spine specialists consider physical therapy sooner, particularly if the pain is severe.) In general, the goals of physical therapy are to decrease back pain, increase function, and provide education on a maintenance program to prevent further recurrences.

There are many different forms of physical therapy. Acutely, the therapist may focus on decreasing pain with passive physical therapy (modalities). These are considered passive therapies because they are done to the patient. Examples of modalities include:

- Heat/ice packs
- TENS units
- Iontophoresis
- Ultrasound

In addition to passive therapies, active physical therapy (exercise) is also necessary to rehabilitate the spine. Generally, a patient's exercise program should encompass a combination of the following:

- Stretching
- Strengthening/pain relief exercises
- Low-impact aerobic conditioning

Even patients with a very busy schedule should be able to maintain a moderate exercise regimen that encompasses stretching, strengthening, and aerobic conditioning.

Stretching

Almost every individual who has suffered from low back pain should stretch their hamstring muscles once or twice daily. Simple hamstring stretching does not take much time, although it can be difficult to remember, especially if there is little or no pain. Therefore, hamstring stretching is best done at the same time every day so it becomes part of a person's daily routine.

Strengthening

To strengthen the back muscles, 15 to 20 minutes of dynamic lumbar stabilization or other prescribed exercises should be done every other day.

Low-Impact Aerobic Conditioning

Low impact aerobics (such as walking, bicycling or swimming) should be done for 30 to 40 minutes three times weekly on alternate days from the strengthening exercises.

Passive Physical Therapy (Passive PT)

Multiple modalities are commonly employed to reduce low back pain. They are especially useful in alleviating acute low back pain (e.g., an intense, debilitating episode of low back pain) for the patient. Physical therapists or chiropractors usually use passive modalities.

Heat/Ice Packs

Heat and/or ice are easily available and are the most commonly used type of modality. Each helps reduce muscle spasm and inflammation.

Some patients find more pain relief with heat and others with ice. The two may also be alternated. They are generally applied for 10 to 20 minutes once every two hours, and are more useful early on (the first few days) in the course of an episode of pain.

Iontophoresis

Iontophoresis is a means of delivering steroids through the skin. The steroid is applied to the skin and then an electrical current is applied that causes it to migrate under the skin. The steroids then produce an anti-inflammatory effect in the general area that is causing pain. This modality is especially effective in relieving acute episodes of pain.

TENS Units

A transcutaneous electrical nerve stimulator (TENS) unit uses electrical stimulation to modulate the sensation of low back pain by overriding the painful signals that are sent to the brain. A trial is usually done first, and if the patient experiences substantial pain relief, a TENS unit may be used at home for low back pain relief on a long-term basis.

Ultrasound

Ultrasound is a form of deep heating in which sound waves are applied to the skin and penetrate into the soft tissues. Ultrasound is especially useful in relieving acute episodes of pain and may enhance tissue healing.

Section 51.2

How Physical Therapy Can Help Your Back

Adapted from "Taking Care of Your Back," with permission of the American Physical Therapy Association. This material is copyrighted, and any further reproduction or distribution is prohibited. Revised by David A. Cooke, M.D., on March 20, 2004.

By standing on their hind legs, human beings freed their hands for work and gained the dexterity to create civilizations. Since ancient days, though, people have paid the price of walking erect—with their backs.

In our modern, industrial society, back pain is the most common cause of loss of activity among adults under 45. It's estimated that over 80% of all American workers suffer back pain at some time during their careers.

And the cost, to all of us, is staggering. American industry loses billions in productivity, and consumers and insurers pay billions more for treatment.

But there's good news, too. Most bad backs respond well to rest and conservative treatment. And most injuries can be prevented. This article tells how and why backs go bad, and how a licensed, professional physical therapist can help you put it right again.

Your Back

Your body depends on the spinal column for structural stability. The shoulders, rib cage, and pelvis are anchored to the spine for strength and support. You also depend on the spine for mobility—the ability to twist, bend, and flex your body for different activities.

The spine is constructed of 24 jointed bones, or vertebrae, stacked from the pelvis to the skull in a gentle S-curve. Between the vertebrae are spongy disks that cushion the bones and bond the stack together. Pairs of bony projections, called facets, connect the rear of each vertebra to form a series of interlocking joints. The column is wrapped tightly in ligaments and supported by muscle.

Openings in each vertebra align to form a protective tube, the vertebral canal, for the spinal cord. Major nerves, connecting the spinal cord with other parts of the body, pass through spaces between the vertebrae.

Your Bad Back

By far the most common site of back pain and injury is the lumbar region—the low back. Your lumbar spine bears the brunt of bending, stooping, sitting, and worst of all, lifting.

Low back pain is a complex process. In some cases, it seems to be primarily an injury to muscles and ligaments in the low back. In others, the intervertebral disks can rupture, spilling its spongy pulp and pushing on adjacent nerve roots. In still other cases, pain may relate to arthritic changes in the small joints connecting one vertebrae to the next. More than one problem may be present at a time. In most cases it is difficult to determine a precise cause for a given person's back pain, even with the use of x-rays or MRI studies. However, effective prevention and treatment does exist that works for most cases of pain.

Avoiding Back Injury

Everyone is vulnerable to back injury, but certain occupations present added risk. Truck drivers sit for long periods while being jostled by vibration; they lead in back injuries. Nurses are also at high risk; bending over bedsides and lifting and moving patients is hazardous to their health.

Everyday activities can be dangerous, as well: even sitting puts an added load on the lumbar spine! Expectant mothers find their backs stressed in new ways. Parents lifting babies and toddlers are also at risk.

We can't avoid every stressful activity. The key to avoiding back injury lies in minimizing the risk inherent in any activity by applying these simple principles.

- Work on your posture. Don't slouch. Maintain the natural arch in your lower back whether standing or sitting.

- Lift with your legs. Don't bend over the object; bend your legs and keep your back straight. And most important, don't twist as you lift!

- Sit with care. Prolonged sitting in one position is a back hazard you might not suspect. Lumbar support and periodic breaks to move around are essential.

- Control your weight. Being overweight, especially if you have a potbelly, puts added stress on your lower back. The important benefits of conditioning are discussed in the next section.

Conditioning Your Back

The muscles of your back provide structure as well as mobility—they help hold your spinal column together. That's why maintaining healthy back muscles is so important in avoiding or recovering from injury.

But recent studies indicate that the most important factor in avoiding back injury may be your general conditioning, not the power of your back muscles. This suggests that regular aerobic exercise, such as walking or swimming, may provide all the conditioning a healthy back needs.

After injury, the first step in getting your back healthy is gentle exercise to improve flexibility. When you've recovered and are free from pain, your physical therapist may recommend mobilization and strengthening exercises.

Treatments for Bad Backs

For thousands of years, back sufferers have sought a cure in vain. Cave drawings depict early patients and attempts to treat their ailment.

Medical science is still searching for more effective therapies; unfortunately, there is as yet no simple cure for low back pain.

While there is disagreement about specific treatments, most experts prefer a conservative approach to treating acute back pain.

- **Bed Rest.** This may be helpful, but should last no more than 24 hours. If your bed sags in the middle, add a board under your mattress. Heat or ice may help ease muscle spasm and aid circulation.

- **Pain Medication.** Pain medication prescribed by your physician will help get you through the period of most severe pain, but it won't help you get better.

- **Traction.** Most experts agree that short applications of lumbar traction in a clinical, outpatient setting can be an effective treatment.

- **Manipulation.** Manual mobilization of the lumbar region may assist recovery by restoring range of motion, reducing spasm, and stimulating circulation.

- **Epidural Injection.** Epidural injection of anti-inflammatory or pain medication has been shown to be an effective treatment for many patients with low back symptoms.

- **Surgery.** Surgery should be considered only with the failure of conservative treatment to control severe, chronic pain or neurological symptoms. While laminectomy (a procedure that allows removal of disk material) enjoys a good success rate, there are risks. It may be wise to talk with several orthopaedic or neurosurgeons before taking this serious step.

Fortunately, the vast majority of cases of back pain DO get better. Only a small minority of patients develop problems with long-lasting or permanent low back pain. However, once you've had a back injury, you maybe vulnerable in that area for the rest of your life. Any successful treatment approach must include a program for preventing reinjury.

How Physical Therapy Can Help Your Back

The licensed physical therapist brings a unique perspective to caring for your back: The patient is the most important participant in the healing and prevention process.

It is, after all, your back. And whatever treatment you receive from others, it can't overcome treatment you give your back, day in and day out.

Your physical therapist will involve you in your care, teaching you to be, in a way, your own therapist. So that as you go about the routine of daily life, you'll be healing yourself, not causing reinjury. It all starts with a careful evaluation.

- **Evaluation.** Physical therapy places greatest emphasis on this process. Your therapist will take the time to talk with you and perform a thorough physical evaluation to identify the dysfunction that causes your pain.

- **Therapy.** Your physical therapist will plan a treatment regimen suited to your individual problem, and begin working to restore flexibility and ease discomfort. Treatment may include heat, cold, massage, traction, manipulation and exercises for relaxation, conditioning, and restoring range of motion.

- **Teaching.** You don't need to become an expert to avoid or overcome injury, but you may need to learn some new habits. Your physical therapist will help you continue therapy on your own with a home program designed to fit your needs.

- **Aftercare.** The goal of physical therapy is to return you to normal life as soon as possible, with the skills you need to prevent reinjury. You won't need to visit your therapist again unless you have an acute injury.

As respected members of the professional health care community, licensed physical therapists work in hospitals, industrial and sports setting, home care, schools, and in private practice.

Chapter 52

Back and Neck Braces

Introduction

If you are diagnosed with a spinal disorder, deformity, or potential problem that can by helped through the use of external structural support, your physician may recommend the use of a back or neck brace. Braces offer a safe, non-invasive way to prevent future problems or to help you heal from a current condition.

The use of braces is widely accepted. They are effective tools in the treatment of spine disorders. In fact, more than 99% of orthopedic physicians advocate using them.

Braces are really nothing new. They have actually been around for centuries. Lumbosacral corsets (for the lower back) were used as far back as 2000 B.C. Bandage and splint braces were used in 500 A.D. in an effort to correct scoliosis (a spine with a sideways curve). Recently, braces have become a popular way to actually help prevent primary and secondary lower back pain from ever occurring.

There are more than 30 types of back supports available for spine disorders. This chapter will discuss several common types and why they are used.

Neck Braces

Neck braces are used to provide stability of the cervical spine after neck surgery, a trauma to the neck, or as an alternative to surgery. They are probably the type of spinal brace you most commonly see people wearing. There are several types available, including:

- Soft Collar—This flexible brace is placed around the neck. It is typically used after a more rigid collar has been worn for the major healing. It is used as a transition to wearing no collar.

- Philadelphia Collar—This is a more rigid/stiff collar that has a front and back piece that attaches with Velcro on the sides. It is usually worn 24 hours a day until your physician instructs you to remove it. This collar is used for conditions such as: a relatively stable cervical (upper spine) fracture, cervical fusion surgery, or a cervical strain. Another similar type is the Miami cervical brace.

- Sterno-Occipital Mandibular Immobilization Device (SOMI)—A SOMI is a brace that holds your neck in a straight line that matches up with your spine. It offers rigid support to a damaged neck and prevents the head from moving around. With this brace, you are unable to bend or twist your neck. The restriction of motion helps the muscles and bones to heal from injury or surgery. If you look at what the name means, you will better understand what a SOMI does: sterno means your upper and middle chest, occipital is the base of your skull, mandibular refers to your jaw and chin, and immobilization describes the support and movement restriction the brace offers. The SOMI is worn on the parts of the body for which it is named. First, there is a chin piece that the lower jaw rests on. Second, the chin piece connects by straps to a headband that is worn across the forehead. Third, the chin piece connects to a chest piece by a front metal extension. Finally, the chest piece then rests on the upper and middle chest—sort of like a vest. This connects to the occipital piece, which supports the base of the head. This brace is obviously a bit more complicated and cumbersome than some of the others, but it provides excellent support for an injured neck.

- Halo—The main purpose of the halo is to immobilize the head and neck. This is the most rigid of the cervical braces. It is only used after complex cervical spine surgery or if there is an unstable cervical fracture. The halo looks a lot like the word sounds. It has a titanium ring (halo) that goes around your head, secured to the skull by four metal pins. The ring then attaches by four bars to a vest that is worn on the chest. The vest offers the weight to hold the ring and neck steadily in place. The halo is worn 24 hours a day until the spine injury heals.

Trochanteric Belts

The trochanteric belt is usually prescribed for sacroiliac joint pain or pelvic fractures. The belt fits around the pelvis, between the trochanter (a bony portion below the neck of your thigh bone) and the iliac (pelvis) ridges/crests. It is about five to eight centimeters wide and it buckles in front, just like a regular belt.

Sacroiliac and Lumbosacral Belts

The lumbosacral belt helps to stabilize the lower back. These belts are usually made of heavy cotton reinforced by lightweight stays. The pressure can be adjusted through laces on the side or back of the belt. These belts range in widths between 10 to 15 centimeters and 20 to 30 centimeters. The sacroiliac belt is used to prevent motion by putting a compressive force on the joints between the hipbone and sacrum (base of the spine).

Corsets

Corsets provide rigidity and support for the back. Corsets can vary in length. A shorter or longer corset will be prescribed, depending upon your condition. A short corset is typically used for low back pain, whereas a longer one is used for problems in the mid to lower thoracic spine. When people think of corsets, they usually conjure up images of women from earlier centuries who used them to make their waists look smaller. Today, in the treatment of back problems, corsets refer to a type of back brace that extends over the buttocks and is often held up by shoulder straps. Like the corsets of old, these lace up from the back, side, or front. There are metal stays that provide the appropriate rigidity and support for the back.

Rigid Braces

These braces are typically prescribed for low back pain and instability. If greater rigidity is needed to support the spine than can be found in standard back supports, rigid frame spinal bracing is often prescribed. These are stiff braces. They usually consist of rear uprights that contour to the lumbar (lower) spine and pelvis, along with thoracic bands. There are also fabric straps on the braces that provide pressure in the front. Common types of rigid models are:

- Williams Brace—This type of brace has no vertical uprights in the middle so that flexion/bending is allowed.

- Chair-Back Brace—This type immobilizes the lumbar spine in the neutral position. The chair-back is designed to reduce sideways and revolving movement of the lower spine.

- Raney Flexion Jacket—This type reduces lumbar lordosis by holding the patient in a neutral tilt.

Hyperextension Braces

This brace is designed to prevent excessive bending, and it is often prescribed to treat frontal compression fractures that have occurred around the junction of the thoracic and lumbar spine. The brace can also be used for post-surgery healing from a spinal fusion.

These braces offer support that allows anterior (front) pressure unloading of the thoracic vertebrae by restricting flexion (bending) of the thoracic and lumbar spine.

Hyperextension braces have a front rectangular metal frame that puts pressure over the upper sternum and the pubis/pubic bone. This encourages spinal extension. There is opposing pressure applied over the T-10 level (the tenth vertebra in your thoracic spine). The braces offer what is called three-point stabilization to the spine through a front abdominal pad, a chest pad, and a rear pad at the level of the fracture.

By applying pressure in three-points—sternal, pubis, and rear lumbosacral—the spine is extended/stretched. The sternum is the narrow, flat bone in the front middle of thorax. The thorax is the portion of body between the base of the neck and the lower diaphragm.

The most common types of hyperextension braces are Knight Taylor and Jewett.

Molded Jackets

These jackets are designed to distribute pressure widely over a large area. By immobilizing the patient from the neck to the hips, pressure is distributed evenly, taking excess pressure off overloaded or unstable areas. These jackets were originally made of plaster of paris, but now are typically made out of molded plastic.

Lifting Belts

These belts are designed to reduce low back strain and muscle fatigue that can occur when you are lifting heavy objects. The belt circles around the waist, covering the lumbar region of the spine, and closes in front. These belts are usually made of cloth or canvas and do not have stays. Some models also have lordosis pads.

Clinical Uses

The braces/supports are most frequently used to treat: low back pain, trauma, infections, muscular weakness, neck conditions, and osteoporosis. Braces, belts, and jackets are designed to immobilize and support the spine when there is a condition that needs to be treated. Depending on the model that is used, they can put the spine in a: neutral, upright, hyper-extended, flexed, or lateral-flexed position.

Goals of Spinal Bracing

Spinal bracing is used for a variety of reasons such as to: control pain, lessen the chance of further injury, allow healing to take place, compensate for muscle weakness, or prevent or correct a deformity. More specifically, lumbar corsets and braces compress the abdomen, which increases the intra-abdominal pressure. This act allows pressure on the vertebral column to unload, providing some relief.

There are other reasons bracing is used. One is the theory that they insulate the skin, producing increased warmth that decreases the sensation of pain—much like a heating pad. Another reason is that the increase in abdominal pressure produces hydraulic support for the back. Finally, certain types of movement may cause stress to the pain generators in the back. The decrease in range of movement by using bracing may relieve this type of pain.

Possible Drawbacks

Though the effects of bracing are primarily positive, they can lead to a loss of muscle function, due to inactivity. Bracing can sometimes lead to psychological addiction, so that even when the patient is healed and ready to be taken off the back brace, he or she feels dependent upon it for physical support.

Chapter 53

How to Do an Ice Massage

An ice massage is quick, free, easy to do, and it can provide significant pain relief for many types of back pain. In a world of sophisticated medical care, a simple ice massage can still be one of the more effective, proven methods to treat a sore back or neck.

Most episodes of back pain are caused by muscle strain. The large paired muscles in the low back (erector spinae) help hold up the spine, and with an injury the muscles can become inflamed and spasm, causing low back pain and significant stiffness.

Common causes of muscle strain of the large back muscles include:

- A sudden movement

- An awkward fall

- Lifting a heavy object (using the back muscles)

- A sports injury

While it sounds like a simple injury, a muscle strain can create a surprising amount of pain. In fact, this type of injury is one of the most common reasons people go to the emergency room. However, not much can be done for a strained back muscle except for rest (e.g., for up to two days), pain relief medications, and ice and/or heat application. This

451

chapter discusses how and to apply ice for quick relief of back pain caused by muscle strain.

How Ice Provides Pain Relief

Ice can help provide relief for back pain in a number of ways, including:

- Ice application slows the inflammation and swelling that occurs after injury. Most back pain is accompanied by some type of inflammation, and addressing the inflammation helps reduce the pain.

- Numbs sore tissues (providing pain relief like a local anesthetic)

- Slows the nerve impulses in the area, which interrupts the pain-spasm reaction between the nerves

- Decreases tissue damage

Ice is most effective if it is applied soon after the injury occurs. The cold makes the veins in the tissue contract, reducing circulation. Once the cold is removed, the veins overcompensate and dilate and blood rushes into the area. The blood brings with it the necessary nutrients to allow the injured back muscles, ligaments, and tendons to heal.

As with all pain relief treatments, there are some cautions with ice. Never apply ice directly to the skin. Instead, be sure that there is a protective barrier between the ice and skin, such as a towel. Additionally, ice should also not be used for patients who have rheumatoid arthritis, Raynaud syndrome, cold allergic conditions, paralysis, or areas of impaired sensation.

How to Do an Ice Massage

While any form of applying cold to the injured area—such as a bag of ice wrapped in a towel or a commercial ice pack—should be helpful, combining massage with ice application is a nice alternative for pain relief.

To do an ice massage, a regular ice cube may be used, but it's better to use a larger piece of ice. One easy way to do this is to freeze water in a paper or Styrofoam cup, then peel the top inch or two of the cup to expose the ice surface.

Someone else can give the ice massage, with the patient lying on his or her stomach in a comfortable position with a pillow under the hips to keep stress off the back. Patients can also give themselves ice massages by lying on their side.

Ice should be gently applied to the lower back as follows:

- Apply the ice gently and massage in a circular motion.

- Focus on the six-inch area of the back where the pain is felt.

- Avoid applying the ice directly on the bony portion of the spine.

- Limit the massage to about 5 minutes at a time (to avoid an ice burn).

In general, one should never apply ice directly to the skin to avoid burning the skin. However, with ice massage it is okay to apply the ice to the skin because the ice doesn't stay in one place for long.

The key is to achieve numbness in the area of injury without burning the skin. Once this numbness has been reached, gentle, minimal stress movements can be made. When the numbness has worn off, the ice can be applied again for another cycle. This can be repeated two to three times a day.

Heat Is Good, Too

Ice is generally most helpful during the first 48 hours following an injury that strains the back muscles. After this initial period, heat is probably more beneficial to the healing process. For some people, alternating heat with cold application provides the most pain relief.

Moist heat, such as a warm bath or whirlpool, is thought to aid the healing process by increasing circulation and relaxing muscle spasms. Whether one uses moist heat or dry heat, the desired effect is for the heat to penetrate down into the muscles, providing relaxation and pain relief, and facilitating stretching the injured tissues to reduce stiffness.

As with ice application, when applying heat care should be taken to avoid burning the skin. Warm is the correct temperature for any type of heat source (such as a heating pad, hot water bottle, gel pack, etc.). Also, never to fall asleep with the heating pad on.

There is no exact prescription for ice and heat application, and many physicians and physical therapists will recommend trying different forms of heat and cold application to see which approach provides the most pain relief.

Chapter 54

How to Apply Heat Therapy

Introduction to Heat Therapy for Lower Back Pain

While the overall qualities of warmth and heat have long been associated with comfort and relaxation, heat therapy goes a step further and can provide both pain relief and healing benefits for many types of lower back pain. In addition, heat therapy for lower back pain—in the form of heating pads, heat wraps, hot baths, warm gel packs, etc.—is both inexpensive and easy to do.

This chapter provides an examination of how heat therapy interacts with the body to alleviate pain as well as options on how to apply heat therapy to help alleviate many types of lower back pain.

How Heat Therapy Works

Many episodes of lower back pain result from strains and overexertions, creating tension in the muscles and soft tissues around the lower spine. As a result, this restricts proper circulation and sends pain signals to the brain.

Muscle spasm in the lower back can create sensations that may range from mild discomfort to excruciating lower back pain. Heat therapy can help relieve pain from the muscle spasm and related tightness in the lower back.

"Benefits of Heat Therapy for Back Pain," by Vert Mooney, M.D., is reprinted with permission from www.Spine-health.com. © March 20, 2003 Spine-health.com. All rights reserved. For more information, please see http://www.Spine-health.com.

Heat therapy application can help provide lower back pain relief through several mechanisms:

- Heat therapy dilates the blood vessels of the muscles surrounding the lumbar spine. This process increases the flow of oxygen and nutrients to the muscles, helping to heal the damaged tissue.

- Heat stimulates the sensory receptors in the skin, which means that applying heat to the lower back will decrease transmissions of pain signals to the brain and partially relieve the discomfort.

- Heat application facilitates stretching the soft tissues around the spine, including muscles, connective tissue, and adhesions. Consequently, with heat therapy, there will be a decrease in stiffness as well as injury, with an increase in flexibility and overall feeling of comfort. Flexibility is very important for a healthy back.

There are several other significant benefits of heat therapy that make it so appealing. Compared to most therapies, heat therapy is quite inexpensive (and in many circumstances it's free—such as taking a hot bath). Heat therapy is also easy to do—it can be done at home while relaxing, and portable heat wraps also make it an option while at work or in the car.

For many people, heat therapy works best when combined with other treatment modalities, such as physical therapy and exercise. Relative to most medical treatments available, heat therapy is appealing to many people because it is a non-invasive and non-pharmaceutical form of lower back pain relief.

How to Apply Heat Therapy

The most effective heat therapy products are the ones that can maintain their heat at the proper temperature. Warm is the proper temperature. Patients should not have their heat source be hot to the point of burning the skin. The desired effect is for the heat to penetrate down into the muscles. Simply increasing the temperature of the skin will do little to decrease discomfort.

In many instances, the longer the heat is applied, the better. The duration that one needs to apply the heat, though, is based on the type of and/or magnitude of the injury. For very minor back tension, short amounts of heat therapy may be sufficient (such as 15 to 20 minutes).

For more intense injuries, longer sessions of heat may be more beneficial (such as 30 minutes to 2 hours, or more).

Two options of heat therapy include moist heat and dry heat.

- Dry heat, such as electric heating pads and saunas, draw out moisture from the body and may leave the skin dehydrated. However, some people feel that dry heat is the easiest to apply and feels the best.

- Moist heat, such as hot baths, steamed towels, or moist heating packs can aid in the heat's penetration into the muscles, and some people feel that moist heat provides better pain relief.

A specific type of heat therapy may feel better for one person than for another, and it may require some experimentation to figure out which one works best. There are many different manners for heat to be applied to the lower back. Some common options include:

- Hot water bottle—tends to stay warm for 20 to 30 minutes.

- Electric heating pad—maintains a constant level of heat as long as it is plugged in.

- Heated gel packs—may be microwaved, or sometimes heated in water, and tend to say warm for about 30 minutes. Certain types of gel packs provide moist heat, which some people prefer.

- Heat wraps—wraps around the lower back and waist and may be worn against the skin under clothing, providing convenience and several hours of low level of heat application.

- Hot bath, hot tub, sauna, steam bath—tend to stimulate general feelings of comfort and relaxation that may help reduce muscle spasm and pain. A whirlpool jet directed at the lower back may provide the added benefit of a light massage.

Finally, it is important to use enough insulation between the heat source and the skin to avoid overheating or burning the skin.

Please note that heat should not be used in certain circumstances. For example, if the lower back is swollen or bruised, heat should not be used. Patients should consult doctors if they have heart disease or hypertension. Heat application is also not suitable in the following cases:

- Dermatitis

- Deep vein thrombosis

- Diabetes

- Peripheral vascular disease

- Open wound

- Severe cognitive impairment

In general, if the injured area is swollen or bruised it is better to apply ice or a cold pack to reduce the inflammation or swelling.

In summary, heat therapy is an easy and inexpensive option to provide relief from many forms of lower back pain. It may be used alone or in conjunction with other therapies. Because it is so simple, it is often overlooked and physicians may forget to mention it, but heat therapy used in the right way can be a valuable part of many lower back pain treatment programs.

Chapter 55

Water Therapy Exercise Programs

Water therapy (also called pool therapy, hydrotherapy, or aquatic therapy) consists of a variety of aquatic-based treatments that are designed for back pain relief, to condition and strengthen muscles, and increase range of motion in the spine and other affected parts of the body. A water therapy exercise program can be used alone or in conjunction with other forms of physical therapy.

Water therapy offers many of the same benefits associated with a carefully designed land-based program, including development of a treatment plan that is carefully tailored to the individual patient. Water therapy is especially helpful in cases where land-based therapy options are limited due to the patient's pain, decreased bone density, disability, or other factors.

The Benefits of Water during Therapy

The physical properties of water make it a highly desirable medium for treating back pain and other musculoskeletal injuries. Some of the most important properties are:

- **Buoyancy:** water counteracts gravity and helps to support the weight of the patient in a controlled fashion as the patient is immersed.

- **Viscosity:** resists movement by means of friction, allowing strengthening and conditioning of an injury, while reducing the risk of further injury due to loss of balance.

- **Hydrostatic pressure:** produces forces perpendicular to body surfaces at every point, increasing kinesthetic (body motion or position) and proprioceptive (posture self-regulating) awareness in some patients.

Together, these properties allow development of a therapeutic exercise regimen that controls such critical factors as the weight placed on the spine (axial load) and risk of injury due to unintended movements.

Moreover, the patient's pain may be relieved as a result of relaxation and sensory alterations due to water temperature and hydrostatic pressure during water therapy. The buoyancy of water permits a greater range of positions due to the virtual elimination of gravitational forces. Buoyancy can be increased with the use of floats.

Limitations

Water-based exercises should only be performed under the guidance of a qualified health professional. Water therapy should not be used in cases involving fever, cardiac failure, incontinence, infection, and other conditions. Patients with severely limited endurance or range of motion may pose safety issues.

The perception of objects in water is affected by refraction, leading to difficulty in learning specific motor skills in patients with limited kinesthetic or body awareness. Water temperature should be controlled to reduce undesirable cardiac, respiratory, and other physiologic effects.

Water Therapy Exercises

Water-Based Therapy

The techniques used in water therapy include spa therapy, standing or floating pool exercises, swimming, and conditioning using specialized equipment, such as surgical tubing, flotation devices, and resistive devices for the hands or feet. Spa treatments typically involve relaxing in warm, agitated water.

Active techniques for water therapy are diverse and should be tailored to the individual patient. Exercises range from simple routines performed in a shallow pool to conditioning using underwater treadmills and other high-tech equipment.

Some of the basic techniques for pool therapy exercises are as follows (they can be modified for varying degrees of difficulty):

- Knee-to-chest—performed with one hand on the side of the pool or with your back to the wall

- Leg raise—performed with one leg outstretched and the supporting leg slightly bent while one hand holds on to the side of the pool

- Wall-facing leg stretch—stretching exercise in Superman position with hands resting on side of pool

- Pool walking—forward or backward walking therapy

- Quadruped activity—performed in prone position with legs and arms making paddling motions, with trunk supported by therapist or flotation jacket

Combined Water Therapy with Land-Based Methods

Continued water therapy is appropriate if land-based methods worsen symptoms or if the patient prefers water exercises. If their functional status or competitive goals require it, patients may transition to a dry environment once they are successfully performing exercises in water. Some patients may benefit from mixed use of wet and dry physical therapy environments.

Conclusion

Although formal scientific evidence for the specific benefits of water therapy in treating back pain is sparse, the value of appropriate exercise programs is well established. The aquatic medium is ideal for patients for whom land-based options are limited.

Chapter 56

Acupuncture for Back Pain

Chapter Contents

Section 56.1

The Use of Acupuncture to Treat Pain

"Acupuncture" is from the National Center for Complementary and Alternative Medicine (NCCAM), March 2002. Available online at http://nccam.nci.nih.gov/health/acupuncture; accessed May 2004.

Acupuncture is one of the oldest, most commonly used medical procedures in the world. Originating in China more than 2,000 years ago, acupuncture began to become better known in the United States in 1971, when New York Times reporter James Reston wrote about how doctors in China used needles to ease his abdominal pain after surgery. Research shows that acupuncture is beneficial in treating a variety of health conditions.

The term acupuncture describes a family of procedures involving stimulation of anatomical points on the body by a variety of techniques. American practices of acupuncture incorporate medical traditions from China, Japan, Korea, and other countries. The acupuncture technique that has been most studied scientifically involves penetrating the skin with thin, solid, metallic needles that are manipulated by the hands or by electrical stimulation.

In the past two decades, acupuncture has grown in popularity in the United States. A Harvard University study published in 1998 estimated that Americans made more than five million visits per year to acupuncture practitioners.[1] The report from a Consensus Development Conference on Acupuncture held at the National Institutes of Health (NIH) in 1997 stated that acupuncture is being "widely" practiced—by thousands of physicians, dentists, acupuncturists, and other practitioners—for relief or prevention of pain and for various other health conditions.[2]

NIH has funded a variety of research projects on acupuncture. These grants have been awarded by the National Center for Complementary and Alternative Medicine (NCCAM), the Office of Alternative Medicine (OAM, NCCAM's predecessor), and other NIH Institutes and Centers.

This section provides general information about acupuncture, research summaries, and a resource section.

Acupuncture Theories

Traditional Chinese medicine theorizes that there are more than 2,000 acupuncture points on the human body, and that these connect with 12 main and 8 secondary pathways called meridians. Chinese medicine practitioners believe these meridians conduct energy, or qi (pronounced "chee"), throughout the body.

Qi is believed to regulate spiritual, emotional, mental, and physical balance and to be influenced by the opposing forces of yin and yang. According to traditional Chinese medicine, when yin and yang are balanced, they work together with the natural flow of qi to help the body achieve and maintain health. Acupuncture is believed to balance yin and yang, keep the normal flow of energy unblocked, and maintain or restore health to the body and mind.

Traditional Chinese medicine practices (including acupuncture, herbs, diet, massage, and meditative physical exercise) all are intended to improve the flow of qi.[3]

Western scientists have found meridians hard to identify because meridians do not directly correspond to nerve or blood circulation pathways. Some researchers believe that meridians are located throughout the body's connective tissue;[4] others do not believe that qi exists at all.[5,6] Such differences of opinion have made acupuncture an area of scientific controversy.

Mechanisms of Action

Several processes have been proposed to explain acupuncture's effects, primarily those on pain. Acupuncture points are believed to stimulate the central nervous system (the brain and spinal cord) to release chemicals into the muscles, spinal cord, and brain. These chemicals either change the experience of pain or release other chemicals, such as hormones, that influence the body's self-regulating systems. The biochemical changes may stimulate the body's natural healing abilities and promote physical and emotional well-being.[7] There are three main mechanisms:

1. **Conduction of electromagnetic signals:** Western scientists have found evidence that acupuncture points are strategic conductors of electromagnetic signals. Stimulating points along these pathways through acupuncture enables electromagnetic signals to be relayed at a greater rate than under normal conditions. These signals may start the flow

of pain-killing biochemicals, such as endorphins, and of immune system cells to specific sites in the body that are injured or vulnerable to disease.[8,9]

2. **Activation of opioid systems:** Research has found that several types of opioids may be released into the central nervous system during acupuncture treatment, thereby reducing pain.[10]

3. **Changes in brain chemistry, sensation, and involuntary body functions:** Studies have shown that acupuncture may alter brain chemistry by changing the release of neurotransmitters and neurohormones. Acupuncture also has been documented to affect the parts of the central nervous system related to sensation and involuntary body functions, such as immune reactions and processes whereby a person's blood pressure, blood flow, and body temperature are regulated.[3,11,12]

Preclinical studies have documented acupuncture's effects, but they have not been able to fully explain how acupuncture works within the framework of the Western system of medicine.[13,14,15,16,17,18]

According to the NIH Consensus Statement on Acupuncture: "Acupuncture as a therapeutic intervention is widely practiced in the United States. While there have been many studies of its potential usefulness, many of these studies provide equivocal results because of design, sample size, and other factors. The issue is further complicated by inherent difficulties in the use of appropriate controls, such as placebos and sham acupuncture groups. However, promising results have emerged, for example, showing efficacy of acupuncture in adult postoperative and chemotherapy nausea and vomiting and in postoperative dental pain. There are other situations such as addiction, stroke rehabilitation, headache, menstrual cramps, tennis elbow, fibromyalgia, myofascial pain, osteoarthritis, low back pain, carpal tunnel syndrome, and asthma, in which acupuncture may be useful as an adjunct treatment or an acceptable alternative or be included in a comprehensive management program. Further research is likely to uncover additional areas where acupuncture interventions will be useful."[7]

Increasingly, acupuncture is complementing conventional therapies. For example, doctors may combine acupuncture and drugs to control surgery-related pain in their patients.[19] By providing both acupuncture and certain conventional anesthetic drugs, some doctors have found it possible to achieve a state of complete pain relief for some patients.[10] They also have found that using acupuncture lowers the need for conventional pain-killing drugs and thus reduces the risk of side effects for patients who take the drugs.[20,21]

Currently, one of the main reasons Americans seek acupuncture treatment is to relieve chronic pain, especially from conditions such as arthritis or lower back disorders.[22,23] Some clinical studies show that acupuncture is effective in relieving both chronic (long-lasting) and acute or sudden pain, but other research indicates that it provides no relief from chronic pain.[24] Additional research is needed to provide definitive answers.

FDA's Role

The U.S. Food and Drug Administration (FDA) approved acupuncture needles for use by licensed practitioners in 1996. The FDA requires manufacturers of acupuncture needles to label them for single use only.[25] Relatively few complications from the use of acupuncture have been reported to the FDA when one considers the millions of people treated each year and the number of acupuncture needles used. Still, complications have resulted from inadequate sterilization of needles and from improper delivery of treatments. When not delivered properly, acupuncture can cause serious adverse effects, including infections and punctured organs.[26]

Research Sponsored by NCCAM and OAM

NCCAM and OAM have supported scientific research to find out more about acupuncture. Examples of recent NCCAM-supported projects include:

- Studying the safety and effectiveness of acupuncture treatment for osteoarthritis of the knee.

- Investigating whether electroacupuncture works for chronic pain and inflammation (and, if so, how).

- Finding out how acupuncture affects the nervous system, by using MRI (magnetic resonance imaging) technology.

- Bringing together leaders from the Oriental medicine and conventional medicine communities to collaboratively study the safety and effectiveness of acupuncture and further develop the standards for clinical trials.

- Studying whether acupuncture can decrease the release of adrenaline in heart patients and improve their survival and quality of life. Adrenaline can make the heart beat faster and can thereby contribute to heart failure.

- Looking at the effectiveness of acupuncture for treating high blood pressure.

- Studying the effects of acupuncture on the symptoms of advanced colorectal cancer.

- Testing the safety and effectiveness of acupuncture for a type of depression called major depression.

With regard to earlier findings, researchers at the University of Maryland in Baltimore, with the support of OAM, conducted a randomized controlled clinical trial and found that patients treated with acupuncture after dental surgery had less intense pain than patients who received a placebo.[19] Scientists at the university also found that older people with osteoarthritis experienced significantly more pain relief after using conventional drugs and acupuncture together than those using conventional therapy alone.[27] OAM also funded several preliminary studies on acupuncture:

- In one small randomized controlled clinical trial, more than half of 11 women with a major depressive episode who were treated with acupuncture improved significantly.[28]

- In another controlled clinical trial, nearly half of the seven children with attention deficit hyperactivity disorder who underwent acupuncture treatment showed some improvement in their symptoms. Researchers concluded that acupuncture was a useful alternative to standard medication for some children with this condition.[29]

- In a third small controlled study, eight pregnant women were given a type of acupuncture treatment called moxibustion to reduce the rate of breech births, in which the fetus is positioned for birth feet-first instead of the normal position of head-first. Researchers found the treatment to be safe, but they were uncertain whether it was effective.[30] Then, researchers reporting in the November 11, 1998, issue of the *Journal of the American Medical Association* conducted a larger randomized controlled clinical trial using moxibustion for breech births. They found that moxibustion applied to 130 pregnant women presenting breech significantly increased the number of normal head-first births.[31]

Acupuncture and You

The use of acupuncture, like the use of many other complementary and alternative medicine (CAM) treatments, has produced a good deal of anecdotal evidence. Much of this evidence comes from people who report their own successful use of the treatment. If a treatment appears to be safe and patients report recovery from their illness or condition after using it, others may decide to use the treatment. However, scientific research may not support the anecdotal reports.

Lifestyle, age, physiology, and other factors combine to make every person different. A treatment that works for one person may not work for another who has the very same condition. You as a health care consumer (especially if you have a preexisting medical condition) should discuss any CAM treatment, including acupuncture, with your health care practitioner. Do not rely on a diagnosis of disease by an acupuncture practitioner who does not have substantial conventional medical training. If you have received a diagnosis from a doctor and have had little or no success using conventional medicine, you may wish to ask your doctor whether acupuncture might help.

Finding a Licensed Acupuncture Practitioner

Health care practitioners can be a resource for referral to practitioners of acupuncture, as more are becoming aware of this CAM therapy. More medical doctors, including neurologists, anesthesiologists, and specialists in physical medicine, are becoming trained in acupuncture, traditional Chinese medicine, and other CAM therapies. In addition, national organizations (consult your local library or search with a Web browser) may provide referrals to practitioners, although some organizations may encourage the use of their practices.

- **Check a practitioner's credentials.** A practitioner who is licensed and credentialed may provide better care than one who is not. About 40 states have established training standards for acupuncture certification, but states have varied requirements for obtaining a license to practice acupuncture.[32] Although proper credentials do not ensure competency, they do indicate that the practitioner has met certain standards to treat patients through the use of acupuncture.

- **Check treatment cost and insurance coverage.** A practitioner should inform you about the estimated number of treatments needed and how much each will cost. If this information is not provided, ask for it. Treatment may take place over a few days or for several weeks or more. Physician acupuncturists may charge more than non-physician practitioners. Check with your insurer before you start treatment as to whether acupuncture will be covered for your condition, and if so, to what extent. Some plans require preauthorization for acupuncture.

- **Check treatment procedures.** Ask about the treatment procedures that will be used and their likelihood of success for your condition or disease. You also should make certain that the practitioner uses a new set of disposable needles in a sealed package every time. The FDA requires the use of sterile, non-toxic needles that bear a labeling statement restricting their use to qualified practitioners. The practitioner also should swab the puncture site with alcohol or another disinfectant before inserting the needle.

During your first office visit, the practitioner may ask you at length about your health condition, lifestyle, and behavior. The practitioner will want to obtain a complete picture of your treatment needs and behaviors that may contribute to the condition. Inform the acupuncturist about all treatments or medications you are taking and all medical conditions you have.

The Sensation of Acupuncture

Acupuncture needles are metallic, solid, and hair-thin. People experience acupuncture differently, but most feel no or minimal pain as the needles are inserted. Some people are energized by treatment, while others feel relaxed.[33] Improper needle placement, movement of the patient, or a defect in the needle can cause soreness and pain during treatment.[34] This is why it is important to seek treatment from a qualified acupuncture practitioner.

Definitions

Anecdotal evidence: Data based on reports of usually unscientific observation. Anecdotes are often accounts of an individual's personal experience.

Attention deficit hyperactivity disorder: A group of disorders of behavior. Symptoms often include a tendency to act on impulse and problems with paying attention.

Clinical trial: Tests of a treatment's effects in humans. Clinical trials help researchers find out whether a promising treatment is safe and effective for people. They also tell scientists which treatments are more effective than others.

Complementary and alternative medicine: Health care practices and products that are not presently considered to be part of conventional medicine. Complementary medicine is used together with conventional medicine. Alternative medicine is used in place of conventional medicine. Conventional medicine is medicine as practiced by holders of M.D. (Doctor of Medicine) or D.O. (Doctor of Osteopathic Medicine) degrees and by their allied health professionals, such as physical therapists, psychologists, and registered nurses. Other terms for conventional medicine include allopathy; Western, mainstream, orthodox, and regular medicine; and biomedicine.

Depression: An illness that involves the body, mood, and thoughts. Among its symptoms are persistent sad, anxious, or "empty" feelings and changes in sleeping and/or eating patterns. Depression comes in various types.

Electroacupuncture: A variation of traditional acupuncture treatment in which acupuncture or needle points are stimulated electronically.

Electromagnetic signal: The minute electrical impulse that transmit information through and between nerve cells. For example, electromagnetic signals convey information about pain and other sensations within the body's nervous system.

Fibromyalgia: A complex chronic condition having multiple symptoms, including muscle pain, fatigue, and tenderness in precise, localized areas, particularly in the neck, spine, shoulders, and hips. People with this syndrome may also experience sleep disturbances, morning stiffness, irritable bowel syndrome, anxiety, and other symptoms.

Major depressive episode: A period of depression during which a person experiences a combination of symptoms that interfere with the ability to work, study, sleep, eat, and enjoy once pleasurable activities. Symptoms vary, but may include persistent feelings of sadness, anxiety, "emptiness," hopelessness, guilt, restlessness, or suicidal thoughts. People may also experience persistent physical symptoms that do not respond to treatment, such as headaches, digestive disorders, and chronic pain.

Meridian: A traditional Chinese medicine term for the 20 pathways throughout the body for the flow of qi, or vital energy, accessed through acupuncture points.

Moxibustion: The use of dried herbs in acupuncture. Generally, moxibustion in the United States involves the use of sticks of compressed herb(s) and is an adjunct to acupuncture rather than a part of acupuncture.

Neurohormone: A chemical substance made by tissue in the body's nervous system that can change the structure or function or direct the activity of an organ or organs.

Neurotransmitter: A biochemical substance that stimulates or inhibits nerve impulses in the brain that relay information about external stimuli and sensations, such as pain.

Opioid: A synthetic or naturally occurring chemical in the brain that may reduce pain and induce sleep.

Placebo: An inactive pill or sham procedure given to a participant in a research study as part of a test of the effects of another substance or treatment. Scientists use placebos to get a true picture of how the substance or treatment under investigation affects participants. In recent years, the definition of placebo has been expanded to include such things as aspects of interactions between patients and their health care providers that may affect their expectations and the study's outcomes.

Preclinical study: A study done to obtain information about a treatment's safety and side effects when given at different doses to animals or to cells grown in the laboratory.

Qi: The Chinese term for vital energy or life force. It is pronounced "chee."

Randomized controlled clinical trial: A type of clinical trial using two groups of people; one group (treatment group) receives the treatment and the other (control group) does not. Participants are assigned to either the treatment group or the control group at random, to prevent bias in the research.

Traditional Chinese medicine: Traditional Chinese medicine (TCM) is the current name for an ancient system of health care from China. TCM is based on a concept of balanced qi (pronounced "chee"), or vital energy, that is believed to flow throughout the body. Qi is proposed to regulate a person's spiritual, emotional, mental, and physical balance and to be influenced by the opposing forces of yin (negative energy) and yang (positive energy). Disease is proposed to result from the flow of qi being disrupted and yin and yang becoming imbalanced. Among the components of TCM are herbal and nutritional therapy, restorative physical exercises, meditation, acupuncture, and remedial massage.

Yang: The Chinese concept of positive energy and forces in the universe and human body. Acupuncture is believed to remove yang imbalances and bring the body into balance.

Yin: The Chinese concept of negative energy and forces in the universe and human body. Acupuncture is believed to remove yin imbalances and bring the body into balance.

References

1. Eisenberg, D.M., Davis, R.B., Ettner, S.L., Appel, S., Wilkey, S., Van Rompay, M., and Kessler, R.C. "Trends in Alternative Medicine Use in the United States, 1990-1997: Results of a Follow-Up National Survey." *Journal of the American Medical Association.* 1998. 280(18):1569–75.

2. Culliton, P.D. "Current Utilization of Acupuncture by United States Patients." National Institutes of Health Consensus Development Conference on Acupuncture, Program & Abstracts (Bethesda, MD, November 3-5, 1997). Office of Alternative Medicine and Office of Medical Applications of Research. Bethesda: National Institutes of Health, 1997.

3. Beinfield, H. and Korngold, E.L. *Between Heaven and Earth: A Guide to Chinese Medicine.* New York: Ballantine Books, 1991.

4. Brown, D. "Three Generations of Alternative Medicine: Behavioral Medicine, Integrated Medicine, and Energy Medicine." Boston University School of Medicine Alumni Report. Fall 1996.

5. Senior, K. "Acupuncture: Can It Take the Pain Away?" *Molecular Medicine Today.* 1996. 2(4):150–3.

6. Raso, J. *Alternative Health Care: A Comprehensive Guide.* Buffalo: Prometheus Books, 1994.

7. National Institutes of Health Consensus Panel. Acupuncture. National Institutes of Health Consensus Development Statement (Bethesda, MD, November 3-5, 1997). Office of Alternative Medicine and Office of Medical Applications of Research. Bethesda: National Institutes of Health, 1997.

8. Dale, R.A. "Demythologizing Acupuncture. Part 1. The Scientific Mechanisms and the Clinical Uses." *Alternative & Complementary Therapies Journal.* April 1997. 3(2):125–31.

9. Takeshige, C. "Mechanism of Acupuncture Analgesia Based on Animal Experiments." *Scientific Bases of Acupuncture.* Berlin: Springer-Verlag, 1989.

10. Han, J.S. "Acupuncture Activates Endogenous Systems of Analgesia." National Institutes of Health Consensus Conference on Acupuncture, Program & Abstracts (Bethesda, MD, November 3-5, 1997). Office of Alternative Medicine and Office of Medical Applications of Research. Bethesda: National Institutes of Health, 1997.

11. Wu, B., Zhou, R.X., and Zhou, M.S. "Effect of Acupuncture on Interleukin-2 Level and NK Cell Immunoactivity of Peripheral Blood of Malignant Tumor Patients." Chung Kuo Chung Hsi I Chieh Ho Tsa Chich. 1994. 14(9):537–9.

12. Wu, B. "Effect of Acupuncture on the Regulation of Cell-Mediated Immunity in the Patients with Malignant Tumors." Chen Tzu Yen Chiu. 1995. 20(3):67–71.

13. Eskinazi, D.P. "National Institutes of Health Technology Assessment Workshop on Alternative Medicine: Acupuncture." *Journal of Alternative and Complementary Medicine.* 1996. 2(1):1–253.

14. Tang, N.M., Dong, H.W., Wang, X.M., Tsui, Z.C., and Han, J.S. "Cholecystokinin Antisense RNA Increases the Analgesic Effect Induced by Electroacupuncture or Low Dose Morphine: Conversion of Low Responder Rats into High Responders." *Pain.* 1997. 71(1):71–80.

15. Cheng, X.D., Wu, G.C., He, Q.Z., and Cao, X.D. "Effect of Electroacupuncture on the Activities of Tyrosine Protein Kinase in Subcellular Fractions of Activated T Lymphocytes from the Traumatized Rats." *Acupuncture and Electro-Therapeutics Research.* 1998. 23(3-4):161–170.

16. Chen, L.B. and Li, S.X. "The Effects of Electrical Acupuncture of Neiguan on the PO2 of the Border Zone between Ischemic and Non-Ischemic Myocardium in Dogs." *Journal of Traditional Chinese Medicine.* 1983. 3(2):83–8.

17. Lee, H.S. and Kim, J.Y. "Effects of Acupuncture on Blood Pressure and Plasma Renin Activity in Two-Kidney One Clip Goldblatt Hypertensive Rats." *American Journal of Chinese Medicine.* 1994. 22(3-4):215–9.

18. Okada, K., Oshima, M., and Kawakita, K. "Examination of the Afferent Fiber Responsible for the Suppression of Jaw-Opening Reflex in Heat, Cold and Manual Acupuncture Stimulation in Anesthetized Rats." *Brain Research.* 1996. 740(1-2):201–7.

19. Lao, L., Bergman, S., Langenberg, P., Wong, R., and Berman, B. "Efficacy of Chinese Acupuncture on Postoperative Oral Surgery Pain." *Oral Surgery, Oral Medicine, Oral Pathology.* 1995. 79(4):423–8.

20. Lewith, G.T. and Vincent, C. "On the Evaluation of the Clinical Effects of Acupuncture: A Problem Reassessed and a Framework for Future Research." *Journal of Alternative and Complementary Medicine.* 1996. 2(1):79–90.

21. Tsibuliak, V.N., Alisov, A.P., and Shatrova, V.P. "Acupuncture Analgesia and Analgesic Transcutaneous Electroneurostimulation in the Early Postoperative Period." *Anesteziologiia i Reanimatologiia.* 1995. 2:93–7.

22. Bullock, M.L., Pheley, A.M., Kiresuk, T.J., Lenz, S.K., and Culliton, P.D. "Characteristics and Complaints of Patients Seeking Therapy at a Hospital-Based Alternative Medicine Clinic." *Journal of Alternative and Complementary Medicine.* 1997. 3(1):31–7.

23. Deihl, D.L., Kaplan, G., Coulter, I., Glik, D., and Hurwitz, E.L. "Use of Acupuncture by American Physicians." *Journal of Alternative and Complementary Medicine.* 1997. 3(2):119–26.

24. Ter Reit, G., Kleijnen, J., and Knipschild, P. "Acupuncture and Chronic Pain: A Criteria-Based Meta-Analysis." *Clinical Epidemiology.* 1990. 43:1191–9.

25. U.S. Food and Drug Administration. "Acupuncture Needles No Longer Investigational." *FDA Consumer Magazine.* June 1996. 30(5).

26. Lytle, C.D. An Overview of Acupuncture. 1993. Washington: U.S. Department of Health and Human Services, Health Sciences Branch, Division of Life Sciences, Office of Science and Technology, Center for Devices and Radiological Health, Food and Drug Administration.

27. Berman, B., Lao, L., Bergman, S., Langenberg, P., Wong, R., Loangenberg, P., and Hochberg, M. "Efficacy of Traditional Chinese Acupuncture in the Treatment of Osteoarthritis: A Pilot Study." *Osteoarthritis and Cartilage.* 1995. (3):139–42.

28. Allen, John J.B. "An Acupuncture Treatment Study for Unipolar Depression." *Psychological Science.* 1998. 9:397–401.

29. Sonenklar, N. Acupuncture and Attention Deficit Hyperactivity Disorder. National Institutes of Health, Office of Alternative Medicine Research grant R21 RR09463. 1993.

30. Milligan, R. Breech Version by Acumoxa. National Institutes of Health, Office of Alternative Medicine Research grant R21 RR09527. 1993.

31. Cardini, F. and Weixin, H. "Moxibustion for Correction of Breech Presentation: A Randomized Controlled Trial." *Journal of the American Medical Association.* 1998. 280:1580–4.

32. White House Commission on Complementary and Alternative Medicine Policy. Interim Progress Report: White House Commission on Complementary and Alternative Medicine Policy. Washington: White House Commission on Complementary and Alternative Medicine Policy, 2001.

33. American Academy of Medical Acupuncture. *Doctor, What's This Acupuncture All About? A Brief Explanation for Patients.* Los Angeles: American Academy of Medical Acupuncture, 1996.

34. Lao, L. "Safety Issues in Acupuncture." *Journal of Alternative and Complementary Medicine.* 1996. 2(1):27–9.

Section 56.2

Acupuncture and Low Back Pain

Back pain is one of the most common reasons people see a health care provider. It has been estimated that up to 80% of the world's population will suffer from back pain at some point in their lives, with the lower back as the most common location of pain. Although most episodes of low back pain last less than two weeks, research has shown that recurrence rates for low back pain can reach as high as 50% in the first few months following an initial episode.[1,2]

While there is no definitive way to resolve lower back pain, the use of acupuncture to treat this condition has increased dramatically in the past few decades, based in a large extent to placebo-controlled studies that have validated it as a reliable method of pain relief. The results of a recent study published in the *Clinical Journal of Pain*[3] provide further proof that acupuncture is a safe and effective procedure for low back pain, and that it can maintain positive outcomes for periods of six months or longer without producing the negative side effects that often accompany more traditional pain remedies.

Drs. Christer Carlsson and Bengt Sjolund of the Lund University Hospital in Sweden recruited 50 patients (33 women, 17 men) from a tertiary level pain clinic for their study. The median age of the participants was 49.8; each patient had been suffering chronic low back pain for a minimum of six months and had tried a variety of other therapies (such as corsets, nerve blocks, drugs, and physiotherapy) to treat their condition, but to no avail.

Subjects were randomly assigned to a manual acupuncture group, an electroacupuncture group, or a placebo group. Treatment sessions lasted a total of 20 minutes each and were delivered once per week for eight weeks, with the same amount of time and care given to all patients in each group. A followup treatment was given after two months, and a tenth and final treatment was given after an additional two months.

In the manual group, local points on the lower back and distal points on the lower limbs, forearms, and hands were used. The number of needles used per patient increased from an average of eight during the first session to as many as 18 during the third or fourth session. Needles were stimulated three times during each session to attain *de qi*. [Editor's Note: *De qi* occurs when acupuncture patients typically experience an aching sensation. It is traditionally believed to be essential in achieving acupuncture's therapeutic effect.]

A slightly different protocol was used on patients receiving electroacupuncture. Patients in this group received manual stimulation only during the first few sessions, followed by electrical stimulation of four needles in the low back in subsequent sessions. A similar number of needles as used in the manual acupuncture group were inserted and activated by hand.

The placebo group was given mock stimulation using what the researchers termed an "impressive"—but disconnected—stimulator attached to two large electrodes. The electrodes were placed on the skin over the most painful areas in the lower back. During mock stimulation, flashing lamps from the machine were displayed and made visible to the patient to give the illusion that treatment was being delivered.

Throughout the study, patients recorded pain levels and other measurements in small booklets called pain diaries. Among the variables measured were pain intensity (recorded twice daily on a visual analog scale from 0 to 100, 100 being severe as possible); intake of analgesics (recorded daily); sleep quality (scored on a scale of "good," "slightly disturbed by pain," or "badly disturbed by pain"); and activity level. These diaries were compiled and their results analyzed by a nurse practitioner at the end of the study.

In addition, assessments were performed by an independent observer who did not know which type of acupuncture each patient received. These assessments were taken at four intervals: baseline, one month, three months, and six months after the treatment period. These assessments consisted of a clinical interview and physical examination, after which the observer classified the patient's pain as improved, unchanged, or worse.

"Significant" Changes Observed in Acupuncture Patients

Analysis of the pain diaries revealed "significant" differences between acupuncture and placebo patients at the one-, three-, and six-month intervals following treatment, all of which favored acupuncture as a more effective form of pain relief. For example, in the acupuncture group, both morning and evening pain scores were lower than baseline measurements and continued to decrease for the duration of treatment. In the placebo group, however, pain scores were several points higher after one month than they were at baseline, and continued to remain higher than the baseline scores throughout the study.

Activity levels were also markedly improved in the acupuncture group. Fourteen acupuncture patients and seven placebo patients had been on sick leave (either part-time or full-time) prior to the start of the study. By the time the tenth acupuncture treatment was delivered, six of the acupuncture patients on sick leave had returned to part-time or full-time work; another six were retired but still reported improved activity levels. In comparison, only one patient in the placebo group showed an improvement in activity; another patient actually regressed to being put on full sick leave.

Furthermore, acupuncture patients experienced less episodes of sleep disturbance than their placebo-treated counterparts. Before the study, 30 acupuncture patients and 12 placebo patients reported sleep disturbances due to pain. The researchers reported that the sleep pattern was "significantly less disturbed after the treatment period" in the acupuncture group, but that there was "no significant difference in sleep disturbance" in the placebo patients.

Finally, total intake of analgesics dropped dramatically in the acupuncture group, but not the placebo group. At the start of the study, patients in the acupuncture group consumed an average of 31 pills per week; those in the placebo group consumed an average of 23 pills. At the six-month follow-up, the number of pills taken by placebo patients remained almost identical (21.5 per person per week), but had dropped more than 28% to 21.4 pills per week in acupuncture patients.

Independent examination by the blinded observer appeared to corroborate the patients' pain estimates. One month after the initial treatment period, 16 acupuncture patients (but only two placebo patients) were judged to be improved. After six months, 14 acupuncture patients (and only two placebo patients) were still improved. Both types of acupuncture worked effectively; of the 14 patients who showed improvement after six months, eight received manual acupuncture and six received electrical stimulation.

One interesting result of the study was that acupuncture appeared to be most effective in women. Of the 16 acupuncture patients judged to be "improved" at the one-month follow-up, 15 were women. At the six-month follow-up, all 14 patients who were still improved were women. The researchers were at a loss to explain this phenomenon, but hypothesized that it may be linked to estrogen receptors in the central nervous system.

Treatment Works Best with Specific Types of Pain

In their discussion, Carlsson and Sjolund stated that the trial "demonstrated a long-term pain-relieving effect of needle acupuncture compared with true placebo in some patients with chronic low back pain." To substantiate this claim, they highlighted several components that had been built into the study to help validate its results. Among them:

- Only acupuncture naive patients (those who had never received acupuncture before) were selected for inclusion;

- Patients were informed at the start of the study that the treatment might not be felt;

- An equal amount of time and care was spent on each patient from every treatment group;

- The placebo treatment used in the trial (mock stimulation) was preferred because, unlike sham acupuncture, needles were not inserted, which might have inadvertently skewed the results from the placebo group; and

- The independent observer who performed assessments was never made aware of which group each subject was in and specifically avoided asking any questions about the type of treatment subjects received.

Taken together, the researchers concluded that these factors "seem sufficient to establish a true placebo treatment in the current study." They added that based on their latest study, in conjunction with the results of acupuncture trials on other disorders, "there is now reasonable evidence that acupuncture has a clinically relevant pain-relieving effect on certain forms of chronic pain."

Carlsson and Sjolund also advised practitioners that just because acupuncture works on certain types of back pain, it may not produce the same results on every type. "It would be as correct to assess the effect of acupuncture on all types of pain," they observed, "as it would be to study the effect of common penicillin on all types of bacterial infections and calculate some form of 'average.' "

As to the specific type of pain, the researchers believe that based on previously published papers, acupuncture may be most effective for low back pain that is nociceptive (caused by an injury or disease outside the nervous system) in origin. Determining the cause of pain, they feel, is paramount to using a particular therapy for relief. As the scientists stated in their conclusion:

"Acupuncture does not seem to be a suitable treatment modality for neuropathic pain. However, the clinical use of acupuncture is sometimes indicated for the treatment of chronic nociceptive pain. Our study is the first to show that acupuncture may have a long-term effect on chronic low back pain superior to that of placebo. Therefore, it is vital that before acupuncture is applied, a thorough analysis of the pain condition is performed to preclude the indiscriminate, unnecessary, and costly use of this treatment technique."

References

1. Moffett JK, Torgerson D, Bell-Syer S, et al. Randomised controlled trial of exercise for low back pain: clinical outcomes, cost and preferences. *British Medical Journal* July 31, 1999;319(7205):279–283.

2. Nyiendo J, Haas M, Goodwin P. Patient characteristics, practice activities, and one-month outcomes for chronic, recurrent low-back pain treated by chiropractors and family medical physicians: a practice-based feasibility study. *Journal of Manipulative and Physiological Therapeutics* May 2000; 23(4):239–245.

3. Carlsson C, Sjolund B. Acupuncture for chronic low back pain: a randomized placebo-controlled study with long-term follow-up. *Clinical Journal of Pain* 2001;17(4):296–305.

Chapter 57

Prolotherapy and Chronic Back Pain

Prolotherapy Introduction

Prolotherapy is a non-surgical injection procedure used to treat connective tissue injuries of the musculoskeletal system that have not healed by either rest or conservative therapy in order to relieve back pain. The injections promote a healing response in small tears and weakened tissue, with the goal of alleviating back pain and improving function. Prolotherapy is also referred to as sclerosant therapy, sclerotherapy, regenerative injection therapy, proliferative injection therapy, and nonsurgical ligament reconstruction.

Prolotherapy has been used in pain management and treatment of numerous conditions, including back pain and neck pain due to spine related conditions such as:

- Degenerative disk disease
- Sacroiliac problems
- Sciatica
- Whiplash

A theory behind prolotherapy is that back pain is related to activation of pain receptors in tendon or ligament tissues, which are sensitive to stretching, pressure, etc. It is thought that the cause of back pain is from ligamentous laxity.

With the prolotherapy procedure, the substance injected into the soft tissue causes an inflammatory response at the site, which in turn causes natural healing to take place (formation or proliferation of new blood vessels), with the goal of strengthening the torn or injured soft tissue and reducing the back pain.

While a history of the prolotherapy treatment approach has been traced back to ancient times, it is not yet widely practiced in the United States and many practitioners consider it an alternative therapy. Prolotherapy as a means of pain management is not taught in medical school or residency training programs.

There currently are few studies that show the effectiveness of the prolotherapy procedure for alleviating back pain. Patients considering prolotherapy for back pain should ask their physician if he or she is trained and experienced in the procedure.

Who Does Prolotherapy for Back Pain?

A physician who has specific training in prolotherapy should perform the prolotherapy injection procedure. Physicians (either M.D.s or D.O.s) who typically perform prolotherapy for spine conditions include physiatrists, anesthesiologists, orthopedic surgeons, and neurosurgeons.

A number of organizations provide educational programs and training on prolotherapy for doctors, including:

- American Association of Orthopaedic Medicine
- American Academy of Sclerotherapy

Other organizations that may be contacted about the procedure and doctors who perform prolotherapy for back pain include:

- International Spinal Injection Society
- American Academy of Physical Medicine and Rehabilitation

What Is Known about Prolotherapy Outcomes for Back Pain?

Reported success rates range from 80% to 90% when performed by a physician trained in the prolotherapy procedure. Many of these reports are based on anecdotal evidence from the physicians themselves. Studies have not yet connected positive outcomes for back pain and healing to prolotherapy.

The anecdotal reports suggest improvements such as:

- Reduction or elimination of back pain

- Increased strength of the ligament, tendon, or joint capsule

- Reduced recurrence of injury to the treated site

- Improved or return to normal function

Factors that may be key for a successful outcome include:

- Proper diagnosis of the location of the sprain or strain

- Willingness of the patient to complete follow-up therapy

- Clinical skill of the physician in performing the injection

Finally, it is important to note that nobody knows exactly what happens in prolotherapy. There is no objective medical evidence, and no histology has been published as to what goes on when injection is placed into the painful soft tissues.

What Is Prolotherapy?

In prolotherapy treatment, a substance is injected using a slender needle next to the site where soft tissue (ligament, tendon, muscle, fascia, joint capsule) is injured or has torn away from the bone.

The substance used in the injection is a natural irritant agent. Examples include:

- Sugar (dextrose or glucose) alone or in combination with glycerin and phenol

- Sodium morrhuate (a purified derivative of cod liver oil)

The agent is typically used with a local anesthetic (lidocaine, procaine, or Marcaine). Prolotherapy involves a series of injections, reportedly ranging from 3 to 30 (average 4 to 10), depending on the condition and the individual being treated. The injection series may cover 3 to 6 months with injections at 2- to 3-week intervals.

Most reports suggest physicians recommending prolotherapy provide substantial counseling for their patients to prepare them for both the procedure and the side effects.

485

To counteract the painful, swollen injection site experienced by most patients for 2 to 3 days following the procedure, physicians may recommend:

- Taking acetaminophen or hydrocodone bitartrate plus acetaminophen for pain, but not aspirin or anti-inflammatory medications which would inhibit the healing response.

- Applying ice to the area 3 to 5 times a day for 20 minutes each as needed.

- Doing moderate exercise such as walking but avoid strenuous exercise or work with heavy lifting.

- Following up the injections with a good physical therapy program.

What Are Current Indications for Prolotherapy?

There are currently no treatment guidelines or protocol for prolotherapy. It is most commonly used for patients with back pain caused by chronic ligament and tendon sprains and strains. Some physicians do use it as a first-line therapy.

It is important to note that approximately 90% of people with acute back pain get better with standard conservative treatments within 6 to 8 weeks and do not require additional treatment.

Candidates for prolotherapy might include patients with back pain who:

- Take medication on the recommendation of their physician (aspirin, ibuprofen, oral steroids) for ligament, tendon, or joint problems

- Have ligament, tendon, or joint pain or weakness/instability lasting over 6 weeks

- Get only temporary relief from manual or physical therapy

- Have had surgery with no pain relief

- Experience joint pain that is worse with exercise and better with rest

Relative Contraindications for Prolotherapy Include

- Unclear diagnosis of the location of the injury (sprains, strains and weakened ligament do not show up on diagnostic imaging studies)
- Lack of training by the selected physician on the solutions used and how to perform the injections

Potential Risks and Complications of Prolotherapy

The injection technique involved in prolotherapy requires skill and care on the part of the physician. Training and experience are important.

Possible side effects may last a few days to a couple weeks and include:

- Swelling

- Intense pain and stiffness

- Headache

- Allergic reaction

Reports of more serious complications have been rare, but could include:

- Spinal fluid leak

- Permanent nerve damage or paralysis

- Pneumothorax

Part Seven

Information about Spinal Surgeries

Chapter 58

Questions to Ask Your Doctor before You Have Surgery

Are you facing surgery? You are not alone. Millions of Americans have surgery each year. Most operations are not emergencies. This means you have time to ask your surgeon questions about the operation and time to decide whether to have it, and if so, when and where. The information presented here does not apply to emergency surgery.

The most important questions to ask about elective surgery are why the procedure is necessary for you and what alternatives there are to surgery. If you do not need to have the operation, then you can avoid any risks that might result. All surgeries and alternative treatments have risks and benefits. They are only worth doing if the benefits are greater than the risks.

Your primary care doctor, that is, your regular doctor, may be the one who suggests that you have surgery and may recommend a surgeon. You may want to identify another independent surgeon to get a second opinion. Check to see if your health insurance will pay for the operation and the second opinion. If you are eligible for Medicare, it will pay for a second opinion. You should discuss your insurance questions with your health insurance company or your employee benefits office.

"Be Informed: Questions To Ask Your Doctor Before You Have Surgery." Agency for Healthcare Research and Quality (formerly Agency for Health Care Policy and Research), Rockville, MD. Publication No. 95-0027, January 1995. Available online at http://www.ahrq.gov; accessed March 2004. Reviewed by David A. Cooke, M.D., on April 11, 2004.

Overview

Following are 12 questions to ask your primary care doctor and surgeon before you have surgery and the reasons for asking them. The answers to these questions will help you be informed and help you make the best decision. Sources are listed at the end of these questions to help you get more information from other places.

Your doctors should welcome questions. If you do not understand the answers, ask the doctors to explain them clearly. Patients who are well informed about their treatment tend to be more satisfied with the outcome or results of their treatment.

What Operation Are You Recommending?

Ask your surgeon to explain the surgical procedure. For example, if something is going to be repaired or removed, find out why it is necessary to do so. Your surgeon can draw a picture or a diagram and explain to you the steps involved in the procedure.

Are there different ways of doing the operation? One way may require more extensive surgery than another. Ask why your surgeon wants to do the operation one way over another.

Why Do I Need the Operation?

There are many reasons to have surgery. Some operations can relieve or prevent pain. Others can reduce a symptom of a problem or improve some body function. Some surgeries are performed to diagnose a problem. Surgery also can save your life. Your surgeon will tell you the purpose of the procedure. Make sure you understand how the proposed operation fits in with the diagnosis of your medical condition.

Are There Alternatives to Surgery?

Sometimes, surgery is not the only answer to a medical problem. Medicines or other nonsurgical treatments, such as a change in diet or special exercises, might help you just as well or more. Ask your surgeon or primary care doctor about the benefits and risks of these other choices. You need to know as much as possible about these benefits and risks to make the best decision.

One alternative may be "watchful waiting," in which your doctor and you check to see if your problem gets better or worse. If it gets worse, you may need surgery right away. If it gets better, you may be able to postpone surgery, perhaps indefinitely.

What Are the Benefits of Having the Operation?

Ask your surgeon what you will gain by having the operation. For example, a hip replacement may mean that you can walk again with ease.

Ask how long the benefits are likely to last. For some procedures, it is not unusual for the benefits to last for a short time only. There might be a need for a second operation at a later date. For other procedures, the benefits may last a lifetime.

When finding out about the benefits of the operation, be realistic. Sometimes patients expect too much and are disappointed with the outcome, or results. Ask your doctor if there is any published information about the outcomes of the procedure.

What Are the Risks of Having the Operation?

All operations carry some risk. This is why you need to weigh the benefits of the operation against the risks of complications or side effects.

Complications can occur around the time of the operation. Complications are unplanned events, such as infection, too much bleeding, reaction to anesthesia, or accidental injury. Some people have an increased risk of complications because of other medical conditions.

In addition, there may be side effects after the operation. For the most part, side effects can be anticipated. For example, your surgeon knows that there will be swelling and some soreness at the site of the operation.

Ask your surgeon about the possible complications and side effects of the operation. There is almost always some pain with surgery. Ask how much there will be and what the doctors and nurses will do to reduce the pain. Controlling the pain will help you be more comfortable while you heal, get well faster, and improve the results of your operation.

What If I Don't Have This Operation?

Based on what you learn about the benefits and risks of the operation, you might decide not to have it. Ask your surgeon what you will gain—or lose—by not having the operation now. Could you be in more pain? Could your condition get worse? Could the problem go away?

Where Can I Get a Second Opinion?

Getting a second opinion from another doctor is a very good way to make sure having the operation is the best alternative for you. Many health insurance plans require patients to get a second opinion before they have certain non-emergency operations. If your plan does not require a second opinion, you may still ask to have one. Check with your insurance company to see if it will pay for a second opinion. If you get one, make sure to get your records from the first doctor so that the second one does not have to repeat tests.

What Has Been Your Experience in Doing the Operation?

One way to reduce the risks of surgery is to choose a surgeon who has been thoroughly trained to do the procedure and has plenty of experience doing it. You can ask your surgeon about his or her recent record of successes and complications with this procedure. If it is more comfortable for you, you can discuss the topic of surgeons' qualifications with your regular or primary care doctor.

Where Will the Operation Be Done?

Most surgeons practice at one or two local hospitals. Find out where your operation will be performed. Have many of the operations you are thinking about having been done in this hospital? Some operations have higher success rates if they are done in hospitals that do many of those procedures. Ask your doctor about the success rate at this hospital. If the hospital has a low success rate for the operation in question, you should ask to have it at another hospital.

Until recently, most surgery was performed on an inpatient basis and patients stayed in the hospital for one or more days. Today, a lot of surgery is done on an outpatient basis in a doctor's office, a special surgical center, or a day surgery unit of a hospital. Outpatient surgery is less expensive because you do not have to pay for staying in a hospital room.

Ask whether your operation will be done in the hospital or in an outpatient setting. If your doctor recommends inpatient surgery for a procedure that is usually done as outpatient surgery, or just the opposite, recommends outpatient surgery that is usually done as inpatient surgery, ask why. You want to be in the right place for your operation.

What Kind of Anesthesia Will I Need?

Anesthesia is used so that surgery can be performed without unnecessary pain. Your surgeon can tell you whether the operation calls for local, regional, or general anesthesia, and why this form of anesthesia is recommended for your procedure.

Local anesthesia numbs only a part of your body for a short period of time, for example, a tooth and the surrounding gum. Not all procedures done with local anesthesia are painless.

Regional anesthesia numbs a larger portion of your body, for example, the lower part of your body for a few hours. In most cases, you will be awake with regional anesthesia.

General anesthesia numbs your entire body for the entire time of the surgery. You will be unconscious if you have general anesthesia.

Anesthesia is quite safe for most patients and is usually administered by a specialized physician (anesthesiologist) or nurse anesthetist. Both are highly skilled and have been specially trained to give anesthesia.

If you decide to have an operation, ask to meet with the person who will give you anesthesia. Find out what his or her qualifications are. Ask what the side effects and risks of having anesthesia are in your case. Be sure to tell him or her what medical problems you have including allergies and any medications you have been taking, since they may affect your response to the anesthesia.

How Long Will It Take Me to Recover?

Your surgeon can tell you how you might feel and what you will be able to do or not do the first few days, weeks, or months after surgery. Ask how long you will be in the hospital. Find out what kind of supplies, equipment, and any other help you will need when you go home. Knowing what to expect can help you cope better with recovery.

Ask when you can start regular exercise again and go back to work. You do not want to do anything that will slow down the recovery process. Lifting a 10-pound bag of potatoes may not seem to be too much a week after your operation, but it could be. You should follow your surgeon's advice to make sure you recover fully as soon as possible.

How Much Will the Operation Cost?

Health insurance coverage for surgery can vary, and there may be some costs you will have to pay. Before you have the operation, call your insurance company to find out how much of these costs it will pay and how much you will have to pay yourself.

Ask what your surgeon's fee is and what it covers. Surgical fees often also include several visits after the operation. You also will be billed by the hospital for inpatient or outpatient care and by the anesthesiologist and others providing care related to your operation.

Surgeons' Qualifications

You will want to know that your surgeon is experienced and qualified to perform the operation. Many surgeons have taken special training and passed exams given by a national board of surgeons. Ask if your surgeon is board certified in surgery. Some surgeons also have the letters F.A.C.S. after their name. This means they are Fellows of the American College of Surgeons and have passed another review by surgeons of their surgical practices.

Chapter 59

Complications of Spinal Surgery

Introduction

With any surgery, there is the risk of complications. When surgery is done near the spine and spinal cord these complications can be very serious—if they occur. The chance that any of these complications will occur during your surgery or during your recovery is usually very small. You should discuss these complications with your doctor before surgery if you have any questions that are not answered here. This is not intended to be a complete list of the possible complications, but these are the most common.

General Complications

- Anesthesia complications
- Bleeding
- Blood clots
- Dural tear
- Lung problems
- Infection
- Persistent pain

Nerve Complications

- Nerve injury
- Spinal cord injury
- Sexual dysfunction

Implant and Fusion Complications

- Delayed union or nonunion
- Hardware fracture
- Implant migration
- Pseudarthrosis
- Transitional syndrome

General Complications

Anesthesia Complications

Most spinal operations require general anesthesia. A very small number of patients may have problems from it. These problems can arise from reactions to the drugs used, other medical conditions you may have, or problems with the anesthesia. Anesthesia affects how the lungs work and can pose problems with lung infections. Nausea and vomiting can occur and are usually treated with medications. The tube inserted into your throat may cause soreness after surgery. In rare cases the tube can harm the vocal cords. Be sure to talk to your doctor and anesthesiologist about possible complications.

Bleeding

Surgery on the spine involves the risk of unexpected bleeding. Spine surgeries performed through the abdominal cavity require the surgeon to move the abdominal aorta and large vessels going to the legs out of the way. Doctors take extra care while performing surgery to avoid harming nearby blood vessels.

Blood Clots

Deep venous thrombosis (DVT) (or thrombophlebitis) is the medical name to describe blood clots formed in the veins of the legs. This is a common problem following many types of surgical procedures.

These blood clots form in the large veins of the calf. They may continue to grow and extend up into the veins of the thigh, and in some cases into the veins of the pelvis.

It is true that some people develop DVT even though they have not undergone any recent surgery. But the risk is much higher following surgery—especially surgery involving the pelvis or the lower extremities. There are logical reasons why the risk is increased. The body is trying to stop bleeding associated with surgery, so the body's clotting mechanism becomes very active during this period. Also injury to blood vessels around the surgical site from normal tugging and pulling during surgery can set off the clotting process. Blood that does not move well sits in the veins and becomes stagnant. If it sits too long in one spot it may begin to clot.

The prevention of DVT is a serious matter. Blood clots that fill the deep veins of the legs stop the normal flow of venous blood from the legs back to the heart. This causes swelling and pain in the affected leg. If the blood clot inside the vein does not dissolve, the swelling may become chronic and can cause permanent discomfort. While the discomfort is unpleasant, the blood clot actually poses much more serious danger. If a portion of the forming blood clot breaks free inside the veins of the leg, it may travel through the veins to the lung. There it can lodge itself in the tiny vessels of the lung, cutting off the blood supply to the blocked portion of the lung. This blocked portion cannot survive and may collapse. This is called a pulmonary embolism. If a pulmonary embolism is large enough, and the portion of the lung that collapses is large enough, it can cause death.

Reducing the risk of developing DVT is a high priority following any type of surgery. Preventative measures fall into two categories—mechanical involves getting the blood moving better, and medical involves using drugs to slow the clotting process.

Mechanical

Blood that is moving is less likely to clot. Getting you moving so that your blood is circulating is perhaps the most effective treatment against developing DVT. Once you begin walking, your leg muscles will contract and keep the blood in the veins of the legs moving. But you can still do things while you are in bed to increase the circulation of blood from the legs back to the heart. Simply pumping your feet up and down (like pushing on the gas pedal) contracts the muscles of the calf, squeezes the veins in the calf, and pushes the blood back to the heart. You should do these exercises as often as you can.

Pulsatile stockings are very effective. They are special stockings that wrap around each calf and thigh. A pump inflates them every few minutes, squeezing the veins in the legs and pushing blood back to the heart. Support hose, sometimes called TED hose, are still commonly used following surgery. The hose work by squeezing the veins of the leg shut. This reduces the amount of stagnant blood that is pooling in the veins of the leg and lowers the risk of blood clotting.

Medical

Medications that slow down the body's clotting mechanism can reduce the risk of DVT. They are widely used following surgery of the hip and knee. Aspirin can be used in very low risk situations. Heparin shots may be given twice a day in moderately risky situations. When there is a high risk for developing DVT, several potent drugs are available that can slow the clotting mechanism very effectively. Heparin can be given by intravenous injection, a new drug called Lovenox can be given in shots administered twice a day, and Coumadin can be given by mouth. Coumadin is the drug of choice when the clotting mechanism must be slowed for more than a few days because it can be taken orally.

In most cases of spinal surgery, both mechanical and medical measures are used simultaneously. It has become normal practice to use pulsatile stockings and place patients on some type of medication to slow the blood clotting mechanism. You are encouraged to get out of bed as soon as possible and begin exercises immediately after surgery.

Dural Tear

A watertight sac of tissue (dura mater) covers the spinal cord and the spinal nerves. A tear in this covering can occur during surgery. It is not uncommon to have a dural tear during any type of spine surgery. If noticed during the surgery, the tear is simply repaired and usually heals uneventfully. If it is not recognized, the tear may not heal and may continue to leak spinal fluid, which can cause problems later. The leaking spinal fluid may cause a spinal headache. It can also increase the risk of infection of the spinal fluid (spinal meningitis). If the dural leak does not seal itself off fairly quickly on its own, a second operation may be necessary to repair the tear in the dura.

Lung Problems

It is important that your lungs are working at their best following surgery to ensure that you get plenty of oxygen to the tissues of the body that are trying to heal. Lungs that are not exercised properly after surgery can lead to poor blood oxygen levels and can even develop pneumonia.

There are several reasons why your lungs may not work normally after surgery. If you were put to sleep with a general anesthetic, the medications used may temporarily cause the lungs to not function as well as normal. This is one reason that a spinal type anesthetic is recommended whenever possible. Lying in bed prevents completely normal function of the lungs, and the medications you take for pain may cause you to not breathe as deeply as you normally would.

After surgery you will need to do several things to keep your lungs working at their best. Your nurse will encourage you to take frequent deep breaths and cough often. Getting out of bed, even upright in a chair, allows the lungs to work much better. You will be allowed to get up and into a chair as soon as possible. Respiratory therapists have tools to help maintain optimal lung function. The incentive spirometer is a small device that measures how hard you are breathing and gives you a tool to help improve your deep breathing. If you have any other lung disease, such as asthma, the respiratory therapist may also use medications that are given through breathing treatments to help open the air pockets in the lungs.

Infection

There is a risk of infection any time surgery is performed. Surgeons take every precaution to prevent infections. You will probably be given antibiotics right before surgery—especially if bone graft, metal screws, or plates will be used. Infections occur in less than 1% of spinal surgeries.

An infection can be in the skin incision only, or it can spread deeper to involve the areas around the spinal cord and the vertebrae. A wound infection that involves only the skin incision is considered superficial. It is less serious and easier to treat than a deeper infection. A superficial wound infection can usually be treated with antibiotics, and perhaps removing the skin stitches. The deeper wound infections can be very serious and will probably require additional operations to drain the infection. In the worst cases, any bone graft, metal screws, or plates that were used may need to be removed. Contact your doctor immediately if you suspect that you have an infection. Some indications of infection include:

- surgical wound that is red, hot, swollen, and does not heal

- clear liquid or yellow pus oozing from the wound

- wound drainage that smells bad

- increasing pain

- fever and shaking chills

Persistent Pain

Some spinal operations are simply unsuccessful. One of the most common complications of spinal surgery is that it does not get rid of all of your pain. Some pain after surgery is expected. If you experience chronic pain well after the operation, you should let your doctor know.

In some cases the procedure may actually increase your pain. Be aware of this risk before surgery and discuss it at length with your surgeon. He or she will be able to give you some idea of your chances of not getting the relief that you expect.

Nerve Complications

Nerve Injury

Any time surgery is done on the spine, there is some risk of injuring the spinal cord, which can lead to nerve damage. The nerves in each area of the spinal cord connect to specific parts of your body. This is why damage to the spinal cord can cause paralysis in certain areas and not others; it depends on which spinal nerves are affected.

Spinal Cord Injury

Operations on the spine have some risk of injuring the spinal cord or spinal nerves. This can occur from instruments used during surgery, from swelling, or from scar formation after surgery. Damage to the spinal cord can cause paralysis in certain areas and not others. Injured nerves can cause pain, numbness, or weakness in the area supplied by the nerve.

Sexual Dysfunction

The spinal cord and spinal nerves carry the nerve signals that allow the rest of your body to function and to feel sensation. Damage to the spinal cord and the nerves around the spinal cord can cause many problems. If a nerve is damaged that connects to the pelvic region, it may cause sexual dysfunction.

Implant and Fusion Complications

Delayed Union or Nonunion

A certain number of fusions simply do not heal as planned. This type of problem case is called a nonunion. A nonunion may require a second operation to try to get the bones to heal. Some fusions will take longer than expected to heal. This type of problem case is called a delayed union.

Hardware Fracture

Metal screws, plates, and rods are used in many different types of spinal operations as part of the procedure to hold the vertebrae in alignment while the surgery heals. These metal devices are called hardware. Once the bone heals, the hardware is usually not doing much of anything. Sometimes the hardware can either break or move from the correct position before the surgery is completely healed. This is called a hardware fracture. If this occurs it may require a second operation to either remove or replace the hardware.

Implant Migration

Implant migration is a term used to describe an intervertebral fusion cage that has moved out of place. When this happens, it usually occurs soon after surgery, before the healing process has progressed to the point where the cage is firmly attached by scar tissue or bone growth.

If the cage moves too far, it may not be doing its job of stabilizing the two vertebrae. If it moves in a direction toward the spine or large vessels, it may damage those structures. A problem with implant migration may require a second operation to replace the cage that has moved. Your doctor will check the status of the hardware with x-rays taken during your follow-up office visits.

Pseudarthrosis

The term "pseud" means false and "arthrosis" refers to joint. The term pseudarthrosis then means false joint. A surgeon uses this term to describe either a fractured bone that has not healed or an attempted fusion that has not been successful. A pseudarthrosis usually means that there is motion between the two bones that should be healed (or fused together).

There is usually continued pain when the vertebrae involved in a surgical fusion do not heal. The pain may increase over time. The spinal motion can also stress the metal hardware used to hold the fusion—possibly causing them to break. You may need additional surgery for a pseudarthrosis. Your surgeon might want to add more bone graft, replace the metal hardware, or add an electrical stimulator to try to get the fusion to heal.

Transitional Syndrome

The spine behaves like a chain of repeating segments. When the entire spine is healthy, each segment works together to share the load throughout the spinal column. Each segment works with its neighboring segment to share the stresses imposed by movements and forces. When one or two segments are not working properly, the neighboring segments have to take on more of the load. It is the segment closest to the non-working segment that gets most of the extra stress. This means that if one or more levels are fused anywhere in the spine, the spinal segment next to where the surgery was performed begins to take on more stress. Over time this can lead to increased wear and tear to this segment, eventually causing pain from the damaged segment. This is called a transitional syndrome because it occurs where the transition from a normal area of the spine to the abnormal area that has been fused.

Chapter 60

Minimally Invasive Spinal Surgery: The Benefits

Thoracoscopic, laparoscopic, endoscopic, "through the scope", minimally invasive? These terms describe recently popularized approaches to spine surgery. In order to understand how these approaches may have a role in your spinal surgery, the terminology must be understood.

Endoscope

An endoscope is an instrument used for the examination of a hollow viscus such as the bladder or a cavity such as the chest. The endoscope is basically a camera mounted on a long thin lens with a cable and a light source. The light source is mounted onto the lens and provides light to illuminate the field to be visualized. The cable mounted on the camera connects to a TV screen, which displays the camera's field of focus.

Endoscopy, Thoracoscopy, Laparoscopy

Endoscopy is the visual inspection of any cavity or hollow viscus by means of an endoscope. Thoracoscopy is the visualization of the thoracic cavity or the chest. Thoracoscopy is used to assist in procedures on the heart and lungs. Laparoscopy is the visualization of the abdominal cavity. Laparoscopy is used to assist in procedures on the intestines, stomach, or removal of the gallbladder.

Reprinted with permission from, "Basic Introduction to Minimally Invasive Spine Surgery," by George D. Picetti, M.D., Associate Clinical Professor, Department of Orthopaedics, University of California, San Francisco. © 2004. This article is also available at http://www.spineuniverse.com.

What is the purpose of utilizing the endoscope? The endoscope allows the surgeon to have an illuminated and magnified view of the operating field without having to make a large incision. With the assistance of the endoscope, surgeons can utilize several small incisions to perform the same procedure they would otherwise perform using a single large incision.

Laparoscopic and thoracoscopic surgery are not new techniques. Dr. Jacobaeus was the first to publish his work in 1910 on both of these topics. In the 1980s laparoscopic cholecystectomy or removal of the gallbladder became very wide spread. However, it was not until the early 1990s when the application of these techniques became utilized in the field of spinal surgery. Early uses were for biopsy, removal of thoracic disk herniations, and releasing or mobilizing the anterior spine for scoliosis and kyphosis. The applications rapidly expanded to many aspects of spinal surgery.

Instrument Availability

Unfortunately just the existence of the endoscope does not automatically allow the spine surgeon to perform surgery endoscopically. First, the surgeon must first recognize if the surgery can be performed without a formal incision. Currently only a small number of spinal surgeries can be performed utilizing an endoscopic approach. Once deciding to perform the surgery endoscopically, the surgeon must determine if all of the instruments and implants (screws, rods, and cages) are available to perform the surgery. You may ask, if the surgery is now being performed with a formal incision, are not all of the tools and implants needed to perform the surgery already available? The answer to this is unfortunately no. Instruments used for endoscopic surgery differ from the instruments used to perform surgery through a formal incision.

Endoscopic Instruments

When a surgery is performed with a large incision, the dissection leads the surgeon directly to the spine. The approach enables the surgeon to touch the spine and manipulate the spine manually as is often necessary. Instruments for performing open surgery are traditionally made short allowing the surgeon better control and tactile feel. The implants and the tools used to insert the implants are often very large and bulky, because the incision size allows a large access.

In developing the endoscopic approach for spinal surgery, the first task was to develop longer streamlined instruments. New and different instruments needed to be developed to perform tasks that were normally done with the surgeon's hands on the spine, but now must be performed at a significant distance from the spine. As these instruments were developed basic procedures could now be performed endoscopically. As the technique progressed, the desire to instrument the spine became the next step. We needed to develop implants that could fit through small incisions and the instruments to insert and manipulate the implants that would fit through the same portals.

Endoscopic Portals

Portals are devices that provide a passage through which the surgeon operates. The incisions for endoscopic surgery are usually a centimeter in length. Once the skin incision is made an instrument is used to continue the dissection into the cavity, usually the chest or abdomen, depending the incision location and the patient's body this can be a fairly long distance. When the instrument is removed all the tissue falls back into place and the opening into the cavity can be very difficult to find. In order to avoid damaging the tissue by moving instruments in and out of the passage, a portal is placed into the incision to hold the tissue apart.

There are two main designs of portals, open or sealed. The open portal is an open tube that allows for the passage of air from outside of the body to inside the cavity and acts only as a spacer. The sealed portal limits the passage of air or gas into or out of the cavity. This type of portal is often used in the abdominal cavity, this allows for the cavity to be expanded allowing the surgeon space to operate. The portals used in the thoracic spine tend to be 11 to 12 millimeters, while portals used in the abdominal cavity tend to be larger. All of the instruments and implants had to be made to not only fit through these small passages, but also perform their function once inside the cavity.

Operating Space

In the thoracic spine the space to operate through is provided by deflating the lung. The anesthesiologist performs this by placing a special breathing tube down the trachea into the large airway of each lung. Once in place the patient is asleep and breathing with only one lung, which is very safe and commonly done. This allows the opposite lung to deflate and falls out of the way of the spine. The portals are placed and the procedure to be performed on the spine is begun. While in the thoracic cavity the lung is collapsed for space, in the abdomen the cavity is filled with CO_2 gas creating the operating space.

The goal of endoscopic surgery must be the same as surgery performed with a formal open procedure. The incision and tissue dissection to the spine may be less, but the surgical procedure cannot be less. Advantages of endoscopic surgery include: improved postoperative recovery, decreased pain, and faster return to activities. These findings have been demonstrated in many, but not all endoscopic procedures. Even today only a small percentage of spinal conditions are suitable for endoscopic surgery. Do not hesitate to discuss with your spine surgeon whether your particular condition is amenable to an endoscopic approach.

Chapter 61

Neck Surgery

Chapter Contents

509

Section 61.1

The Basics of Cervical Spinal Surgery

Cervical spinal surgery is used to correct the part of the spine in the neck, including problems with the bones (vertebrae), disks, and nerves.

Description

The spinal column is composed of 33 bones (called vertebrae) spanning from the base of the skull to the pelvis. Each vertebra has a round, solid body and a bony arch. The spinal cord runs through the hole between the arch and the body of the vertebra and is thus protected by bone on all sides.

A pair of spinal nerves (one on the right and one on the left) runs out between every vertebra. Soft intervertebral disks separate the bodies of the vertebrae, and the arches are connected to one another through joints called facets.

The part of the spine in the neck is called the cervical spine and consists of 7 vertebrae and 8 pairs of spinal nerves (called C1 to C8 for cervical nerves 1 through 8). The two most common problems people have with the cervical spine are disk herniation and stenosis.

Normally a vertebral disk has a fibrous outer "rind" and a soft interior, somewhat like a thick-skinned orange. When a disk herniates, the soft inside material squeezes out through a break in the rind and can pinch the nerves as they exit the spinal column. This will cause pain and sometimes weakness and numbness in the neck and arm.

Spinal stenosis occurs when the facet joints develop arthritis and start to grow excess bone around them (a typical response of a joint to arthritis). The extra bone narrows the space through which the spinal nerve exits the spinal column. This can lead to weakness and pain in the neck and arms.

By physical examination, a doctor (usually a neurologist, orthopedist, or neurosurgeon) can often determine the exact location of the trouble. The physician will test sensation, muscle strength and reflexes, and perform a number of other special tests to determine where the problem lies.

The treating doctor will also usually order x-rays and an MRI, which will help confirm the diagnosis and will help the physician develop an appropriate treatment plan.

Other less common conditions that can cause problems in the cervical spine include fractures, tumors, and infections.

The specific surgery depends on the exact nature of the problem. The surgery is conducted while the patient is under general anesthesia (unconscious and pain-free).

If there is a single herniated disk, then the disk may simply be excised through an incision either through the front or back of the neck.

If there is more than one disk that needs to be excised, then the spine usually needs to be fused to keep it from becoming unstable. For surgery from the front that means that bone is placed in the space where the disk was removed and plates are screwed into the vertebrae to keep them from moving. Rods are sometimes used to connect the vertebrae if the surgery is done from the back.

Spinal stenosis is a more difficult problem to treat and generally requires more extensive surgery. The spinal nerves and cord need to be decompressed and this can again be done from either the front or the back. Again, if there is enough bone taken away that the cervical spine becomes unstable, it will be necessary to fuse the remaining bone together with bone and plates, rods, or metal cages. The bone may be taken from the patient's body, usually from either the hip or the lower leg.

Indications

For most cervical spine problems, the initial treatment will be non-operative and may consist of rest and anti-inflammatory medications. Some people with cervical problems may benefit from neck braces. As the pain improves, physical therapy will have a role in preventing recurrence of pain.

Surgery is generally used when conservative therapy fails, if the pain and weakness become progressively worse, or if there is evidence that the spinal cord itself is being compressed.

Risks

Risks for any anesthesia include the following:

- Reactions to medications
- Problems breathing

Risks for any surgery include the following:

- Bleeding
- Infection

Additional risks specific to spinal surgery include injury to the spinal nerves or spinal cord, injury to the blood vessels feeding the spine, and failure of the bone to fuse. Fortunately, these complications are rare but they are serious and you should discuss them with your doctor before undergoing surgery.

Expectations after Surgery

With surgery on a single herniated disk, more than 90% of patients experience total or near-total relief from their symptoms.

More complex surgeries on multiple disks vary in outcome, depending on the technique and the particular case.

Spinal stenosis is more difficult to treat and results from this surgery are not as good as for disk excision. From 50% to 90% of patients can expect good to excellent results.

Convalescence

The hospital stay is about 7 days. You will be encouraged to walk the first or second day after surgery to reduce the risk of blood clots (deep venous thrombosis).

Complete recovery takes about five weeks. Heavy work is not recommended until several months after surgery or not at all.

Section 61.2

Cervical Corpectomy and Fusion

About the Operation

Your doctor has recommended surgery on your neck. This surgery is called an anterior cervical corpectomy and fusion. Displaced bony disk material will be removed from your neck. This displaced material is causing a problem by pressing on nerves. It will be replaced with bone taken from your hip or the fibula bone in your lower leg.

During the operation, an incision (cut) will be made on your neck. The size of this incision will depend on the extent of your problem. A second incision will be made on the front of your hip or leg. Bone will be removed from your hip or leg and will be placed in your neck. This transfer is called a bone graft. The surgery may take about four hours.

If you have one or two vertebrae repaired (a single-level corpectomy), you will probably be sent directly to a general patient unit after surgery. Your hospital stay will be two to three days.

If you have two or more bones removed (a multiple-level corpectomy), you will probably be sent to the intensive care unit (ICU). During surgery a plastic breathing tube will be inserted down your throat, to keep your airway open. This is necessary because of swelling in your neck. You will remain in the ICU while you have a breathing tube. Most patients stay in the ICU one to two days. Then you will be sent to a general patient unit for two to five days.

Incisions are usually closed with stitches and may be secured with Steri-Strip tapes, which are paper-like strips that stick to your skin and help keep the sides of the incision from shifting. The stitches will dissolve completely. The Steri-Strips will fall off by themselves, usually within two weeks of surgery.

After the Operation

After the operation, your throat may be sore from the surgery and the breathing tube. You will be given ice chips or clear liquids. After the breathing tube is removed, ice chips are helpful until normal bowel function returns. Usually, you can eat a soft diet by the time you go home. Your hip or leg may feel sore for several weeks following surgery.

You will wear a Dennison brace or the Miami-J collar, which was placed on your neck in the operating room, for about six weeks. You will wear the brace or collar from the time of surgery until your doctor removes it. You will receive instructions about wearing your brace.

On your first day after surgery, you will be able to sit in a chair as often as you like. Physical therapy will begin on that day. If you need to stay in the ICU, physical therapy will begin your first day in the general patient unit. A staff member or physical therapist will help you get a cane or walker if needed after surgery.

At Home

- Do not return to work until your doctor says you may.

- Do not drive while you are wearing your brace or collar—usually for six weeks. The brace does not allow peripheral, or side, vision while driving. This is a safety concern as well as a legal issue. In addition, your reaction time may be slower due to pain or certain prescribed medications.

- You may ride in a car from the hospital to your home. However, you should not take car trips until your doctor says you may.

- Walking is good for you, but you should rest as needed. Do not get overtired. Try to limit going up and down stairs to once a day for one to two weeks.

- Avoid strenuous exercise or activities like swimming, golfing, or running until you check with your doctor.

- Do not bend from the waist to pick up things. This movement strains your back muscles. You should bend your knees and squat.

- Do not carry heavy items, such as groceries or laundry. Do not lift anything heavier than a gallon of milk. Do not try to move heavy furniture until your doctor says you may. Do not lift anything over your head.

- Keep the incision dry. Take sponge baths; do not take tub baths until your doctor says you may. Showering is usually allowed seven to 10 days after surgery, if the incision is not red or draining. Before showering, remove the brace and cover the incision with plastic wrap, to keep water from hitting the incision. Be sure to use a rubber mat in the shower, to prevent slipping. Be careful not to move your neck from side to side while the brace is off.

- Usually you may sleep in any position that is comfortable.

- You may resume sexual activities when you feel comfortable.

- Incisions may be numb or tender for a few weeks after surgery. Some redness around the incision is common and usually disappears within one to three weeks. Ask a family member to help you check your incision regularly.

- A raised toilet seat will be provided for you. If necessary, other assistive devices will be arranged for you by hospital staff or your primary care physician.

When to Call the Doctor

If you notice any of the following signs of infection, call your doctor or nurse immediately:

- increased redness at the incision site
- increased pain at the site
- increased swelling at the site
- pus-like drainage from the site
- black tissue around the site
- fever of 101 degrees Fahrenheit (38.3 degrees Celsius) or above for more than 24 hours
- chills

Use common sense in judging what you can and cannot do. If you have any questions or concerns, please feel free to call your doctor or nurse.

515

Section 61.3

Posterior Cervical Laminectomy

Introduction

The spinal cord needs adequate space inside the spinal canal. The spinal canal is a protective ring of bone that surrounds the spinal cord. Conditions such as fractures, dislocations, tumors, or degenerative changes in the disks and joints of the neck can put pressure on the spinal cord. This is because the protective ring of bone around the spinal cord does not expand to accommodate more space. Extra pressure within the confined space of the spinal canal can place the entire spinal cord in danger. Surgery to open the back of the spinal cord is one way to relieve pressure that is on the spinal cord. This procedure is called laminectomy.

Learn about cervical laminectomy including

- how the cervical spine is affected

- why a laminectomy is performed

- what you can expect from this procedure including possible complications

- how rehabilitation can improve your results

Anatomy

In order to understand your symptoms and treatment choices, it is helpful to start with a basic understanding of the anatomy of the neck. This includes becoming familiar with the various parts that make up the cervical spine and how they work together.

The bones of the spinal column protect the spinal cord. The vertebral body at each level of the spine protects the front of the spinal cord. The pedicle and lamina bones form a protective ring of bone that surrounds the sides and back of the spinal cord. The pedicles connect to the vertebral body. The lamina bones attach to the pedicles. The lamina bones cover the back surface of the spinal canal, forming a protective roof over the spinal cord.

Rationale

Bone spurs or a herniated disk can take up space inside the spinal canal and put pressure on the spinal cord. This condition is called spinal stenosis. If spinal stenosis is the main cause of your symptoms, the spinal canal may need to be enlarged. Bone spurs that are pressing on the nerves may need to be removed. This can be achieved with a complete laminectomy. Laminectomy means to remove the lamina.

Removing the lamina gives more room for the spinal cord and spinal nerves and relieves the pressure. Surgeons may also remove bone spurs that may be causing irritation and inflammation around the spinal nerves.

Procedure

The surgeon begins by making an incision down the center of the back of the neck. The neck muscles are then moved to the side.

Upon reaching the back surface of the spine, the surgeon uses an x-ray to identify the problem vertebra. The lamina is removed, taking the pressure off the back part of the spinal cord and nerves.

Removing the entire lamina in the cervical spine may cause problems with the stability of cervical spine. If the facet joints are damaged during the laminectomy, the spine may become unstable and cause problems later. One way that spine surgeons try to prevent this problem is not to actually remove the lamina. Instead they simply cut one side of the lamina and fold it back slightly. The other side of the lamina opens like a hinge. This makes the spinal canal larger, giving the spinal cord more room. The cut area of the lamina eventually heals to keep the spine from tilting forward.

Complications

Like all surgical procedures, operations on the neck may have complications. Because the surgeon is operating around the spinal cord, neck operations are always considered extremely delicate and potentially dangerous. Take time to review the risks associated with cervical spine surgery with your doctor. Make sure you are comfortable with both the risks and the benefits of the procedure planned for your treatment.

Rehabilitation

You'll be able to get up and begin moving within a few hours after surgery. Your doctor may have placed you in a neck collar after surgery. Limit your activities to avoid doing too much too soon. Most patients are able to return home when their medical condition is stabilized, usually within a few days after surgery.

Your doctor may have you attend physical therapy beginning four to six weeks after surgery. A well-rounded rehabilitation program assists in calming pain and inflammation, improving your mobility and strength, and helping you do your daily activities with greater ease and ability. Therapy sessions may be scheduled two to three times each week for up to six weeks.

The goals of physical therapy are to help you:

- learn how to manage your condition and control symptoms

- improve flexibility and strength

- learn correct posture and body movements to reduce neck strain

- return to work safely.

Chapter 62

Low Back Surgery

Chapter Contents

Section 62.1

What Is Lumbar Spinal Surgery?

Lumbar spinal surgery is used to correct problems with the spinal bones (vertebrae), disks, or nerves of the lower back (lumbar spine).

Description

The spine consists of bones (vertebrae) separated by soft cushions (disks). Pressure on the nerves that branch off the spinal cord can produce pain, numbness, tingling, or weakness and may be caused by the following:

- Injured disks that bulge out (slipped disk) between the vertebrae

- Bone injuries (fractures)

- Narrowing of the space between vertebrae (spinal stenosis)

- Growths (tumors)

- Pockets of infection (abscesses)

- Pockets of blood (hematomas)

Patients with spinal pain in the neck or back are usually treated conservatively before surgery is considered. Bedrest, traction, anti-inflammatory medications (nonsteroid and steroid), physical therapy, braces, and exercise are often prescribed.

Maintaining good health, muscle strength, and body posture with appropriate rest and exercise help prevent unnecessary strain on the spine and muscles.

Lumbar spinal surgery is done while the patient is under general anesthesia (unconscious and pain-free). An incision is made over the troubled area. The bone that curves around and covers the spinal cord (lamina) is removed (laminectomy) and the tissue that is causing pressure on the nerve or spinal cord is removed.

The hole through which the nerve passes may be enlarged to prevent further pressure on the nerve. Sometimes, a piece of bone (bone graft) or metal rods (such as Harrington rods) may be used to strengthen the area of surgery.

Occasionally, strong screws (pedicle screws) are used to stabilize the rods to the bones.

Indications

Symptoms of lumbar spine problems include:

- Pain that extends (radiates) from the back to the buttocks or back of thigh
- Pain that interferes with daily activities
- Weakness of legs or feet
- Numbness of legs, feet, or toes
- Loss of bowel or bladder control

Risks

Risks for any anesthesia include the following:

- Reactions to medications
- Problems breathing

Risks for any surgery include the following:

- Bleeding
- Infection

Additional risks of spinal surgery include the following:

- Nerve damage leading to paralysis
- Blood clots
- Muscle weakness
- Loss of bowel or bladder control

Expectations after Surgery

The outcome depends on the source of the problem or the extent of the injury but most patients do very well after surgery.

Convalescence

The hospital stay is about 7 days. You will be encouraged to walk the first or second day after surgery to reduce the risk of blood clots (deep venous thrombosis).

Complete recovery takes about five weeks. Heavy work is not recommended until several months after surgery or not at all.

Section 62.2

Facts about Low Back Surgery

"Low Back Surgery," © 2000 American Academy of Orthopaedic Surgeons. Reprinted with permission from *Your Orthopaedic Connection*, the patient education website of the American Academy of Orthopaedic Surgeons located at http://orthoinfo.aaos.org.

Low back problems may make it difficult for you to perform daily activities and may affect your ability to move freely. You may even feel pain while resting or lying down.

Medication, changes in daily activity, and exercise may all play a role in improving your mobility and relieving your pain. Most low back pain problems, such as that caused by improper lifting, will disappear in a few days or weeks with care that doesn't require surgery.

Other pain, caused by the wear and tear of daily living that affects the vertebrae and disks in your back, may require surgery. You and your orthopaedic surgeon will discuss what is the best treatment for you.

This section will help you understand how your spine works, the causes of some back and leg pain, and the benefits and limitations of surgery to relieve pressure on nerves in your spine and/or to stabilize your spine. You'll learn what is involved in making the decision for surgery, what to expect during and after surgery, and how to avoid complications after surgery.

How the Normal Spine Works

Normal body movement—walking, standing, sitting, twisting, and bending—is possible because of the unique structure of the spinal column.

There are 24 vertebrae in three upper segments of the spinal column. These three segments create three natural curves of the back: the curves of the neck area (cervical), chest area (thoracic), and lower back (lumbar). The lower segments of the spine (sacrum and coccyx) are made up of a series of vertebrae that are fused together.

Between the vertebrae are disks, which are cushioning pads that absorb pressure and allow spine movement.

The spinal column is held in alignment or balance by ligaments, cartilage, and muscles that surround and protect the spinal cord membranes and the nerves that branch out to your legs, arms, and all parts of your body.

Displacement (herniation) of the disk can lead to low back pain as well as pain and numbness in the legs (sciatic pain) and weakness of the muscles in one or both legs.

When the vertebrae are aligned, a canal is formed by the vertebral arch (lamina) that contains the spinal cord. Nerves pass through openings (foramina) of the adjoining vertebrae and into your arms and legs.

The muscles and ligaments attached to the vertebrae need to be kept in good condition to enable the spine to withstand the stresses of daily activity. A well-balanced, flexible spine is less likely to develop low back pain and is less likely to require medical treatment.

Common Causes of Low Back Pain

As a result of wear and tear on the spine, ligaments, and disks, the disk may begin to protrude or collapse and put pressure on the nerve root leading to a leg or foot, causing pain in those areas (sciatica).

The problem can be aggravated by associated conditions, such as narrowing (stenosis) of the canal or shifting of the vertebra (spondylolisthesis), one upon the other.

You also may have low back pain from improper lifting of an object, a fall, or sudden twisting. Most back pain from these causes is due to overuse of muscles and disappears in a few weeks.

Is Low Back Surgery for You?

If you have persistent back pain or pain in your thigh, buttock, or leg; numbness or tingling in your leg; and/or weakness in your leg, and it doesn't respond to conservative, nonoperative treatment, your family doctor can refer you to an orthopaedic surgeon for an evaluation.

You and your orthopaedic surgeon will determine whether you would benefit from low back surgery, which relieves pressure on the nerves in the spinal cord and/or stabilizes the spine.

The Orthopaedic Evaluation

The orthopaedic evaluation consists of four components:

- A medical history, in which your orthopaedic surgeon gathers information about your general health and asks about your symptoms.

- A physical examination to assess the stability, strength, alignment, and motion of your back, as well as a neurological evaluation.

- Diagnostic tests such as x-rays, which may be obtained to evaluate the bones and structure of your spine. An MRI (magnetic resonance imaging) may be arranged to provide more detailed information about the spine. MRIs are not x-rays and use no radiation to create images. A myelogram also may be requested. (A myelogram uses x-ray imaging and an injected dye to define bony and soft tissue structures affecting the nerve root.) Other imaging studies such as a CAT scan also may be ordered that provides details about the bones and soft tissues not seen on regular x-rays.

- Discussion by you and your orthopaedic surgeon of the findings of the physical and diagnostic examination and the treatment for your condition. Initially, medication and physical therapy may be prescribed to reduce inflammation at the site of the pain and to strengthen the muscles supporting the spinal column. If you are overweight, a weight reduction program may be suggested. In addition, you will be encouraged to begin a regular aerobic exercise program once your problem has been corrected.

Preparing for Surgery

You may be asked to stop taking certain medicine or to stop smoking. Depending on your age and general medical fitness, you may be asked to undergo a general medical checkup by your family doctor.

Medication

Some medicines may interfere with or affect the results of your surgery. They may cause bleeding or may interfere with the effects of your anesthesia. These medications include aspirin and nonsteroidal anti-inflammatory drugs. Your doctor may ask you to stop taking the medication before your surgery.

Donating Blood

Donating blood usually is not necessary for most low back surgery that does not include fusing vertebrae together. However, there is always a chance that some blood loss will occur during surgery. Your doctor will discuss the advantages and disadvantages of donating your own blood compared with using someone else's blood. If you decide to donate your own blood, your doctor may prescribe an iron supplement to help build up your blood before surgery.

Advance Planning

You will be able to walk after surgery, but you may need to arrange for some help with washing, dressing, and household activities, such as cleaning, laundry, and shopping, for a few days after your return home. Your orthopaedic surgeon will probably recommend that you don't drive a car for a period of time after surgery. You will need to arrange for transportation to and from your hospital appointments and to other places that you need to go during this time. You should consult your doctor before taking car trips.

Your Surgery

Patients usually are admitted to the hospital on the day of surgery. After admission, you will be taken to the preoperative preparation area where you will be interviewed by a doctor from the anesthesia department, who will review your medical history and physical examination reports. You and your doctor will discuss the type of anesthesia to be used. (Sometimes this is done during an outpatient visit up to seven days before your surgery.) The most common types of anesthesia used for low back surgery are general (you are asleep for the entire operation) or spinal (you may be awake but have no feeling from your waist down).

The surgical procedure usually takes one to three hours, depending on your problem. Your orthopaedic surgeon will remove a portion of bone and ligament overlying the nerve roots and will remove displaced disk material to relieve pressure on the nerve roots. Fusion is sometimes done at the same time, if an instability (spondylolisthesis) is present.

When your surgery is completed, you will be moved to the recovery room, where you will be observed and monitored by a nurse until you awake from your anesthesia. You will have an intravenous (IV) line inserted into a vein in your arm. You also may have a catheter inserted into your bladder to make urination easier.

When you are fully awake and alert, you will be taken to your hospital room. Your IV and catheter will be removed soon after.

Your Hospital Stay

You will feel some pain at the site of your surgery. Your doctor will prescribe pain medicines to help reduce this discomfort. You will be encouraged to breathe deeply and to cough frequently to avoid fluid buildup in your lungs. You may be given a small machine called an incentive spirometer (blow bottle) to help you.

You will be encouraged to begin walking on the same evening after your surgery or the next day to help speed your recovery. If your doctor orders a brace or support, you and your family members will be taught how to put it on and take it off.

Physical Therapy

A physical therapist may instruct you on how to walk up and down stairs without assistance, how to sit properly, and how to maintain good spinal balance. You also should exercise your legs in bed to help prevent blood clots. A follow-up program of physical therapy may be prescribed, depending on the situation.

Possible Complications after Surgery

The incidence of complications after low back surgery is low. Major complications that can occur include, but are not limited to, infection, heart attack, stroke, blood clots, and recurrent disk herniations. Although rare, new nerve damage can occur as a result of this surgery. These complications may result in pain and prolonged recovery time.

Your Recovery at Home

After your discharge from the hospital, you will need to follow your doctor's orders exactly to ensure a successful recovery. You should arrange for transportation home that will allow you to ride in a leaning back or lying down position. You may do as much for yourself as you can as long as you maintain a balanced position of your spine. You shouldn't stay in bed during the day. Don't hesitate to ask for help from your family members or friends if it is needed. If necessary, arrangements can be made for a home health aide.

Wound Care

Your wound may be closed with stitches (sutures) or staples, which will be removed approximately two weeks after surgery. If the wound is clean and dry, no bandage is needed. If drainage continues after you are home, the wound should be covered with a bandage and a call made to your surgeon.

Diet

Some loss of appetite is common. Eating well-balanced meals and drinking plenty of fluids is important. Your doctor may recommend iron supplement pills or vitamins before and after your surgery.

Activity

Loss of energy is frequently experienced after major surgery, but this improves over time. An exercise program designed to gradually increase your strength and stamina may be prescribed. Initially, your doctor will recommend that you should only participate in walking. Later, he or she will encourage you to swim or use an exercise bike or treadmill to improve your general physical condition.

Avoiding Problems after Surgery

It is important that you carefully follow any instructions from your doctor relating to warning signs of blood clots and infection. These complications are most likely to occur during the first few weeks after surgery.

Warning signs of possible blood clots include the following:

- Swelling in the calf, ankle, or foot
- Tenderness or redness, which may extend above or below the knee
- Pain in the calf

Occasionally, a blood clot will travel through the bloodstream and may settle in your lungs. If this happens, you may experience a sudden chest pain and shortness of breath or cough. If you experience any of these symptoms, you should notify your doctor immediately. If you cannot reach your doctor, someone should take you to the hospital emergency room or call 911.

Infection following spine surgery occurs very rarely. Warning signs of infection include:

- Redness, tenderness, and swelling around the wound edges
- Drainage from the wound
- Pain or tenderness
- Shaking chills
- Elevated temperature, usually above 100 degrees if taken with an oral thermometer

If any of these symptoms develop, you should contact your doctor or go to the nearest emergency room immediately.

After Recovery

After you have recovered from your low back surgery, you may continue to have some achy pain in your lower back; this may be persistent. You can reduce the pain by staying in good physical condition. If you are overweight, you should enroll in a program to help you lose weight and keep it off.

Your doctor will evaluate you after your surgery to make sure that your recovery is progressing as expected.

Your orthopaedic surgeon is a medical doctor with extensive training in the diagnosis and nonsurgical and surgical treatment of the musculoskeletal system, including bones, joints, ligaments, tendons, muscles, and nerves.

This information has been prepared by the American Academy of Orthopaedic Surgeons and is intended to contain current information on the subject from recognized authorities. However, it does not represent official policy of the Academy and its text should not be construed as excluding other acceptable viewpoints. Persons with questions about a medical condition should consult a physician who is informed about the condition and the various modes of treatment available.

Chapter 63

Spinal Fusion Surgery

Chapter Contents

Section 63.1

Facts about Spinal Fusion Surgery

What Is Spinal Fusion?

The spine is made up of a series of bones called vertebrae; between each vertebra are strong connective tissues that hold one vertebra to the next and act as cushions between the vertebrae. The disk allows for movements of the vertebrae and lets people bend and rotate their neck and back. The type and degree of motion varies between the different levels of the spine: cervical (neck), thoracic (chest), or lumbar (low back). The cervical spine is a highly mobile region that permits movement in all directions. The thoracic spine is much more rigid due to the presence of ribs and is designed to protect the heart and lungs. The lumbar spine allows mostly forward and backward bending movements (flexion and extension).

Fusion is a surgical technique in which one or more of the vertebrae of the spine are united together (fused) so that motion no longer occurs between them. The concept of fusion is similar to that of welding in industry. Spinal fusion surgery, however, does not weld the vertebrae during surgery. Rather, bone grafts are placed around the spine during surgery. The body then heals the grafts over several months—similar to healing a fracture—which joins, or welds, the vertebrae together.

When Is Fusion Needed?

There are many potential reasons for a surgeon to consider fusing the vertebrae. These include: treatment of a fractured (broken) vertebra; correction of deformity (spinal curves or slippages); elimination of pain from painful motion; treatment of instability; and treatment of some cervical disk herniations.

One of the less controversial reasons to do spinal fusion is vertebral fracture. Although not all spinal fractures need surgery, some fractures—particularly those associated with spinal cord or nerve injury—generally require fusion as part of the surgical treatment.

Certain types of spinal deformity, such as scoliosis, are commonly treated with spinal fusion. Scoliosis is an S-shaped curvature of the spine that sometimes occurs in children and adolescents. Fusion is indicated for very large curves or for smaller curves that are getting worse.

Sometimes a hairline fracture allows vertebrae to slip forward on top of each other. This condition is called spondylolisthesis and can be treated by fusion surgery.

Another condition that is treated by fusion surgery is actual or potential instability. Instability refers to abnormal or excessive motion between two or more vertebrae. It is commonly believed that instability can either be a source of back or neck pain or cause potential irritation or damage to adjacent nerves. Although there is some disagreement on the precise definition of instability, many surgeons agree that definite instability of one or more segments of the spine is an indication for fusion.

Cervical disk herniations that require surgery usually need not only removal of the herniated disk (discectomy), but also fusion. With this procedure, the disk is removed through an incision in the front of the neck (anteriorly) and a small piece of bone is inserted in place of the disk. Although disk removal is commonly combined with fusion in the neck, this is not generally true in the low back (lumbar spine).

Spinal fusion is sometimes considered in the treatment of a painful spinal condition without clear instability. A major obstacle to the successful treatment of spine pain by fusion is the difficulty in accurately identifying the source of a patient's pain. The theory is that pain can originate from painful spinal motion, and fusing the vertebrae together to eliminate the motion will get rid of the pain. Unfortunately, current techniques to precisely identify which of the many structures in the spine could be the source of a patient's back or neck pain are not perfect. Because it can be so hard to locate the source of pain, treatment of back or neck pain alone by spinal fusion is somewhat controversial. Fusion under these conditions is usually viewed as a last resort and should be considered only after other conservative (nonsurgical) measures have failed.

How Is Fusion Done?

There are many surgical approaches and methods to fuse the spine, and they all involve placement of a bone graft between the vertebrae. The spine may be approached and the graft placed either from the back (posterior approach), from the front (anterior approach), or by a combination of both. In the neck, the anterior approach is more common; lumbar and thoracic fusion is usually performed posteriorly.

The ultimate goal of fusion is to obtain a solid union between two or more vertebrae. Fusion may or may not involve use of supplemental hardware (instrumentation) such as plates, screws, and cages. Instrumentation is sometimes used to correct a deformity, but usually is just used as an internal splint to hold the vertebrae together to while the bone grafts heal.

Whether or not hardware is used, it is important that bone or bone substitutes be used to get the vertebrae to fuse together. The bone may be taken either from another bone in the patient (autograft) or from a bone bank (allograft). Fusion using bone taken from the patient has a long history of use and results in predictable healing. Autograft is currently the gold standard source of bone for a fusion. Allograft (bone bank) bone may be used as an alternative to the patient's own bone. Although healing and fusion is not as predictable as with the patient's own bone, allograft does not require a separate incision to take the patient's own bone for grafting, and therefore is associated with less pain. Smoking, medications you are taking for other conditions, and your overall health can affect the rate of healing and fusion, too.

Currently, there is promising research being done involving the use of synthetic bone as a substitute for either autograft or allograft. It is likely that synthetic bone substitutes will eventually replace the routine use of autograft or allograft bone.

With some of the newer minimally invasive surgical techniques currently available, fusion may sometimes be done through smaller incisions. The indications for minimally invasive surgery (MIS) are identical to those for traditional large incision surgery; however, it is important to realize that a smaller incision does not necessarily mean less risk involved in the surgery.

How Long Will It Take to Recover?

The immediate discomfort following spinal fusion is generally greater than with other types of spinal surgeries. Fortunately, there are excellent methods of postoperative pain control available, including oral pain medications and intravenous injections. Another option is a patient-controlled postoperative pain control pump. With this technique, the patient presses a button that delivers a predetermined amount of narcotic pain medication through an intravenous line. This device is frequently used for the first few days following surgery.

Recovery following fusion surgery is generally longer than for other types of spinal surgery. Patients generally stay in the hospital for three or four days, but a longer stay after more extensive surgery is not uncommon. A short stay in a rehabilitation unit after release from the hospital is often recommended for patients who had extensive surgery or for elderly or debilitated patients.

It also takes longer to return to a normal active lifestyle after spinal fusion than many other types of surgery. This is because you must wait until your surgeon sees evidence of bone healing. The fusion process varies in each patient as the body heals and incorporates the bone graft to solidly fuse the vertebrae together. The healing process after fusion surgery is very similar to that after a bone fracture. In general, the earliest evidence of bone healing is not apparent on x-ray until at least six weeks following surgery. During this time, the patient's activity is generally restricted. Substantial bone healing does not usually take place until three or four months after surgery. At that time activities may be increased, although continued evidence of bone healing and remodeling may continue for up to a year after surgery.

The length of time required you must be off of work will depend upon both the type of surgery and the kind of job you have. It can vary anywhere from approximately 4 to 6 weeks for a single level fusion in a young, healthy patient with a sedentary job to as much as 4 to 6 months for more extensive surgery in an older patient with a more physically demanding occupation.

In addition to some restrictions in activity, a brace is sometimes used for the early post-operative period. There are many types of braces that might be used. Some are very restrictive and are designed to severely limit motion, whereas others are intended mainly for comfort and to provide some support. The decision to use a brace or not, and the optimal type of brace, depends upon your surgeon's preference and other factors related to the type of surgery.

Following spinal fusion surgery, a postoperative rehabilitation program may be recommended by your surgeon. The rehabilitation program may include back strengthening exercises and possibly a cardiovascular (aerobic) conditioning program, and a comprehensive program custom-designed for the patient's work environment to safely get the patient back to work. The decision to proceed with a postoperative rehabilitation program depends upon many factors. These include factors related to the surgery (such as the type and extent of the surgery) as well as factors related to the patient (age, health, and anticipated activity level.) Active rehabilitation may begin as early as 4 weeks postoperatively for a young patient with a single level fusion.

What Can I Expect in the Long Run?

Although fusion can be a very good treatment for some spinal conditions, it does not return your spine to "normal." The normal spine has some degree of motion between vertebrae. Fusion surgery eliminates the ability to move between the fused vertebrae, which can put added strain on the vertebrae above and below the fusion.

Fortunately, once a fusion has healed it rarely, if ever, breaks down. However, it does place more stress on the vertebrae next to the fusion. This has some potential to accelerate degeneration of those segments, but this risk varies between individuals. Many surgeons therefore recommend that spinal fusion patients avoid repetitive strenuous activities that involve combined lifting and twisting maneuvers to minimize the stress on the areas around the fusion.

The decision whether to undergo spinal fusion is complex and involves many factors related to the condition being treated, the age and health of the patient, and the patient's anticipated level of function following surgery. This decision must therefore be made carefully and should be discussed thoroughly with your surgeon.

Section 63.2

The Use of Pedicle Screws and Rods in Spinal Fusion Surgery

Rationale

A combination of metal screws and rods (hardware) creates a solid brace that holds the vertebrae in place. These devices are intended to stop movement from occurring between the vertebrae. These metal devices give more stability to the fusion site and allow the patient to be out of bed much sooner.

Procedure

Special screws called pedicle screws are placed through the pedicle bone on the back of the spinal column. The screw inserts through the pedicle and into the vertebral body, one on each side. The screws grab into the bone of the vertebral body, giving them a good solid hold on the vertebra. Once the screws are placed they are attached to metal rods that connect all the screws together. When everything is bolted together and tightened, this creates a stiff metal frame that holds the vertebrae still so that healing can occur. The bone graft is then placed around the back of the vertebrae.

Chapter 64

What's a Bone Graft?

Bone grafts are bone that is transplanted from one area of the skeleton to another to aid in healing, strengthening, or improving function. Bone or bone-like materials used in bone grafts may come from you, from a donor, or from a manmade source. In many cases they are used to fill in an empty space that may have been created in or between the bones of the spine by disease, injury, deformity, or during a surgical procedure such as spinal fusion.

What types of bone grafts are there?

Bone grafts that are transplanted directly from one area of an individual's skeleton into his or her own spine are called autogenous bone grafts, or bone autografts. In most cases, these are the preferred bone grafts to use. The graft bone is harvested, or taken, from the bones of the hip, the ribs, or the leg. Autograft bone is one of the safest to use due to the low risk of disease transmission. It also offers a better chance of acceptance and effectiveness in the transplant site, since it contains the greatest amount of the patient's own bone-growing cells and proteins.

Autograft bone provides a strong framework for the new bone to grow into. The downsides of autograft bone are the facts that it adds another surgical site to a spine procedure (and therefore another location to feel postoperative pain and discomfort) and it can increase the cost of the spinal procedure.

Bone graft that comes from a donor is called allograft bone. Allograft bone usually comes from bone banks that harvest the bone from cadavers. The types of allograft bone used for spine surgery include fresh frozen and lyophilized (freeze dried). The bone is cleaned and disinfected to reduce the possibility of disease transmission from donor to recipient. Allograft, like autograft, provides a framework for the new bone to grow on and into. Unlike autograft bone, allograft bone does not always have the same strength properties or the cells and proteins that can influence the growth of new bone. The advantages of allograft bone are the elimination of the harvesting surgical site, the related postoperative pain, and the added expense of a second operative procedure. Disadvantages of allograft bone are the slight chance of disease transmission and a lessened effectiveness since the bone growth cells and proteins are removed during the cleansing and disinfecting process.

How safe is allograft bone?

As bone grafting using allograft bone has become more widely used, the methods of screening donors, bone preparation, and storage have been vastly improved in regards to diminishing the chances of disease transmission. Studies indicate that the risk of contacting HIV infection through the use of allograft bone is less than 1 per 1 million uses.

Who needs bone grafting?

Your surgeon may want to use bone grafting for a number of reasons. Possible reasons include situations where healing may be difficult due to the use of nicotine (which has been shown in medical studies to limit healing of the spine) or the presence of diseases such as diabetes or autoimmune deficiencies. Other possible reasons include a large amount of bone or disk material that is removed during surgery or spinal procedures that span many levels of vertebrae.

One of the most common uses of bone grafts in spine surgery is during spinal fusion. The use of autogenous bone grafts for spinal fusion has been a standard in the spine community for many years and is considered to be the standard by which other bone grafts are measured. Spinal fusions are performed to relieve pain and provide stability to spines in people who have experienced a vertebral fracture or motion between the vertebrae that causes pain, have a spinal deformity, or who have some types of disk herniations. In certain types of spinal fusion, bone grafts or bone graft alternatives are used to replace the cushioning disk material that lies between the vertebrae. When the bone graft is placed between the vertebrae it creates a framework and support that eventually aids in joining the two bones together. Once the bone bridge between the vertebrae is in place, the spine is stabilized and movement and pressure on nerve roots is relieved, thus easing pain.

Bone grafts can also be used in surgical procedures to stabilize the spine after a fracture or to correct deformity.

What are bone graft substitutes?

Since both allograft and autograft have drawbacks, scientists have long searched for materials that could be used in place of the transplanted bone. Although most of the substitutes available possess some of the positive properties of autograft, none yet have all the benefits of one's own bone. Investigators hope one day to use these substitutes to simultaneously be able to stimulate bone healing and provide a strong and biologically compatible framework for the new bone to grow into.

Some of these bone graft alternatives include:

- **Demineralized Bone Matrix (DBM)**—a product of processed allograft bone. DMB contains collagen, proteins, and growth factors that are extracted from the allograft bone. It is available in the form of a powder, crushed granules, putty, chips, or as a gel that can be injected through a syringe. DBM is extensively processed and therefore has little risk for disease transmission; however, because of the form it takes it does not provide strength to the surgical site.

- **Ceramics**—Ceramics are also used as a substitute for bone grafts. Ceramics offer no possibility for disease transmission, although they may be associated with inflammation in some patients. They are available in many forms such as porous and mesh. Although ceramics may provide a framework for bone growth, they contain none of the natural proteins that influence bone growth.

- **Coral**—Bone implants made from coral have shown to be useful in the treatment of bone defects due to trauma, tumors, and cysts. It is also used for spinal surgery as either a graft additive, or extender, or as an implant to provide a framework for bone to grow into. The use of these substitutes, under certain conditions, has had promising outcomes.

- **Graft Composites**—A newer area of bone graft substitutes, graft composites use combinations of other bone grafting materials and/or bone growth factors to gain the benefits of a variety of substances. Among the combinations in use are a collagen/ceramic composite, which closely reproduces the composition of natural bone; DBM combined with bone marrow cells, which aid in the growth of new bone; and a collagen/ceramic/autograft composite.

- **Bone Morphogenetic Proteins**—Bone morphogenetic proteins (BMPs) are produced in our bodies and regulate bone formation and healing. Scientists have discovered that these proteins can speed up healing as well as limit the negative reaction some people have to donor bone and the nonbone substitutes. Scientists have also discovered how to extract these substances from human or cow bones and even produce them in the laboratory. Currently, the United States Food and Drug Administration has not yet approved these therapies; however, extensive research is being undertaken in both humans and animals to determine their safety and effectiveness.

Which type of bone graft is right for me?

The determination if bone graft is to be used and the type to be used is best made by your surgeon. Different surgical situations may call for different types of bone grafting and unique bone graft materials. If your surgeon says that he or she would like to use a bone graft on your spine, you should discuss this decision with him or her to determine which bone graft material is best suited for your situation.

As with any medical procedure, you should ask your surgeon about any questions or concerns you may have and make sure all of your questions are answered.

Chapter 65

Promising Alternatives to Traditional Surgical Treatments for Back and Neck Pain

Chapter Contents

Section 65.1

Artificial Disk Replacement

Reprinted with permission from, "Artificial Disc Replacement," by
Howard S. An, M.D., and Kristen Karl Juarez, RN, MSN, Rush-Presby-
terian St. Luke's Medical Center, Chicago, IL. © 2004. This article is
also available at http://www.spineuniverse.com.

Individuals with degenerated disks in the lower (lumbar) spine
sometimes suffer from disabling, chronic low back pain. Most patients
with symptomatic degenerative conditions in the spine are treated
non-surgically with anti-inflammatory medications, physical therapy,
and injections. Most of these individuals will favorably respond to
non-surgical methods of treatment, but a subset of individuals will
continue to experience pain. The chronic nature of back pain often interferes with the ability to work and participate in regular daily activities. As a result, surgical treatment may become necessary.

There are multiple conservative and minimally invasive treatment
options available to manage symptomatic degenerative disk disease.
However, if surgery is indicated the surgical treatment of choice has
traditionally consisted of a lumbar spinal fusion. Unfortunately, there
are a number of drawbacks to undergoing a spinal fusion. First, the
ability of the bone to heal or fuse varies. The average success rate of
a lumbar spinal fusion is approximately 75% to 80%. Failure of the fusion to heal may be associated with continued symptoms. Second, a spinal fusion at one or more levels will cause stiffness and decreased motion
of the spine. Third, having a spinal fusion at one or more levels will cause
more stress to be transferred to adjacent levels. The problem with the
transferred stress is that it may cause new problems to develop at the
other levels, which may also lead to additional back surgery.

For these reasons, neurosurgeons and orthopedic surgeons have
engaged in research to offer an alternative to lumbar spinal fusion
surgery. One promising area of research includes the development of
an artificial spinal disk. In order to better appreciate the advantages
and disadvantages of artificial spinal disk replacement, it is important to have a basic understanding of normal spinal anatomy, including the function of the spinal disks.

The spine is a column that is made of up bones and disks. The blocks of bone (or vertebrae) provide the anterior support and structure of the spine. Posteriorly, the two facet joints at each level provide stability and movement of the motion segment. The spinal disks are in between the bones and act like a cushion or shock absorber between the vertebrae. The disks also contribute to the flexibility and motion of the spinal column. The disks are made up of two parts: 1) the inner portion of the disk is called the nucleus pulposus and is a jelly-like material and 2) the outer part of the disk is a stronger, more fibrous, material called the annulus fibrosus. The annulus fibrosus surrounds and supports the inner jelly material. The annulus is also in contact with nerve fibers or pain receptors, called nociceptors. Disk material is primarily composed of water and other proteins. As a normal part of aging, the water content gradually diminishes, which can cause the disk to flatten out and even develop tears or cracks throughout the annulus fibrosus. These disks are often referred to as degenerative disks and may or may not cause pain.

In the case of a degenerative disk, the inner jelly material can bulge out and press up against the annulus fibrosus. This can stimulate the pain receptors causing back pain to occur. The cracks or tears that develop within the annulus fibrosus can also become a source of pain. Back pain that is caused by the spinal disk is often referred to as discogenic low back pain.

Sir John Charley revolutionized orthopedics in the 1960s with the advent of the total hip replacement. At that time, early research in the development of artificial disk replacement began as well. Despite the early interest, lumbar spinal fusion remained the gold standard treatment for back pain. Because of the complications associated with lumbar spinal fusion, a renewed interest in artificial disk replacement resurfaced in the 1990s. The purpose and advantage of artificial disk replacement is to replace the worn-out disk, while preserving the motion at the operated spinal level. This could potentially not only treat the underlying back pain, but also protect patients from developing problems at an adjacent level of the spine.

Currently, artificial disk replacement is considered experimental and is not approved by the Food and Drug Administration (FDA). Most of the research that has been conducted on artificial disks has been carried out in Europe. Different models have been developed, but the most widely used and known artificial disk is the LINK SB Charite III prosthesis made by Waldemar Link GmbH & Company, Hamburg, Germany. The model consists of two metal metallic plates that have teeth to anchor the implant between the bones or vertebral bodies.

Between the two plates is a rubber core made up of polyethylene that allows for motion. A metal ring surrounds the outside of the rubber core so that it can be located on x-ray.

In order to avoid complications that may arise from artificial disk replacement surgery, careful selection of patients by the surgeon is critical. At present, it is thought that the best candidates for spinal disk replacement are adults with a one level symptomatic degenerative disk. Patients whose bone may not be as strong due to aging, or some other bone disorder, may develop problems if the implant settles into the soft bone. Therefore, these individuals are not considered optimal candidates for this type of procedure. Since there can be movement of the implant, patients with a slippage of one vertebra on another (termed spondylolisthesis) are also not considered candidates for artificial disk replacement. Based on the current research, the clinical diagnoses that seem the most fitting for artificial disk replacement include symptomatic degenerative disk disease and post-discectomy syndrome. Post-discectomy syndrome is persistent back pain following previous surgery to remove a herniated disk.

In addition to the potential complications associated with undergoing surgery and general anesthesia, the complications associated with artificial disk replacement may include breakage of the metal plate, dislocation of the implant, and infection. To help minimize complications associated with the implant itself, proper selection of patients and size of implant is very important. Patients may also not improve following the procedure and may require additional surgery. Finally, like joint replacement surgery, artificial implants may fail over time due to wear of the materials and loosening of the implants. Therefore, long-term studies that track the lifespan of the implants are needed.

Another artificial disk device that is similar to the metal implant is the prosthetic disk nucleus (PDN). Like the metal implant, the purpose of it is to restore disk height and allow for normal spinal motion. However, instead of the whole disk being removed, with the prosthetic disk nucleus, only the inner jelly material, or nucleus, is removed and is then replaced with two mini pillows.

Section 65.2

Intradiscal Electrothermal Annuloplasty (IDET)

Practically everyone suffers from back pain at some point. Sometimes the pain results from pressure on nerves, sometimes from spinal fractures, and sometimes from problems with the cushioning disks that separate the bones of the spine. Depending on the cause of the pain, treatment can be as simple as rest and exercise, or as complex as major surgery. Usually, simpler methods are tried first; if they are not successful in relieving the pain, more aggressive treatments can be used.

A relatively new treatment for back pain resulting from problems within the cushioning disks is intradiscal electrothermal annuloplasty, also called intradiscal electrothermal therapy (IDET). This outpatient procedure applies high heat directly to the inside of the disk. It is a less expensive and less invasive procedure than spinal surgery, but it is not appropriate for everyone who has low back pain.

Disk Anatomy

Disks are cushioning tissues located between each vertebra of the spine. The disk has a soft center (nucleus) surrounded by tougher ligament tissue (annulus). As we age, the outer ligament tissue begins to fray and tear from use or injury. This allows nerves and small blood vessels from the soft center to seep into the injury site, triggering pain receptors in the ligament tissue. The result is discogenic back pain.

Discogenic pain differs from a ruptured or herniated disk because the pain originates within the disk and does not come from nerves or other structures. Discogenic pain is confined to the back and does not radiate down the legs.

Diagnosis

In addition to interviewing you about the pain, the physician will take your medical history and give you a physical examination. Tests that can help determine the source of the pain include x-rays, magnetic resonance imaging (MRI), computed tomography (CT) scans, and discography.

Discography is used to identify the painful disk. In this test, the physician pierces the disk with a thin needle and injects a contrast dye. X-rays show whether the dye enters the disk's outer tissues. Discography is called a provocative test because it will provoke pain in an injured disk.

IDET

IDET is usually reserved only for patients who have tried aggressive, non-operative techniques to relieve their pain without success. Because this is a relatively new procedure, you should make sure that the practitioner you see is adequately trained in using the equipment. The procedure itself takes about one hour to complete. A local anesthetic and intravenous pain relievers are used.

- The physician uses an x-ray machine (fluoroscope) to see the spinal structures.

- A hollow needle is inserted into the painful disk. A thin heating wire (electrothermal catheter) is passed through the needle into the disk, and maneuvered into place around the outer edge of the central nucleus.

- The wire is heated slowly to a temperature of about 194 degrees Fahrenheit (90 degrees Celsius) for about 15 minutes. Heat can potentially contract and shrink the fibers that make up the disk wall, closing any tears. The heat can also potentially cauterize (burn) tiny nerve endings in the disk, making them less sensitive to pain.

- After the wire and needle are removed, there is a short observation period before the patient is released.

Postoperative Treatment

Although IDET is much less invasive than most back surgeries, it will still take several weeks for healing to occur. Pain relief is not immediate; pain may actually increase for a day or two after surgery. But gradually the pain from the procedure itself should diminish.

After the IDET procedure, you will need to rest for a few days and limit the time you spend sitting. You may need to wear a back support for several weeks. You will also need to participate in a physical therapy program. If your job is sedentary does not involve lifting or manual labor, you may be able to return to work in a week or so; otherwise it may be several months before you can resume your activities. You will not be able to participate in rigorous recreational activity or do any heavy lifting or twisting for at least six months after the procedure.

IDET is not recommended if you have severe disk degeneration, nerve compression, spinal instability, and/or narrowing of the spinal column (spinal stenosis). IDET is not yet covered by many insurance plans.

The long-term results of this procedure are still unknown. IDET was introduced in 1997 and case series without controls have reported encouraging results. However, these results need to be confirmed in prospective, randomized trials. Additionally, there is debate about how the procedure actually works. Not every patient will benefit from IDET treatment. Some patients continue to experience back pain and may eventually have other surgical procedures.

Section 65.3

Percutaneous Vertebral Augmentation

Two new techniques have been developed recently that are intended to provide stability to the spine after a fracture. Long-term results are still being followed, and there is the potential for side effects and complications with both. Discuss all of your options with your physician before proceeding with any spinal procedure.

Vertebroplasty

Percutaneous vertebroplasty is a relatively new minimally invasive procedure used to treat compression fractures if traditional conservative therapy fails. Vertebroplasty may be able to offer spine stability to patients with spinal fractures due to osteoporosis and those who have had trauma or tumors of the spine.

After a diagnosis of the compression fracture has been made through an MRI or CT scan, the patient lies prone and is sedated with a mild anesthetic. Under the guidance of an imaging technique called C-arm fluoroscopy, the physician injects a cement-like mixture (polymethylmethacrylate) into the vertebra. The entire process takes one to two hours, although the actual injection usually takes only about 10 minutes. The cement mixture hardens in about half an hour and after a short recovery period the patient is sent home. Painkillers are often given to the patient for the first couple of days to help ease the pain.

Percutaneous vertebroplasty may be preferred to open surgery for osteoporosis patients because of the already brittle bone. However, percutaneous vertebroplasty will not correct the bone lost due to by osteoporosis; it may only stabilize new fractures. The procedure may restore lost height and decrease widow's hump.

Although the long-term prognosis may not be good for patients with spinal tumors, percutaneous vertebroplasty can be used for spine stabilization to improve their quality of life, pain relief, and ability to function.

Percutaneous vertebroplasty is relatively new and long-term results are not known. Patients who have one vertebral fracture are five times more likely to get another adjacent to the damaged one; therefore steps should be taken to limit the effects of osteoporosis. Although complications appear to be less than 1%, percutaneous vertebroplasty can cause infection, bleeding, or embolism if the cement mixture gets into the bloodstream and passes through the heart and lungs. Please discuss with your physician whether vertebroplasty is an appropriate medical option for you.

Kyphoplasty

Kyphoplasty is a new minimally invasive surgical technique for treating fractures of the spine that occur due to osteoporosis, usually in postmenopausal women. Generally, osteoporotic fractures of the spine result in a collapsing of the front portion of the vertebrae causing it to compact into a wedge shape, thus causing pain, a loss of height, and a hunched-over appearance (called dowager's hump or widow's hump.)

Kyphoplasty uses a two-step process of inserting of a special balloon device into the compacted vertebrae to attempt to restore the vertebrae to a more normal shape. Subsequently, a cement-like material (polymethylmethacrylate) is injected into the space created by the balloon to retain the correction. By restoring the vertebrae to a more normal state, alignment of the spine may be improved.

Kyphoplasty is performed through a small incision in the back. It is done in a hospital setting under either a local or general anesthetic, depending upon the severity of the case. The entire procedure takes about an hour for each treated vertebrae and patients may return home the day of surgery, or perhaps stay in the hospital overnight. Pain relief may be seen within two days of surgery.

Kyphoplasty is a new therapy and long-term results are not known, nor are the effects of the therapy on the surrounding vertebrae. As with all medical procedures, kyphoplasty does have risks that should be discussed with your physician prior to considering treatment.

Part Eight

Additional Help and Information

Chapter 66

Glossary of Terms Related to Back and Neck Care

Acupuncture: Puncture with long, fine needles.

Analgesic: A compound capable of producing analgesia, i.e., one that relieves pain by altering perception of nociceptive stimuli without producing anesthesia or loss of consciousness.

Ankylosing spondylitis: Arthritis of the spine, resembling rheumatoid arthritis, that may progress to bony ankylosis with lipping of vertebral margins; the disease is more common in the male.

Annulus: A circular band surrounding a wide central opening; a ring-shaped or circular structure surrounding an opening or level area.

Anterior: In human anatomy, denoting the front surface of the body; often used to indicate the position of one structure relative to another, i.e., situated nearer the front part of the body.

Arthritis: Inflammation of a joint or a state characterized by inflammation of joints.

Bone graft: Bone transplanted from a donor site to a recipient site; bone can be transplanted within the same individual (i.e., autogeneic graft) or between different individuals (i.e., allogeneic graft).

Definitions in this chapter were excerpted and reprinted with permission from *Stedman's Medical Dictionary, 27th Edition.* © 2000, Lippincott Williams & Wilkins. All rights reserved.

Cauda equina: The bundle of spinal nerve roots arising from the lumbosacral enlargement and medullary cone and running through the lumbar cistern (subarachnoid space) within the vertebral canal below the first lumbar vertebra; it comprises the roots of all the spinal nerves below the first lumbar.

Cervical: Relating to a neck, or cervix, in any sense.

Chiropractic: A system that, in theory, uses the recuperative powers of the body and the relationship between the musculoskeletal structures and functions of the body, particularly of the spinal column and the nervous system, in the restoration and maintenance of health.

Chiropractor: One who is licensed and certified to practice chiropractic.

Coccyx: The small bone at the end of the vertebral column in humans, formed by the fusion of four rudimentary vertebrae; it articulates above with the sacrum.

Corticosteroids: A steroid produced by the adrenal cortex (i.e., adrenal corticoid); a corticoid containing a steroid.

Dura mater: A tough, fibrous membrane forming the outer covering of the central nervous system.

Facet joint: The synovial joints between zygapophyses or articular processes of the vertebrae.

Fusion: The joining of two bones into a single unit, thereby obliterating motion between the two.

Herniated disk: Protrusion of a degenerated or fragmented intervertebral disk into the intervertebral foramen with potential compression of a nerve root or into the spinal canal with potential compression of the cauda equina in the lumbar region or the spinal cord at higher levels.

Kyphosis: An anteriorly concave curvature of the vertebral column; excessive forward curvature of the thoracic spine may represent a pathologic condition.

Laminectomy: Excision of a vertebral lamina; commonly used to denote removal of the posterior arch.

Ligament: A band or sheet of fibrous tissue connecting two or more bones, cartilages, or other structures, or serving as support for fasciae or muscles.

Lordosis: An anteriorly convex curvature of the vertebral column; the normal lordoses of the cervical and lumbar regions are secondary curvatures of the vertebral column, acquired postnatally.

Lumbar: Relating to the loins, or the part of the back and sides between the ribs and the pelvis.

Muscle spasm: A sudden involuntary contraction of one or more muscles; includes cramps, contractures.

Nerve root: One of the two bundles of nerve fibers (posterior and anterior roots) emerging from the spinal cord that join to form a single segmental (mixed) spinal nerve; some of the cranial nerves are similarly formed by the union of two roots, in particular the fifth or trigeminal nerve.

Neuralgia: Pain of a severe, throbbing, or stabbing character in the course or distribution of a nerve.

Non-steroidal anti-inflammatory drugs: A large number of drugs exerting anti-inflammatory (and also usually analgesic and antipyretic) actions; examples include aspirin, acetaminophen, diclofenac, indomethacin, ketorolac, ibuprofen, and naproxen. A contrast is made with steroidal compounds (such as hydrocortisone or prednisone) exerting anti-inflammatory activity.

Orthopedics: The medical specialty concerned with the preservation, restoration, and development of form and function of the musculoskeletal system, extremities, spine, and associated structures by medical, surgical, and physical methods.

Orthopedist: One who practices orthopedics.

Osteoarthritis: Arthritis characterized by erosion of articular cartilage, either primary or secondary to trauma or other conditions, which becomes soft, frayed, and thinned with eburnation of subchondral bone and outgrowths of marginal osteophytes; pain and loss of function result; mainly affects weight-bearing joints, is more common in older persons.

Osteoporosis: Reduction in the quantity of bone or atrophy of skeletal tissue; an age-related disorder characterized by decreased bone mass and increased susceptibility to fractures.

Paralysis: Loss of power of voluntary movement in a muscle through injury or disease of it or its nerve supply.

Paraplegia: Paralysis of both lower extremities and, generally, the lower trunk.

Posterior: In human anatomy, denoting the back surface of the body. Often used to indicate the position of one structure relative to another, i.e., nearer the back of the body.

Quadriplegia: Paralysis of all four limbs.

Radiculopathy: Disorder of the spinal nerve roots.

Sacroiliac joint: The synovial joint on either side between the auricular surface of the sacrum and that of the ilium.

Sacrum: The segment of the vertebral column forming part of the pelvis; a broad, slightly curved, spade-shaped bone, thick above, thinner below, closing in the pelvic girdle posteriorly; it is formed by the fusion of five originally separate sacral vertebrae; it articulates with the last lumbar vertebra, the coccyx, and the hip bone on either side.

Sciatica: Pain in the lower back and hip radiating down the back of the thigh into the leg, initially attributed to sciatic nerve dysfunction (hence the term), but now known to usually be due to herniated lumbar disk compromising a nerve root.

Scoliosis: Abnormal lateral and rotational curvature of the vertebral column. Depending on the etiology, there may be one curve, or primary and secondary compensatory curves; scoliosis may be fixed as a result of muscle and/or bone deformity or mobile as a result of unequal muscle contraction.

Spina bifida: Embryologic failure of fusion of one or more vertebral arches; subtypes of spina bifida are based on degree and pattern of malformation associated with neuroectoderm involvement.

Spondylolisthesis: Forward movement of the body of one of the lower lumbar vertebrae on the vertebra below it, or upon the sacrum.

Stinger: Episodes of upper extremity burning pain.

Subluxation: An incomplete luxation or dislocation; though a relationship is altered, contact between joint surfaces remains.

Syringomyelia: The presence in the spinal cord of longitudinal cavities lined by dense, gliogenous tissue, which are not caused by vascular insufficiency.

Thoracic: Relating to the thorax.

Thorax: The upper part of the trunk between the neck and the abdomen; it is formed by the 12 thoracic vertebrae, the 12 pairs of ribs, the sternum, and the muscles and fasciae attached to these; below, it is separated from the abdomen by the diaphragm; it contains the chief organs of the circulatory and respiratory systems.

Torticollis: A contraction, or shortening, of the muscles of the neck, chiefly those supplied by the spinal accessory nerve; the head is drawn to one side and usually rotated so that the chin points to the other side.

Vertebrae: One of the segments of the spinal column; in humans, there are usually 33 vertebrae: 7 cervical, 12 thoracic, 5 lumbar, 5 sacral (fused into one bone, the sacrum), and 4 coccygeal (fused into one bone, the coccyx).

Vertebral column: The series of vertebrae that extend from the cranium to the coccyx, providing support and forming a flexible bony case for the spinal cord.

Whiplash: Forceful application of a forward and backward movement of the unsupported head that may produce an injury to the cervical spine or the brain.

Chapter 67

Directory of Back and Neck Organizations and Resources

Government Agencies and Organizations

Agency for Healthcare Research and Quality
540 Gaither Road
Rockville, MD 20850
Phone: (301) 427-1364
Website: http://www.ahrq.gov
E-mail: info@ahrq.gov

BRAIN
P.O. Box 5801
Bethesda, MD 20824
Toll-Free: (800) 352-9424
Phone: (301) 496-5751
Website: http://
www.ninds.nih.gov

Centers for Disease Control and Prevention
1600 Clifton Road
Atlanta, GA 30333
Toll-Free: (800) 311-3435
Phone: (404) 639-3311
Website: http://www.cdc.gov
E-mail: ccdinfo@cdc.gov

Healthfinder.gov
U.S. Department of Health and
Human Services
P.O. Box 1133
Washington, DC 20013-1133
Website: http://
www.healthfinder.gov
E-mail: healthfinder@nhic.org

Resources in this chapter were compiled from a variety of sources deemed reliable. All contact information was verified in June 2004. Inclusion does not constitute endorsement.

National Center for Alternative and Complementary Medicine
P.O. Box 7923
Gaithersburg, MD 20898
Toll-Free: (888) 644-6226
Phone: (301) 519-3153
TTY: (866) 464-3615
Fax: (866) 464-3616
Website: http://nccam.nih.gov
E-mail: info@nccam.nih.gov

National Institute of Arthritis and Musculoskeletal and Skin Diseases
1 AMS Circle
Bethesda, MD 20892-3675
Toll-Free: (877) 22-NIAMS (226-4267)
Phone: (301) 495-4484
TTY: (301) 565-2966
Fax: (301) 718-6366
Website: http://www.niams.nih.gov
E-mail: niamsinfo@mail.nih.gov

National Institute of Neurological Disorders and Stroke (NINDS)
P.O. Box 5801
Bethesda, MD 20824
Toll-Free: (800) 352-9424
Phone: (301) 496-5751
TTY: (301) 468-5981
Website: http://www.ninds.nih.gov

National Institutes of Health Clinical Trials
8600 Rockville Pike
Bethesda, MD 20894
Toll-Free: (888) 346-3656
Website: http://www.clinicaltrials.gov
E-mail: custserv@nlm.nih.gov

National Institute on Aging
Building 31, Room 5C27
31 Center Drive, MSC 2292
Bethesda, MD 20892
Phone: (301) 496-1752
Website: http://www.nia.nih.gov
E-mail: webmaster@nia.nih.gov

U.S. Food and Drug Administration
5600 Fishers Lane
Rockville, MD 20857-0001
Toll-Free: (888) 463-6332
Website: http://www.fda.gov

U.S. National Library of Medicine
8600 Rockville Pike
Bethesda, MD 20894
Toll-Free: (888) 346-3656
Phone: (301) 594-4983
Fax: (301) 496-2809
Website: http://www.nlm.nih.gov
E-mail: custserv@nlm.nih.gov

Private and Nonprofit Organizations

AllAboutBackandNeckPain.com/ DePuy Spine
325 Paramount Drive
Raynham, MA 02767
Phone: (508) 828-3656
Website: http://
www.allaboutbackandneckpain.com
E-mail:
info@allaboutbackandneckpain.com

American Academy of Neurology
1080 Montreal Avenue
Saint Paul, MN 55116
Toll-Free: (800) 879-1960
Phone: (651) 695-2717
Fax: (651) 695-2791
Website: http://www.aan.com
E-mail: memberservices@aan.com

American Academy of Orthopaedic Surgeons (AAOS)
6300 North River Road
Rosemont, IL 60018-4262
Toll-Free: (800) 346-AAOS
Phone: (847) 823-7186
Fax: (847) 823-8125
Website: http://www.aaos.org
E-mail: custserv@aaos.org

American Academy of Pain Management
13947 Mono Way #A
Sonora, CA 95370
Phone: (209) 533-9744
Fax: (209) 533-9750
Website: http://
www.aapainmanage.org
E-mail: aapm@aapainmanage.org

American Academy of Physical Medicine and Rehabilitation
One IBM Plaza, Suite 2500
Chicago, IL 60611-3604
Phone: (312) 464-9700
Fax: (312) 464-0227
Website: http://www.aapmr.org
E-mail: info@aapmr.org

American Academy of Spine Physicians
1795 Grandstand Place
Elgin, IL 60123-4980
Phone: (847) 697-4660
Fax: (847) 931-7975
Website: http://
www.spinephysicians.org
E-mail:
aasp@spinephysicians.org

American Association of Neurological Surgeons
5550 Meadowbrook Drive
Rolling Meadows, IL 60008
Toll-Free: (888) 566-AANS (2267)
Phone: (847) 378-0500
Fax: (847) 378-0600
Website: http://www.aans.org
E-mail: info@aans.org

American Chiropractic Association
1701 Clarendon Blvd.
Arlington, VA 22209
Toll-Free: (800) 986-4636
Phone: (703) 276-8800
Fax: (703) 243-2593
Website: http://www.amerchiro.org
E-mail: AmerChiro@aol.com

American Chronic Pain Association
P.O. Box 850
Rocklin, CA 95677
Toll-Free: (800) 533-3231
Phone: (916) 632-0922
Fax: (916) 632-3208
Website: http://www.theacpa.org
E-mail: ACPA@pacbell.net

American College of Rheumatology
1800 Century Place, Suite 250
Atlanta, GA 30345-4300
Phone: (404) 633-3777
Fax: (404) 633-1870
Website: http://
www.rheumatology.org

American Medical Association/Medem
649 Mission Street, 2nd Floor
San Francisco, CA 94105
Toll-Free: (877) 926-3336
Phone: (415) 644-3800
Fax: (415) 644-3950
Website: http://www.medem.com
E-mail: info@medem.com

American Occupational Therapy Association
4720 Montgomery Lane
P.O. Box 31220
Bethesda, MD 20824-1220
Phone: (301) 652-2682
TTY: (800) 377-8555
Fax: (301) 652-7711
Website: http://www.aota.org

American Osteopathic Association
142 East Ontario Street
Chicago, IL 60611
Toll-Free: (800) 621-1773
Phone: (312) 202-8000
Fax: (312) 202-8200
Website: http://
www.osteopathic.org
E-mail: info@osteotech.org

American Pain Foundation
201 N. Charles Street, Suite 710
Baltimore, MD 21201-4111
Toll-Free: (888) 615-PAIN (7246)
Website: http://
www.painfoundation.org
E-mail: info@painfoundation.org

American Pain Society
4700 West Lake Avenue
Glenview, IL 60025-1485
Phone: (847) 375-4715
Fax (Toll-Free): (877) 734-8758
http://www.ampainsoc.org
E-mail: info@ampainsoc.org

American Physical Therapy Association
1111 North Fairfax Street
Alexandria, VA 22314-1488
Toll-Free: (800) 999-2782, X2782
Phone: (703) 684-2782
Fax: (703) 684-7343
TDD: (703) 683-6748
Website: http://www.apta.org

American Podiatric Medical Association
9312 Old Georgetown Road
Bethesda, MD 20814
Toll-Free: (800) ASK-APMA
Phone: (301) 571-9200
Fax: (301) 530-2752
Website: http://www.apma.org
E-mail: askapma@apma.org

Arthritis Foundation
1330 West Peachtree Street
Atlanta, GA 30309
Toll-Free: (800) 283-7800
Phone: (404) 872-7100
Website: http://www.arthritis.org
E-mail:
arthritis@finelinesolutions.com

Arthritis Source
University of Washington
Department of Orthopaedics
and Sports Medicine
1959 N.E. Pacific Street
P.O. Box 356500
Seattle, WA 98195-6500
Phone: (206) 543-3690
Fax: (206) 685-3139
Website: http://
www.orthop.washington.edu/
arthritis
E-mail:
sportsmd@u.washington.edu

Athletic Advisor
Phone: (713) 858-3802
Website: http://
www.athleticadvisor.com
E-mail: info@athleticadvisor.com

Cleveland Clinic
9500 Euclid Avenue
Cleveland, OH 44195
Toll-Free: (800) 223-2273, ext.
48950
Phone: (216) 444-2200
TTY: (216) 444-0261
Website: http://
www.clevelandclinic.org

Dynamic Chiropractic
P.O. Box 4109
Huntington Beach, CA 92605-4109
Toll-Free: (800) 359-2289
Phone: (714) 230-3150
Fax: (714) 899-4273
Website: http://
www.chiroweb.com
E-mail: editorial@mpamedia.com

Dystonia Medical Research Foundation
One East Wacker Drive, Ste. 2430
Chicago, Illinois 60601-1905
Toll-Free: (800) 361-8061 (In Canada)
Phone: (312) 755-0198
Fax: (312) 803-0138
Website: http://www.dystonia-foundation.org
E-mail: dystonia@dystonia-foundation.org

Federation of Chiropractic Licensing Boards
901 54th Avenue, Suite 101
Greeley, CO 80634-4400
Phone: (970) 356-3500
Fax: (970) 356-3599
Website: http://www.fclb.org
E-mail: info@fclb.org

*Foundation for
Chiropractic Education
and Research*
380 Wright Road
P.O. Box 400
Norwalk, IA 50211
Toll-Free: (800) 622-6309
Phone: (515) 981-9888
Fax: (515) 981-9427
Website: http://www.fcer.org
E-mail: FCER@fcer.org

*Hospital for Special
Surgery—Rheumatology
Division*
535 East 70th Street
New York, NY 10021
Toll-Free: (866) 749-7047
Phone: (212) 606-1753
Website: http://
www.rheumatology.hss.edu

*International
Chiropractors Association*
1110 N. Glebe Road, Suite 1000
Arlington, VA 22201
Toll-Free: (800) 423-4690
Phone: (703) 528-5000
Fax: (703) 528-5023
Website: http://
www.chiropractic.org
E-mail: chiro@chiropractic.org

*International Intradiscal
Therapy Society*
810 North Street
Belgium, WI 53004-9531
Phone: (262) 285-4487
Fax: (262) 285-4231
Website: http://www.iits.org

*International Spinal
Injection Society*
10 Edgehill Way
San Francisco, CA 94127
Toll-Free: (888) 255-0005
Phone: (415) 661-6177
Fax: (415) 661-6179
Website: http://
www.spinalinjection.com/ISIS
E-mail: isisfiles@email.msn.com

*National Ankylosing
Spondylitis Society*
P.O. Box 179
Mayfield, East Sussex TN20 6ZL
UNITED KINGDOM
Phone: 011-44-1435 873527
Fax: 011-44-1435 873027
Website: http://www.nass.co.uk
E-mail: nass@nass.co.uk

*National Association for
Chiropractic Medicine*
15427 Baybrook Drive
Houston, TX 77062
Phone: (281) 280-8262
Fax: (281) 280-8262
Website: http://
www.chiromed.org

*National Chronic Pain
Outreach Association, Inc.*
7979 Old Georgetown Road,
Suite 100
Bethesda, MD 20814-2429
Phone: (301) 652-4948
Fax: (301) 907-0745
Website: http://
neurosurgery.mgh.harvard.edu/
ncpainoa.htm

National Osteoporosis Foundation
1232 22nd Street NW
Washington, DC 20037-1292
Toll-Free: (877) 868-4520
Phone: (202) 223-2226
Fax: (202) 223-2237
Website: http://www.nof.org
E-mail: customerservice@nof.org

National Pain Foundation
3511 S. Clarkson Street
Englewood, CO 80113
Website: http://
www.painconnection.org
E-mail:
aardrup@painconnection.org

National Scoliosis Foundation
5 Cabot Place
Stoughton, MA 02072
Toll-Free: (800) 673-6922
Fax: (781) 341-8333
Website: http://www.scoliosis.org
E-mail: NSF@scoliosis.org

Nemours Foundation Center for Children's Health Media
1600 Rockland Road
Wilmington, DE 19803
Phone: (302) 651-4000
Fax: (302) 651-4055
Website: http://
www.kidshealth.org
E-mail: info@kidshealth.org

North American Spine Society
22 Calendar Court, 2nd Floor
LaGrange, IL USA 60525
Toll-Free: (877) SPINE-DR
Website: http://www.spine.org
E-mail: info@spine.org

Scoliosis Association, Inc.
P.O. Box 811705
Boca Raton, FL 33481-1705
Toll-Free: (800) 800-0669
Phone: (561) 991-4435
Fax: (561) 994-2455
Website: http://www.scoliosis-assoc.org

Scoliosis Research Society
611 East Wells Street
Milwaukee, WI 53202-3892
Phone: (414) 289-9107
Fax: (414) 276-3349
Website: http://www.srs.org

Spina Bifida Association of America
4590 MacArthur Blvd., NW, Suite 250
Washington, DC 20007-4226
Toll-Free: (800) 621-3141
Phone:(202) 944-3285
Fax:(202) 944-3295
Website: http://www.sbaa.org
E-mail: sbaa@sbaa.org

Spine-health.com
1840 Oak Avenue, Suite 112
Evanston, IL 60201
Website: http://www.spine-health.com
E-mail: admin@spine-health.com

SpineSource.com/John Regan, MD

Cedars-Sinai Institute for
Spinal Disorders
Cedars-Sinai Medical Center
444 San Vicente Blvd., Suite 800
Los Angeles, CA 90048
Toll-Free: (877) 85-SPINE (857-7462)
Phone: (310) 423-9701
Fax: (310) 423-9918
Website: http://
www.spinesource.com
E-mail: regan@spinesource.com

SpineUniverse.com

621 N.W. 53rd Street, Suite 240
Boca Raton, FL 33487
Website: http://
www.spineuniverse.com
E-mail:
feedback@SpineUniverse.com

Spondylitis Association of America

P.O. Box 5872
Sherman Oaks, CA 91413
Toll-Free: (800) 777-8189
Website: http://
www.spondylitis.org
E-mail: info@spondylitis.org

Spinal Cord Injury (SCI) Resources

American Paraplegia Society (APS)

75-20 Astoria Blvd.
Jackson Heights, NY 11370
Toll-Free: (800) 444-0120
Phone: (718) 803-3782
Fax: (718) 803-0414
Website: http://www.apssci.org
E-mail: aps@unitedspinal.org

American Spinal Injury Association

2020 Peachtree Road, NW
Atlanta, GA 30309-1402
Phone: (404) 355-9772
Fax: (404) 355-1826
Website: http://www.asia-spinalinjury.org

Darrell Gwynn Foundation

4850 SW 52nd Street
Davie, FL 33314
Phone: (954) 792-7223 ext. 105
Website: http://
www.darrellgwynnfoundation.org
E-mail:
info@darrellgwynnfoundation.org

Daniel Heumann Fund for Spinal Cord Research

6516 Truman Lane, Suite #100
Falls Church, VA 22043-1821
Phone: (703) 442-8797
Fax: (703) 448-6914
Website: http://
www.heumannfund.org

Geoffrey Lance Foundation for SCI Research and Support
132 S. 10th Street, #375 Main
c/o Regional SCI Center of
Delaware Valley
Philadelphia, PA 19107
Phone: (877) GLANCE1 (452-6231)
Fax: (215) 955-5152
Website: http://
www.geofflance.com
E-mail: info@geofflance.com

Miami Project to Cure Paralysis/Buoniconti Fund
P.O. Box 016960
Miami, FL 33101-6960
Phone: (305) 243-7147
Toll-Free: (800) STANDUP (782-6387)
Fax: (305) 243-6017
Website: http://
www.themiamiproject.org
E-mail:
mpinfo@miamiproject.med.miami.edu

National Spinal Cord Injury Association
6701 Democracy Blvd. #300-9
Bethesda, MD 20817
Toll-Free: (800) 962-9629
Phone: (301) 214-4006
Fax: (301) 881-9817
Website: http://
www.spinalcord.org
E-mail: info@spinalcord.org

Christopher Reeve Paralysis Foundation/Paralysis Resource Center
500 Morris Avenue
Springfield, NJ 07081
Toll-Free: (800) 539-7309
Phone: (973) 379-2690
Fax: (973) 912-9433
Website: http://
www.christopherreeve.org
E-mail: info@crpf.org

Spinal Cord Injury Information Network
Website: http://
www.spinalcord.uab.edu
E-mail: sciweb@uab.edu

Spinal Cord Society
19051 County Highway 1
Fergus Falls, MN 56537
Phone: (218) 739-5252
Phone: (218) 739-5261
Fax: (218) 739-5262
Website: http://
members.aol.com/scsweb

United Spinal Association
75-20 Astoria Boulevard
Jackson Heights, New York
11370
Phone: (718) 803-3782
Fax: (718) 803-0414
Website: http://
www.unitedspinal.org
E-mail: info@unitedspinal.org

Organizations That Provide Information and Assistance for People Disabled by Back and Neck Disorders

Americans with Disabilities Act Home Page
U.S. Department of Justice
950 Pennsylvania Avenue, NW
Civil Rights Division
Disability Rights Section–NYAV
Washington, DC 20530
Toll-Free: (800) 514-0301
Fax: (202) 307-1198
TTY: (800) 514-0383
Website: http://www.ada.gov

Center for Assistive Technology & Environmental Access
490 Tenth Street NW
Atlanta, GA 30332-0156
Toll-Free: (800) 726-9119
Phone: (404) 894-1414
Fax: (404) 894-9320
Website: http://
www.assistivetech.net
E-mail: info@assistivetech.net

Job Accommodation Network
P.O. Box 6080
Morgantown, WV 26506-6080
Toll-Free V/TTY: (800) 526-7234
Phone V/TTY: (304) 293-7186
Fax: (304) 293-5407
Website: http://www.jan.wvu.edu
E-mail: jan@jan.wvu.edu

Medicare Rights Center
1460 Broadway, 17th Floor
New York, NY 10036
Phone: (212) 869-3850
Fax: (212) 869-3532
Website: http://
www.medicarerights.org/
index.html
E-mail: info@medicarerights.org

National Center on Physical Activity and Disability
1640 W. Roosevelt Road
Chicago, IL 60608-6904
Toll-Free V/TTY: (800) 900-8086
Fax: (312) 355-4058
Website: http://www.ncpad.org

National Organization of Social Security Claimants' Representatives
6 Prospect Street
Midland Park, NJ 07432-1691
Toll-Free: (800) 431-2804
Website: http://www.nosscr.org
E-mail: webmaster@nosscr.org

National Organization on Disability
910 Sixteenth Street, NW
Suite 600
Washington, DC 20006
Phone: (202) 293-5960
TTY: (202) 293-5968
Fax: (202) 293-7999
Website: http://www.nod.org
E-mail: ability@nod.org

Office of Disability Employment Policy

Website: http://disabilityinfo.gov

Rehabilitation Services Administration

400 Maryland Avenue, SW
Washington, DC 20202-2551
Phone: (202) 205-5482
Website: http://www.ed.gov/
about/offices/list/osers/rsa

Chapter 68

References and Additional Reading

Books about Back and Neck Disorders

Adams, Michael; Bogduk, Nikolai; Burton, Kim; and Dolan, Patricia. *The Biomechanics of Back Pain.* Oxford, United Kingdom: Churchill Livingstone, 2002. ISBN 0443062072.

Arthritis Foundation. *The Arthritis Foundation's Guide to Good Living with Osteoarthritis.* Atlanta, GA: Arthritis Foundation, 2000. ISBN 0912423250.

Brownstein, Art. *Healing Back Pain Naturally: The Mind-Body Program Proven to Work.* Boyne City, MI: Harbor House, 1999. ISBN 0936197390.

Cristian, Adrian. *Living with Spinal Cord Injury: A Wellness Guide.* New York, NY: Demos Medical Publishing, 2004. ISBN 193260300X.

Cunningham, Chet. *The Sciatica Relief Handbook.* Encinitas, CA: United Research Publishers, 1998. ISBN 1887053093.

Ernst, Edzard. *Back Pain: Practical Ways to Restore Health Using Complementary Medicine.* New York, NY: Sterling Publishing, 1999. ISBN 0806970642.

Resources listed in this chapter were compiled from several sources. Inclusion does not constitute endorsement. This list is not considered complete; it is merely intended to serve as a starting point for readers interested in pursuing additional information. Websites were all verified and accessed in May 2004.

Fehrsen-Du Toit, Renita. *The Good Back Book: A Practical Guide to Alleviating and Preventing Back Pain.* Ontario, Canada: Firefly Books, 2003. ISBN 1552978265.

Fishman, Loren, and Ardman, Carol. *Back Pain: How to Relieve Low Back Pain and Sciatica.* New York, NY: W.W. Norton and Company, 1999. ISBN 039331961X.

Hobden, Jane. *The Back Pack: The Natural Guide to Being Kind to Your Back.* New York, NY: St. Martin's Press, 1999. ASIN 0312243405. (Out of print; check your local library for availability)

Hochschuler, Stephanie, and Resnick, Bob. *Treat Your Back Without Surgery: The Best Non-Surgical Alternatives for Eliminating Back and Neck Pain.* Alameda, CA: Hunter House Inc., Publishers, 1998. ISBN 089793234X.

Klein, Arthur C. *Chronic Pain: The Complete Guide to Relief.* New York, NY: Carroll and Graf, 2001. ISBN 0786708344.

Lenarz, Michael, and St. George, Victoria. *The Chiropractic Way: How Chiropractic Care Can Stop Your Pain and Help You Regain Your Health Without Drugs or Surgery.* New York, NY: Bantam Books, 2003. ISBN 0553381598.

McKenzie, Robin, and Kubey, Craig. *7 Steps to a Pain-Free Life: How to Rapidly Relieve Back and Neck Pain.* New York, NY: Penguin Putnam, Inc., 2000. ISBN 0452282772.

Neuwirth, Michael, and Osborn, Kevin. *The Scoliosis Sourcebook, 2nd edition.* By New York, NY: McGraw-Hill, 2001. ISBN 0737303212.

Palmer, Sara; Kriegsman, Kay Harris; Palmer, Jeffrey B. Spinal *Cord Injury: A Guide for Living.* Baltimore, MD: Johns Hopkins University Press, 2000. ISBN 0801863538.

Sandler, Adrian. *Living with Spina Bifida.* Chapel Hill, NC: University of North Carolina Press, 2004. ISBN 0807855472.

Sarno, John E. *Healing Back Pain: The Mind-Body Connection.* New York, NY: Warner Books, 1991. ISBN 0446392308.

Schatz, Mary Pullig. *Back Care Basics: A Doctor's Gentle Yoga Program for Back and Neck Pain Relief.* Berkeley, CA: Rodmell Press, 1992. ISBN 0962713821.

Schofferman, Jerome. *What to Do for a Pain in the Neck: The Complete Program for Neck Pain Relief.* New York, NY: Fireside Books, 2001. ISBN 068487394X.

Siegel, Ronald; Urdang, Michael H.; and Johnson, Douglas R. *Back Sense: A Revolutionary Approach to Halting the Cycle of Chronic Back Pain.* New York, NY: Broadway Books, 2002. ISBN 0767905814.

Stanmore, Tia. *The Pilates Back Book: Heal Neck, Back, and Shoulder Pain With Easy Pilates Stretches.* Gloucester, MA: Fair Winds Press, 2002. ISBN 1931412898.

Wharton, Jim, and Warton, Phil. *The Wharton's Back Book.* Emmaus, PA: Rodale Press, 2003. ISBN 1579547036.

Magazine and Journal Articles about Back and Neck Disorders

"Spinal Cord Injury: Facts and Figures at a Glance." *Journal of Spinal Cord Medicine,* vol. 27 no. 2, 201–203, 2004.

Agoston, H. "Step Forward for Spinal-Cord Repair." *Lancet Neurology,* vol. 3 no. 6, p. 327, June 2004.

Bogduk, N. "The Anatomy and Pathophysiology of Neck Pain." *Physical Medicine and Rehabilitation Clinics of North America,* vol. 14 no. 3, pp. 455–472, August 2003.

Bono, C.M. "Low-Back Pain in Athletes." *Journal of Bone and Joint Surgery,* vol. 86-A no. 2, pp. 382-396, February 2004.

Bronfort, G.; Haas, M.; Evans, R.L.; Bouter, L.M. "Efficacy of Spinal Manipulation and Mobilization for Low Back Pain and Neck Pain: A Systematic Review and Best Evidence Synthesis." *Spine Journal,* vol. 4 no. 3, pp. 335–356, May-June 2004.

Buttermann, G.R. "Treatment of Lumbar Disc Herniation: Epidural Steroid Injection Compared with Discectomy. A Prospective, Randomized Study." *Journal of Bone and Joint Surgery,* vol. 86-A no. 4, pp. 670–679, April 2004.

Carroll, L.J.; Cassidy, J.D.; Cote, P. "Depression as a Risk Factor for Onset of an Episode of Troublesome Neck and Low Back Pain." *Pain,* vol. 107 nos. 1–2, pp. 134–139, January 2004.

Coggrave, M. "Effective Bowel Management for Patients after Spinal Cord Injury." *Nursing Times,* vol. 100 no. 20, pp. 48–51, May 18, 2004.

Davis, T.T.; Delamarter, R.B.; Sra, P.; Goldstein, T.B. "The IDET Procedure for Chronic Discogenic Low Back Pain." *Spine,* vol. 29 no. 7, pp. 752–756, April 16, 2004.

Ernst, E. "Chiropractic Spinal Manipulation for Neck Pain: A Systematic Review." *Journal of Pain,* vol. 4 no. 8, pp. 417–421, October 2003.

Hartvigsen, J.; Christensen, K.; Frederiksen, H. "Back and Neck Pain Exhibit Many Common Features in Old Age: A Population-Based Study of 4,486 Danish Twins 70–102 Years of Age." *Spine,* vol. 29 no. 5, pp. 576–580, March 2004.

Jackson, R.S.; Banit, D.M.; Rhyne, A.L.; Darden, B.V. "Upper Cervical Spine Injuries." *Journal of the American Academy of Orthopaedic Surgeons,* vol. 10 no. 4, pp. 271–280, July 2002.

Katz, N.; Rodgers, D.B.; Krupa, D.; Reicin, A. "Onset of Pain Relief with Rofecoxib in Chronic Low Back Pain: Results of Two Four-Week, Randomized, Placebo-Controlled Trials." *Current Medical Research and Opinion,* vol. 20 no. 5, pp. 651–658, May 2004.

Kemp, B.J.; Kahan, J.S.; Krause, J.S.; Adkins, R.H.; Nava, G. "Treatment of Major Depression in Individuals with Spinal Cord Injury." *Journal of Spinal Cord Medicine,* vol. 27 no. 1, pp. 22–28, 2004.

Levins, S.M.; Redenbach, D.M.; Dyck, I. "Individual and Societal Influences on Participation in Physical Activity Following Spinal Cord Injury: A Qualitative Study." *Physical Therapy,* vol. 84 no. 6, pp. 496–509, June 2004.

MacPherson, H.; Thorpe, L.; Thomas, K.; Campbell, M. "Acupuncture for Low Back Pain: Traditional Diagnosis and Treatment of 148 Patients in a Clinical Trial." *Complementary Therapies in Medicine,* vol. 12 no. 1, pp. 38–44, March 2004.

McLain, R.F. "Functional Outcomes after Surgery for Spinal Fractures: Return to Work and Activity." *Spine,* vol. 29 no. 4, pp. 470–477 discussion Z6, February 2004.

Minassian, K.; Jilge, B.; Rattay, F; Pinter, M.M.; Binder, H.; Gerstenbrand, F.; Dimitrijevic, M.R. "Stepping-Like Movements in Humans with Complete Spinal Cord Injury Induced by Epidural Stimulation of the Lumbar Cord: Electromyographic Study of Compound Muscle Action Potentials." *Spinal Cord,* May 4, 2004.

Myckatyn, T.M.; Mackinnon, S.E.; McDonald, J.W. "Stem Cell Transplantation and Other Novel Techniques for Promoting Recovery from Spinal Cord Injury." *Transplant Immunology,* vol. 12 nos 3–4, pp. 343–358, April 2004.

Putzke, J.D.; Barrett, J.J.; Richards, J.S.; Underhill, A.T.; Lobello, S.G. "Life Satisfaction Following Spinal Cord Injury: Long-Term Follow-Up." *Journal of Spinal Cord Medicine,* vol. 27 no. 2, pp. 106–110, 2004.

Rodriquez, A.A.; Barr, K.P.; Burns, S.P. "Whiplash: Pathophysiology, Diagnosis, Treatment, and Prognosis." *Muscle and Nerve,* vol. 29 no. 6, pp. 768–781, June 2004.

Speed, C. "Low Back Pain." *British Medical Journal,* vol. 328 no. 7448, pp. 1119–1121, May 2004.

Thonse, R.; Belthur, M. "Rheumatoid Arthritis and Neck Pain." *Postgraduate Medicine Journal,* vol. 79 no. 938, p. 711, December 2003.

Tubach, F.; Beaute, J.; Leclerc, A. "Natural History and Prognostic Indicators of Sciatica." *Journal of Clinical Epidemiology,* vol. 57 no. 2, pp. 174–179, February 2004.

Ugwonali, O.F.; Lomas, G.; Choe, J.C.; Hyman, J.E.; Lee, F.Y.; Vitale, M.G.; Roye, D.P. "Effect of Bracing on the Quality of Life of Adolescents with Idiopathic Scoliosis." *Spine Journal,* vol. 4 no. 3, pp. 254–260, May-June 2004.

Victor, L.; Richeimer, S.M. "Psychosocial Therapies for Neck Pain." *Physical Medicine and Rehabilitation Clinics of North America,* vol. 14 no. 3, pp. 643–657, August 2003.

Yelland, M.; Mar, C.; Pirozzo, S.; Schoene, M.; Vercoe, P. "Prolotherapy Injections for Chronic Low-Back Pain." *Cochrane Database of System Reviews,* vol. 2, p. CD004059, 2004.

Yu, S.W.; Lee, P.C.; Ma, C.H.; Chuang, T.Y.; Chen, Y.J. "Vertebroplasty for the Treatment of Osteoporotic Compression Spinal Fracture: Comparison of Remedial Action at Different Stages of Injury." *Journal of Trauma,* vol. 56 no. 3, pp. 629–632, March 2004.

Websites That Provide Information about Back and Neck Disorders

All About Back and Neck Pain/DePuy Spine
http://www.allaboutbackandneckpain.com

American Academy of Orthopaedic Surgeons (AAOS)
http://www.aaos.org

American Academy of Physical Medicine and Rehabilitation
http://www.aapmr.org

American Association of Neurological Surgeons
http://www.neurosurgerytoday.org

American Association of Spinal Cord Injury Nurses
http://www.aascin.org

American Association of Spinal Cord Injury Psychologists and Social Workers
http://www.aascipsw.org

American Back Society
http://www.americanbacksoc.org

American Board of Physical Medicine and Rehabilitation
http://www.abpmr.org

American Chiropractic Association
http://www.amerchiro.org

American College of Rheumatology
http://www.rheumatology.org

American Pain Society
http://www.ampainsoc.org

American Paraplegia Society
http://www.apssci.org

American Physical Therapy Association
http://www.apta.org

American Society for Bone and Mineral Research
http://www.asbmr.org

American Spinal Injury Association
http://www.asia-spinalinjury.org

Annals of Internal Medicine
http://www.annals.org

Arthritis Foundation
http://www.arthritis.org

BackCare
http://www.backcare.org.uk

Back.com
http://www.back.com

CenterWatch
http://www.centerwatch.com/patient/trials.html

Cervical Spine Research Society
http://www.csrs.org

Christopher and Dana Reeve Paralysis Resource Center
http://www.paralysis.org

Clinical Immunology Society
http://www.clinimmsoc.org

ClinicalTrials.gov
http://www.clinicaltrials.gov

Dangerwood: The Site to Survive Spinal Cord Injury and Paralysis
http://www.survivingparalysis.com

Dynamic Chiropractic
http://www.chiroweb.com

Federation of Chiropractic Licensing Boards
http://www.fclb.org

Foundation for Spinal Cord Injury
http://fscip.org

International Chiropractors Association
http://www.chiropractic.org

International Intradiscal Therapy Society
http://www.iits.org

International Society for the Study of the Lumbar Spine
http://www.issls.org

International Spinal Injection Society
http://www.spinalinjection.com/ISIS

MedlinePLUS Health Information from the National Library of Medicine
http://www.medlineplus.org

National Center for Complementary and Alternative Medicine
http://www.nccam.nih.gov

National Institute of Arthritis and Musculoskeletal and Skin Diseases
http://www.niams.nih.gov

National Institute of Neurological Disorders and Stroke
http://www.ninds.nih.gov

National Spinal Cord Injury Association
http://www.spinalcord.org

NeckReference.com
http://www.neckreference.com

North American Spine Society
http://www.spine.org

Paralyzed Veterans of America
http://www.pva.org

Scoliosis Research Society
http://www.srs.org

Spinal Cord Injury Information Network
http://www.spinalcord.uab.edu

Spinal Cord Injury Network
http://www.spinalcordinjury.net

Spine Dr.
http://www.spine-dr.com

Spine-health.com
http://www.spine-health.com

SpineSource
http://www.spinesource.com

SpineUniverse
http://www.spineuniverse.com

USA TechGuide to Assistive Technology
http://www.usatechguide.org

Journals That Publish Research on Back and Neck Disorders

American Chiropractic Association Today
http://www.amerchiro.org/publications/aca_today.shtml

European Spine Journal
http://springerlink.metapress.com/app/home/
journal.asp?wasp=6cc6l52gun7wqgf4ek0j&referrer=parent&backto
=linkingpublicationresults,1:101557,1

Joint Bone Spine
http://www.elsevier.com/wps/find/journaldescription.cws_home/
621372/description#description

Journal of the American Chiropractic Association
http://www.amerchiro.org/publications

Journal of Bone and Joint Surgery
http://www.jbjs.co.uk

Journal of Manipulative and Physiological Therapeutics
http://www.us.elsevierhealth.com/product.jsp?isbn=01614754

Journal of Spinal Disorders
http://www.jspinaldisorders.com

Journal of the American Academy of Orthopaedic Surgeons
http://www5.aaos.org/jaaos/index.cfm

Journal of Spinal Cord Medicine
http://www.apssci.org/pages.php?catid=28

Seminars in Spine Surgery
http://www.us.elsevierhealth.com/product.jsp?isbn=10407383

Spinal Cord
http://www.nature.com/sc/index.html

Spine
http://www.spinejournal.com

Spine Journal
http://www.spine.org/tsj.cfm

Today's Chiropractic
http://www.todayschiropractic.com

Topics in Spinal Cord Injury Rehabilitation
http://www.thomasland.com/app/home/
main.asp?wasp=088vrkxyqr5e51mlpt6y

Index

Index

583

Health Reference Series
COMPLETE CATALOG

Adolescent Health Sourcebook

Basic Consumer Health Information about Common Medical, Mental, and Emotional Concerns in Adolescents, Including Facts about Acne, Body Piercing, Mononucleosis, Nutrition, Eating Disorders, Stress, Depression, Behavior Problems, Peer Pressure, Violence, Gangs, Drug Use, Puberty, Sexuality, Pregnancy, Learning Disabilities, and More

Along with a Glossary of Terms and Other Resources for Further Help and Information

Edited by Chad T. Kimball. 658 pages. 2002. 0-7808-0248-9. $78.

"It is written in clear, nontechnical language aimed at general readers. . . . Recommended for public libraries, community colleges, and other agencies serving health care consumers."
— *American Reference Books Annual, 2003*

"Recommended for school and public libraries. Parents and professionals dealing with teens will appreciate the easy-to-follow format and the clearly written text. This could become a 'must have' for every high school teacher." — *E-Streams, Jan '03*

"A good starting point for information related to common medical, mental, and emotional concerns of adolescents." — *School Library Journal, Nov '02*

"This book provides accurate information in an easy to access format. It addresses topics that parents and caregivers might not be aware of and provides practical, useable information." — *Doody's Health Sciences Book Review Journal, Sep-Oct '02*

"Recommended reference source."
— *Booklist, American Library Association, Sep '02*

AIDS Sourcebook, 3rd Edition

Basic Consumer Health Information about Acquired Immune Deficiency Syndrome (AIDS) and Human Immunodeficiency Virus (HIV) Infection, Including Facts about Transmission, Prevention, Diagnosis, Treatment, Opportunistic Infections, and Other Complications, with a Section for Women and Children, Including Details about Associated Gynecological Concerns, Pregnancy, and Pediatric Care

Along with Updated Statistical Information, Reports on Current Research Initiatives, a Glossary, and Directories of Internet, Hotline, and Other Resources

Edited by Dawn D. Matthews. 664 pages. 2003. 0-7808-0631-X. $78.

ALSO AVAILABLE: AIDS Sourcebook, 1st Edition. Edited by Karen Bellenir and Peter D. Dresser. 831 pages. 1995. 0-7808-0031-1. $78.

AIDS Sourcebook, 2nd Edition. Edited by Karen Bellenir. 751 pages. 1999. 0-7808-0225-X. $78.

"The 3rd edition of the *AIDS Sourcebook*, part of Omnigraphics' *Health Reference Series*, is a welcome update. . . . This resource is highly recommended for academic and public libraries."
— *American Reference Books Annual, 2004*

"Excellent sourcebook. This continues to be a highly recommended book. There is no other book that provides as much information as this book provides."
— *AIDS Book Review Journal, Dec-Jan 2000*

"Recommended reference source."
— *Booklist, American Library Association, Dec '99*

"A solid text for college-level health libraries."
— *The Bookwatch, Aug '99*

Cited in *Reference Sources for Small and Medium-Sized Libraries, American Library Association, 1999*

Alcoholism Sourcebook

Basic Consumer Health Information about the Physical and Mental Consequences of Alcohol Abuse, Including Liver Disease, Pancreatitis, Wernicke-Korsakoff Syndrome (Alcoholic Dementia), Fetal Alcohol Syndrome, Heart Disease, Kidney Disorders, Gastrointestinal Problems, and Immune System Compromise and Featuring Facts about Addiction, Detoxification, Alcohol Withdrawal, Recovery, and the Maintenance of Sobriety

Along with a Glossary and Directories of Resources for Further Help and Information

Edited by Karen Bellenir. 613 pages. 2000. 0-7808-0325-6. $78.

"This title is one of the few reference works on alcoholism for general readers. For some readers this will be a welcome complement to the many self-help books on the market. Recommended for collections serving general readers and consumer health collections."
— *E-Streams, Mar '01*

"This book is an excellent choice for public and academic libraries."
— *American Reference Books Annual, 2001*

"Recommended reference source."
— *Booklist, American Library Association, Dec '00*

"Presents a wealth of information on alcohol use and abuse and its effects on the body and mind, treatment, and prevention." — *SciTech Book News, Dec '00*

"Important new health guide which packs in the latest consumer information about the problems of alcoholism." — *Reviewer's Bookwatch, Nov '00*

SEE ALSO Drug Abuse Sourcebook, Substance Abuse Sourcebook

Allergies Sourcebook, 2nd Edition

Basic Consumer Health Information about Allergic Disorders, Triggers, Reactions, and Related Symptoms, Including Anaphylaxis, Rhinitis, Sinusitis, Asthma, Dermatitis, Conjunctivitis, and Multiple Chemical Sensitivity

Along with Tips on Diagnosis, Prevention, and Treatment, Statistical Data, a Glossary, and a Directory of Sources for Further Help and Information

Edited by Annemarie S. Muth. 598 pages. 2002. 0-7808-0376-0. $78.

ALSO AVAILABLE: *Allergies Sourcebook, 1st Edition.* Edited by Allan R. Cook. 611 pages. 1997. 0-7808-0036-2. $78.

"This book brings a great deal of useful material together. . . . This is an excellent addition to public and consumer health library collections."
—American Reference Books Annual, 2003

"This second edition would be useful to laypersons with little or advanced knowledge of the subject matter. This book would also serve as a resource for nursing and other health care professions students. It would be useful in public, academic, and hospital libraries with consumer health collections." *—E-Streams, Jul '02*

Alternative Medicine Sourcebook, 2nd Edition

Basic Consumer Health Information about Alternative and Complementary Medical Practices, Including Acupuncture, Chiropractic, Herbal Medicine, Homeopathy, Naturopathic Medicine, Mind-Body Interventions, Ayurveda, and Other Non-Western Medical Traditions

Along with Facts about such Specific Therapies as Massage Therapy, Aromatherapy, Qigong, Hypnosis, Prayer, Dance, and Art Therapies, a Glossary, and Resources for Further Information

Edited by Dawn D. Matthews. 618 pages. 2002. 0-7808-0605-0. $78.

ALSO AVAILABLE: *Alternative Medicine Sourcebook, 1st Edition.* Edited by Allan R. Cook. 737 pages. 1999. 0-7808-0200-4. $78.

"Recommended for public, high school, and academic libraries that have consumer health collections. Hospital libraries that also serve the public will find this to be a useful resource." *—E-Streams, Feb '03*

"Recommended reference source."
—Booklist, American Library Association, Jan '03

"An important alternate health reference."
—MBR Bookwatch, Oct '02

"A great addition to the reference collection of every type of library." *—American Reference Books Annual, 2000*

Alzheimer's Disease Sourcebook, 3rd Edition

Basic Consumer Health Information about Alzheimer's Disease, Other Dementias, and Related Disorders, Including Multi-Infarct Dementia, AIDS Dementia Complex, Dementia with Lewy Bodies, Huntington's Disease, Wernicke-Korsakoff Syndrome (Alcohol-Related Dementia), Delirium, and Confusional States

Along with Information for People Newly Diagnosed with Alzheimer's Disease and Caregivers, Reports Detailing Current Research Efforts in Prevention, Diagnosis, and Treatment, Facts about Long-Term Care Issues, and Listings of Sources for Additional Information

Edited by Karen Bellenir. 645 pages. 2003. 0-7808-0666-2. $78.

ALSO AVAILABLE: *Alzheimer's, Stroke & 29 Other Neurological Disorders Sourcebook, 1st Edition.* Edited by Frank E. Bair. 579 pages. 1993. 1-55888-748-2. $78.

ALSO AVAILABLE: *Alzheimer's Disease Sourcebook, 2nd Edition.* Edited by Karen Bellenir. 524 pages. 1999. 0-7808-0223-3. $78.

"This very informative and valuable tool will be a great addition to any library serving consumers, students and health care workers."
—American Reference Books Annual, 2004

"This is a valuable resource for people affected by dementias such as Alzheimer's. It is easy to navigate and includes important information and resources."
—Doody's Review Service, Feb. 2004

"Recommended reference source."
—Booklist, American Library Association, Oct '99

SEE ALSO Brain Disorders Sourcebook

Arthritis Sourcebook, 2nd Edition

Basic Consumer Health Information about Osteoarthritis, Rheumatoid Arthritis, Other Rheumatic Disorders, Infectious Forms of Arthritis, and Diseases with Symptoms Linked to Arthritis, Featuring Facts about Diagnosis, Pain Management, and Surgical Therapies

Along with Coping Strategies, Research Updates, a Glossary, and Resources for Additional Help and Information

Edited by Amy L. Sutton. 593 pages. 2004. 0-7808-0667-0. $78.

ALSO AVAILABLE: *Arthritis Sourcebook, 1st Edition.* Edited by Allan R. Cook. 550 pages. 1998. 0-7808-0201-2. $78.

". . . accessible to the layperson."
—Reference and Research Book News, Feb '99

Asthma Sourcebook

Basic Consumer Health Information about Asthma, Including Symptoms, Traditional and Nontraditional Remedies, Treatment Advances, Quality-of-Life Aids, Medical Research Updates, and the Role of Allergies, Exercise, Age, the Environment, and Genetics in the Development of Asthma

Along with Statistical Data, a Glossary, and Directories of Support Groups, and Other Resources for Further Information

Edited by Annemarie S. Muth. 628 pages. 2000. 0-7808-0381-7. $78.

"A worthwhile reference acquisition for public libraries and academic medical libraries whose readers desire a quick introduction to the wide range of asthma information." *— Choice, Association of College & Research Libraries, Jun '01*

"Recommended reference source."
—Booklist, American Library Association, Feb '01

"Highly recommended." *— The Bookwatch, Jan '01*

"There is much good information for patients and their families who deal with asthma daily."
—American Medical Writers Association Journal, Winter '01

"This informative text is recommended for consumer health collections in public, secondary school, and community college libraries and the libraries of universities with a large undergraduate population."
— American Reference Books Annual, 2001

Attention Deficit Disorder Sourcebook

Basic Consumer Health Information about Attention Deficit/Hyperactivity Disorder in Children and Adults, Including Facts about Causes, Symptoms, Diagnostic Criteria, and Treatment Options Such as Medications, Behavior Therapy, Coaching, and Homeopathy

Along with Reports on Current Research Initiatives, Legal Issues, and Government Regulations, and Featuring a Glossary of Related Terms, Internet Resources, and a List of Additional Reading Material

Edited by Dawn D. Matthews. 470 pages. 2002. 0-7808-0624-7. $78.

"Recommended reference source."
—Booklist, American Library Association, Jan '03

"This book is recommended for all school libraries and the reference or consumer health sections of public libraries." *— American Reference Books Annual, 2003*

Back & Neck Sourcebook, 2nd Edition

Basic Consumer Health Information about Spinal Pain, Spinal Cord Injuries, and Related Disorders, Such as Degenerative Disk Disease, Osteoarthritis, Scoliosis, Sciatica, Spina Bifida, and Spinal Stenosis, and Featuring Facts about Maintaining Spinal Health, Self-Care, Pain Management, Rehabilitative Care, Chiropractic Care, Spinal Surgeries, and Complementary Therapies

Along with Suggestions for Preventing Back and Neck Pain, a Glossary of Related Terms, and a Directory of Resources

Edited by Amy L. Sutton. 633 pages. 2004. 0-7808-0738-3 $78.

ALSO AVAILABLE: *Back & Neck Disorders Sourcebook, 1st Edition.* Edited by Karen Bellenir. 548 pages. 1997. 0-7808-0202-0. $78.

"The strength of this work is its basic, easy-to-read format. Recommended."
—Reference and User Services Quarterly, American Library Association, Winter '97

Blood & Circulatory Disorders Sourcebook

Basic Information about Blood and Its Components, Anemias, Leukemias, Bleeding Disorders, and Circulatory Disorders, Including Aplastic Anemia, Thalassemia, Sickle-Cell Disease, Hemochromatosis, Hemophilia, Von Willebrand Disease, and Vascular Diseases

Along with a Special Section on Blood Transfusions and Blood Supply Safety, a Glossary, and Source Listings for Further Help and Information

Edited by Karen Bellenir and Linda M. Shin. 554 pages. 1998. 0-7808-0203-9. $78.

"Recommended reference source."
—Booklist, American Library Association, Feb '99

"An important reference sourcebook written in simple language for everyday, non-technical users. "
—Reviewer's Bookwatch, Jan '99

Brain Disorders Sourcebook

Basic Consumer Health Information about Strokes, Epilepsy, Amyotrophic Lateral Sclerosis (ALS/Lou Gehrig's Disease), Parkinson's Disease, Brain Tumors, Cerebral Palsy, Headache, Tourette Syndrome, and More

Along with Statistical Data, Treatment and Rehabilitation Options, Coping Strategies, Reports on Current Research Initiatives, a Glossary, and Resource Listings for Additional Help and Information

Edited by Karen Bellenir. 481 pages. 1999. 0-7808-0229-2. $78.

"Belongs on the shelves of any library with a consumer health collection." *— E-Streams, Mar '00*

"Recommended reference source."
—Booklist, American Library Association, Oct '99

SEE ALSO *Alzheimer's Disease Sourcebook*

Breast Cancer Sourcebook, 2nd Edition

Basic Consumer Health Information about Breast Cancer, Including Facts about Risk Factors, Prevention, Screening and Diagnostic Methods, Treatment Options, Complementary and Alternative Therapies, Post-Treatment Concerns, Clinical Trials, Special Risk Populations, and New Developments in Breast Cancer Research

Along with Breast Cancer Statistics, a Glossary of Related Terms, and a Directory of Resources for Additional Help and Information

Edited by Sandra J. Judd. 595 pages. 2004. 0-7808-0668-9. $78.

ALSO AVAILABLE: Breast Cancer Sourcebook, 1st Edition. Edited by Edward J. Prucha and Karen Bellenir. 580 pages. 2001. 0-7808-0244-6. $78.

"It would be a useful reference book in a library or on loan to women in a support group."
— *Cancer Forum, Mar '03*

"Recommended reference source."
— *Booklist, American Library Association, Jan '02*

"This reference source is highly recommended. It is quite informative, comprehensive and detailed in nature, and yet it offers practical advice in easy-to-read language. It could be thought of as the 'bible' of breast cancer for the consumer." — *E-Streams, Jan '02*

"The broad range of topics covered in lay language make the *Breast Cancer Sourcebook* an excellent addition to public and consumer health library collections."
— *American Reference Books Annual 2002*

"From the pros and cons of different screening methods and results to treatment options, *Breast Cancer Sourcebook* provides the latest information on the subject."
— *Library Bookwatch, Dec '01*

"This thoroughgoing, very readable reference covers all aspects of breast health and cancer.... Readers will find much to consider here. Recommended for all public and patient health collections."
— *Library Journal, Sep '01*

SEE ALSO Cancer Sourcebook for Women, Women's Health Concerns Sourcebook

Breastfeeding Sourcebook

Basic Consumer Health Information about the Benefits of Breastmilk, Preparing to Breastfeed, Breastfeeding as a Baby Grows, Nutrition, and More, Including Information on Special Situations and Concerns Such as Mastitis, Illness, Medications, Allergies, Multiple Births, Prematurity, Special Needs, and Adoption

Along with a Glossary and Resources for Additional Help and Information

Edited by Jenni Lynn Colson. 388 pages. 2002. 0-7808-0332-9. $78.

SEE ALSO Pregnancy & Birth Sourcebook

"Particularly useful is the information about professional lactation services and chapters on breastfeeding when returning to work.... *Breastfeeding Sourcebook* will be useful for public libraries, consumer health libraries, and technical schools offering nurse assistant training, especially in areas where Internet access is problematic."
— *American Reference Books Annual, 2003*

Burns Sourcebook

Basic Consumer Health Information about Various Types of Burns and Scalds, Including Flame, Heat, Cold, Electrical, Chemical, and Sun Burns

Along with Information on Short-Term and Long-Term Treatments, Tissue Reconstruction, Plastic Surgery, Prevention Suggestions, and First Aid

Edited by Allan R. Cook. 604 pages. 1999. 0-7808-0204-7. $78.

"This is an exceptional addition to the series and is highly recommended for all consumer health collections, hospital libraries, and academic medical centers."
— *E-Streams, Mar '00*

"This key reference guide is an invaluable addition to all health care and public libraries in confronting this ongoing health issue."
— *American Reference Books Annual, 2000*

"Recommended reference source."
— *Booklist, American Library Association, Dec '99*

SEE ALSO Skin Disorders Sourcebook

Cancer Sourcebook, 4th Edition

Basic Consumer Health Information about Major Forms and Stages of Cancer, Featuring Facts about Head and Neck Cancers, Lung Cancers, Gastrointestinal Cancers, Genitourinary Cancers, Lymphomas, Blood Cell Cancers, Endocrine Cancers, Skin Cancers, Bone Cancers, Sarcomas, and Others, and Including Information about Cancer Treatments and Therapies, Identifying and Reducing Cancer Risks, and Strategies for Coping with Cancer and the Side Effects of Treatment

Along with a Cancer Glossary, Statistical and Demographic Data, and a Directory of Sources for Additional Help and Information

Edited by Karen Bellenir. 1,119 pages. 2003. 0-7808-0633-6. $78.

ALSO AVAILABLE: Cancer Sourcebook, 1st Edition. Edited by Frank E. Bair. 932 pages. 1990. 1-55888-888-8. $78.

New Cancer Sourcebook, 2nd Edition. Edited by Allan R. Cook. 1,313 pages. 1996. 0-7808-0041-9. $78.

Cancer Sourcebook, 3rd Edition. Edited by Edward J. Prucha. 1,069 pages. 2000. 0-7808-0227-6. $78.

"With cancer being the second leading cause of death for Americans, a prodigious work such as this one, which locates centrally so much cancer-related information, is clearly an asset to this nation's citizens and others." — *Journal of the National Medical Association, 2004*

"This title is recommended for health sciences and public libraries with consumer health collections."
— *E-Streams, Feb '01*

". . . can be effectively used by cancer patients and their families who are looking for answers in a language they can understand. Public and hospital libraries should have it on their shelves."
— *American Reference Books Annual, 2001*

"Recommended reference source."
— *Booklist, American Library Association, Dec '00*

Cited in *Reference Sources for Small and Medium-Sized Libraries*, American Library Association, 1999

"The amount of factual and useful information is extensive. The writing is very clear, geared to general readers. Recommended for all levels." — *Choice*, Association of College & Research Libraries, Jan '97

SEE ALSO Breast Cancer Sourcebook, Cancer Sourcebook for Women, Pediatric Cancer Sourcebook, Prostate Cancer Sourcebook

■

Cancer Sourcebook for Women, 2nd Edition

Basic Consumer Health Information about Gynecologic Cancers and Related Concerns, Including Cervical Cancer, Endometrial Cancer, Gestational Trophoblastic Tumor, Ovarian Cancer, Uterine Cancer, Vaginal Cancer, Vulvar Cancer, Breast Cancer, and Common Non-Cancerous Uterine Conditions, with Facts about Cancer Risk Factors, Screening and Prevention, Treatment Options, and Reports on Current Research Initiatives

Along with a Glossary of Cancer Terms and a Directory of Resources for Additional Help and Information

Edited by Karen Bellenir. 604 pages. 2002. 0-7808-0226-8. $78.

ALSO AVAILABLE: *Cancer Sourcebook for Women, 1st Edition.* Edited by Allan R. Cook and Peter D. Dresser. 524 pages. 1996. 0-7808-0076-1. $78.

"An excellent addition to collections in public, consumer health, and women's health libraries."
— *American Reference Books Annual, 2003*

"Overall, the information is excellent, and complex topics are clearly explained. As a reference book for the consumer it is a valuable resource to assist them to make informed decisions about cancer and its treatments." — *Cancer Forum, Nov '02*

"Highly recommended for academic and medical reference collections." — *Library Bookwatch, Sep '02*

"This is a highly recommended book for any public or consumer library, being reader friendly and containing accurate and helpful information."
— *E-Streams, Aug '02*

"Recommended reference source."
— *Booklist, American Library Association, Jul '02*

SEE ALSO Breast Cancer Sourcebook, Women's Health Concerns Sourcebook

Cardiovascular Diseases & Disorders Sourcebook, 1st Edition

SEE Heart Diseases & Disorders Sourcebook, 2nd Edition

■

Caregiving Sourcebook

Basic Consumer Health Information for Caregivers, Including a Profile of Caregivers, Caregiving Responsibilities and Concerns, Tips for Specific Conditions, Care Environments, and the Effects of Caregiving

Along with Facts about Legal Issues, Financial Information, and Future Planning, a Glossary, and a Listing of Additional Resources

Edited by Joyce Brennfleck Shannon. 600 pages. 2001. 0-7808-0331-0. $78.

"Essential for most collections."
— *Library Journal, Apr 1, 2002*

"An ideal addition to the reference collection of any public library. Health sciences information professionals may also want to acquire the *Caregiving Sourcebook* for their hospital or academic library for use as a ready reference tool by health care workers interested in aging and caregiving." — *E-Streams, Jan '02*

"Recommended reference source."
— *Booklist, American Library Association, Oct '01*

■

Child Abuse Sourcebook

Basic Consumer Health Information about the Physical, Sexual, and Emotional Abuse of Children, with Additional Facts about Neglect, Munchausen Syndrome by Proxy (MSBP), Shaken Baby Syndrome, and Controversial Issues Related to Child Abuse, Such as Withholding Medical Care, Corporal Punishment, and Child Maltreatment in Youth Sports, and Featuring Facts about Child Protective Services, Foster Care, Adoption, Parenting Challenges, and Other Abuse Prevention Efforts

Along with a Glossary of Related Terms and Resources for Additional Help and Information

Edited by Dawn D. Matthews. 620 pages. 2004. 0-7808-0705-7. $78.

■

Childhood Diseases & Disorders Sourcebook

Basic Consumer Health Information about Medical Problems Often Encountered in Pre-Adolescent Children, Including Respiratory Tract Ailments, Ear Infections, Sore Throats, Disorders of the Skin and Scalp, Digestive and Genitourinary Diseases, Infectious Diseases, Inflammatory Disorders, Chronic Physical and Developmental Disorders, Allergies, and More

Along with Information about Diagnostic Tests, Common Childhood Surgeries, and Frequently Used Medications, with a Glossary of Important Terms and Resource Directory

Edited by Chad T. Kimball. 662 pages. 2003. 0-7808-0458-9. $78.

"This is an excellent book for new parents and should be included in all health care and public libraries."
— American Reference Books Annual, 2004

Colds, Flu & Other Common Ailments Sourcebook

Basic Consumer Health Information about Common Ailments and Injuries, Including Colds, Coughs, the Flu, Sinus Problems, Headaches, Fever, Nausea and Vomiting, Menstrual Cramps, Diarrhea, Constipation, Hemorrhoids, Back Pain, Dandruff, Dry and Itchy Skin, Cuts, Scrapes, Sprains, Bruises, and More

Along with Information about Prevention, Self-Care, Choosing a Doctor, Over-the-Counter Medications, Folk Remedies, and Alternative Therapies, and Including a Glossary of Important Terms and a Directory of Resources for Further Help and Information

Edited by Chad T. Kimball. 638 pages. 2001. 0-7808-0435-X. $78.

"A good starting point for research on common illnesses. It will be a useful addition to public and consumer health library collections."
— American Reference Books Annual 2002

"Will prove valuable to any library seeking to maintain a current, comprehensive reference collection of health resources. . . . Excellent reference."
— The Bookwatch, Aug '01

"Recommended reference source."
— Booklist, American Library Association, July '01

Communication Disorders Sourcebook

Basic Information about Deafness and Hearing Loss, Speech and Language Disorders, Voice Disorders, Balance and Vestibular Disorders, and Disorders of Smell, Taste, and Touch

Edited by Linda M. Ross. 533 pages. 1996. 0-7808-0077-X. $78.

"This is skillfully edited and is a welcome resource for the layperson. It should be found in every public and medical library." — Booklist Health Sciences Supplement, American Library Association, Oct '97

Congenital Disorders Sourcebook

Basic Information about Disorders Acquired during Gestation, Including Spina Bifida, Hydrocephalus, Cerebral Palsy, Heart Defects, Craniofacial Abnormalities, Fetal Alcohol Syndrome, and More

Along with Current Treatment Options and Statistical Data

Edited by Karen Bellenir. 607 pages. 1997. 0-7808-0205-5. $78.

"Recommended reference source."
— Booklist, American Library Association, Oct '97

SEE ALSO Pregnancy & Birth Sourcebook

Consumer Issues in Health Care Sourcebook

Basic Information about Health Care Fundamentals and Related Consumer Issues, Including Exams and Screening Tests, Physician Specialties, Choosing a Doctor, Using Prescription and Over-the-Counter Medications Safely, Avoiding Health Scams, Managing Common Health Risks in the Home, Care Options for Chronically or Terminally Ill Patients, and a List of Resources for Obtaining Help and Further Information

Edited by Karen Bellenir. 618 pages. 1998. 0-7808-0221-7. $78.

"Both public and academic libraries will want to have a copy in their collection for readers who are interested in self-education on health issues."
— American Reference Books Annual, 2000

"The editor has researched the literature from government agencies and others, saving readers the time and effort of having to do the research themselves. Recommended for public libraries."
— Reference and User Services Quarterly, American Library Association, Spring '99

"Recommended reference source."
— Booklist, American Library Association, Dec '98

Contagious Diseases Sourcebook

Basic Consumer Health Information about Infectious Diseases Spread by Person-to-Person Contact through Direct Touch, Airborne Transmission, Sexual Contact, or Contact with Blood or Other Body Fluids, Including Hepatitis, Herpes, Influenza, Lice, Measles, Mumps, Pinworm, Ringworm, Severe Acute Respiratory Syndrome (SARS), Streptococcal Infections, Tuberculosis, and Others

Along with Facts about Disease Transmission, Antimicrobial Resistance, and Vaccines, with a Glossary and Directories of Resources for More Information

Edited by Karen Bellenir. 643 pages. 2004. 0-7808-0736-7. $78.

Contagious & Non-Contagious Infectious Diseases Sourcebook

Basic Information about Contagious Diseases like Measles, Polio, Hepatitis B, and Infectious Mononucleosis, and Non-Contagious Infectious Diseases like Tetanus and Toxic Shock Syndrome, and Diseases Occurring as Secondary Infections Such as Shingles and Reye Syndrome

Along with Vaccination, Prevention, and Treatment Information, and a Section Describing Emerging Infectious Disease Threats

Edited by Karen Bellenir and Peter D. Dresser. 566 pages. 1996. 0-7808-0075-3. $78.

Death & Dying Sourcebook

Basic Consumer Health Information for the Layperson about End-of-Life Care and Related Ethical and Legal Issues, Including Chief Causes of Death, Autopsies, Pain Management for the Terminally Ill, Life Support Systems, Insurance, Euthanasia, Assisted Suicide, Hospice Programs, Living Wills, Funeral Planning, Counseling, Mourning, Organ Donation, and Physician Training

Along with Statistical Data, a Glossary, and Listings of Sources for Further Help and Information

Edited by Annemarie S. Muth. 641 pages. 1999. 0-7808-0230-6. $78.

"Public libraries, medical libraries, and academic libraries will all find this sourcebook a useful addition to their collections."
— American Reference Books Annual, 2001

"An extremely useful resource for those concerned with death and dying in the United States."
— Respiratory Care, Nov '00

"Recommended reference source."
— Booklist, American Library Association, Aug '00

"This book is a definite must for all those involved in end-of-life care." *— Doody's Review Service, 2000*

Dental Care & Oral Health Sourcebook, 2nd Edition

Basic Consumer Health Information about Dental Care, Including Oral Hygiene, Dental Visits, Pain Management, Cavities, Crowns, Bridges, Dental Implants, and Fillings, and Other Oral Health Concerns, Such as Gum Disease, Bad Breath, Dry Mouth, Genetic and Developmental Abnormalities, Oral Cancers, Orthodontics, and Temporomandibular Disorders

Along with Updates on Current Research in Oral Health, a Glossary, a Directory of Dental and Oral Health Organizations, and Resources for People with Dental and Oral Health Disorders

Edited by Amy L. Sutton. 609 pages. 2003. 0-7808-0634-4. $78.

ALSO AVAILABLE: *Oral Health Sourcebook, 1st Edition. Edited by Allan R. Cook. 558 pages. 1997. 0-7808-0082-6. $78.*

"This book could serve as a turning point in the battle to educate consumers in issues concerning oral health."
— American Reference Books Annual, 2004

"Unique source which will fill a gap in dental sources for patients and the lay public. A valuable reference tool even in a library with thousands of books on dentistry. Comprehensive, clear, inexpensive, and easy to read and use. It fills an enormous gap in the health care literature." *— Reference and User Services Quarterly, American Library Association, Summer '98*

"Recommended reference source."
— Booklist, American Library Association, Dec '97

Depression Sourcebook

Basic Consumer Health Information about Unipolar Depression, Bipolar Disorder, Postpartum Depression, Seasonal Affective Disorder, and Other Types of Depression in Children, Adolescents, Women, Men, the Elderly, and Other Selected Populations

Along with Facts about Causes, Risk Factors, Diagnostic Criteria, Treatment Options, Coping Strategies, Suicide Prevention, a Glossary, and a Directory of Sources for Additional Help and Information

Edited by Karen Belleni. 602 pages. 2002. 0-7808-0611-5. $78.

"*Depression Sourcebook* is of a very high standard. Its purpose, which is to serve as a reference source to the lay reader, is very well served."
— Journal of the National Medical Association, 2004

"Invaluable reference for public and school library collections alike." *— Library Bookwatch, Apr '03*

"Recommended for purchase."
— American Reference Books Annual, 2003

Diabetes Sourcebook, 3rd Edition

Basic Consumer Health Information about Type 1 Diabetes (Insulin-Dependent or Juvenile-Onset Diabetes), Type 2 Diabetes (Noninsulin-Dependent or Adult-Onset Diabetes), Gestational Diabetes, Impaired Glucose Tolerance (IGT), and Related Complications, Such as Amputation, Eye Disease, Gum Disease, Nerve Damage, and End-Stage Renal Disease, Including Facts about Insulin, Oral Diabetes Medications, Blood Sugar Testing, and the Role of Exercise and Nutrition in the Control of Diabetes

Along with a Glossary and Resources for Further Help and Information

Edited by Dawn D. Matthews. 622 pages. 2003. 0-7808-0629-8. $78.

ALSO AVAILABLE: *Diabetes Sourcebook, 1st Edition. Edited by Karen Bellenir and Peter D. Dresser. 827 pages. 1994. 1-55888-751-2. $78.*

Diabetes Sourcebook, 2nd Edition. Edited by Karen Bellenir. 688 pages. 1998. 0-7808-0224-1. $78.

"This edition is even more helpful than earlier versions. . . . It is a truly valuable tool for anyone seeking readable and authoritative information on diabetes."
— American Reference Books Annual, 2004

"An invaluable reference." *— Library Journal, May '00*

Selected as one of the 250 "Best Health Sciences Books of 1999." *— Doody's Rating Service, Mar-Apr 2000*

"Provides useful information for the general public."
— Healthlines, University of Michigan Health Management Research Center, Sep/Oct '99

". . . provides reliable mainstream medical information . . . belongs on the shelves of any library with a consumer health collection." *— E-Streams, Sep '99*

"Recommended reference source."
— Booklist, American Library Association, Feb '99

Diet & Nutrition Sourcebook, 2nd Edition

Basic Consumer Health Information about Dietary Guidelines, Recommended Daily Intake Values, Vitamins, Minerals, Fiber, Fat, Weight Control, Dietary Supplements, and Food Additives

Along with Special Sections on Nutrition Needs throughout Life and Nutrition for People with Such Specific Medical Concerns as Allergies, High Blood Cholesterol, Hypertension, Diabetes, Celiac Disease, Seizure Disorders, Phenylketonuria (PKU), Cancer, and Eating Disorders, and Including Reports on Current Nutrition Research and Source Listings for Additional Help and Information

Edited by Karen Bellenir. 650 pages. 1999. 0-7808-0228-4. $78.

ALSO AVAILABLE: Diet & Nutrition Sourcebook, 1st Edition. Edited by Dan R. Harris. 662 pages. 1996. 0-7808-0084-2. $78.

"This book is an excellent source of basic diet and nutrition information." *— Booklist Health Sciences Supplement, American Library Association, Dec '00*

"This reference document should be in any public library, but it would be a very good guide for beginning students in the health sciences. If the other books in this publisher's series are as good as this, they should all be in the health sciences collections."
—American Reference Books Annual, 2000

"This book is an excellent general nutrition reference for consumers who desire to take an active role in their health care for prevention. Consumers of all ages who select this book can feel confident they are receiving current and accurate information." *—Journal of Nutrition for the Elderly, Vol. 19, No. 4, '00*

"Recommended reference source."
—Booklist, American Library Association, Dec '99

SEE ALSO Digestive Diseases & Disorders Sourcebook, Eating Disorders Sourcebook, Gastrointestinal Diseases & Disorders Sourcebook, Vegetarian Sourcebook

■

Digestive Diseases & Disorders Sourcebook

Basic Consumer Health Information about Diseases and Disorders that Impact the Upper and Lower Digestive System, Including Celiac Disease, Constipation, Crohn's Disease, Cyclic Vomiting Syndrome, Diarrhea, Diverticulosis and Diverticulitis, Gallstones, Heartburn, Hemorrhoids, Hernias, Indigestion (Dyspepsia), Irritable Bowel Syndrome, Lactose Intolerance, Ulcers, and More

Along with Information about Medications and Other Treatments, Tips for Maintaining a Healthy Digestive Tract, a Glossary, and Directory of Digestive Diseases Organizations

Edited by Karen Bellenir. 335 pages. 2000. 0-7808-0327-2. $78.

"This title would be an excellent addition to all public or patient-research libraries."
—American Reference Books Annual, 2001

"This title is recommended for public, hospital, and health sciences libraries with consumer health collections." *— E-Streams, Jul-Aug '00*

"Recommended reference source."
—Booklist, American Library Association, May '00

SEE ALSO Diet & Nutrition Sourcebook, Eating Disorders Sourcebook, Gastrointestinal Diseases & Disorders Sourcebook

■

Disabilities Sourcebook

Basic Consumer Health Information about Physical and Psychiatric Disabilities, Including Descriptions of Major Causes of Disability, Assistive and Adaptive Aids, Workplace Issues, and Accessibility Concerns

Along with Information about the Americans with Disabilities Act, a Glossary, and Resources for Additional Help and Information

Edited by Dawn D. Matthews. 616 pages. 2000. 0-7808-0389-2. $78.

"It is a must for libraries with a consumer health section." *— American Reference Books Annual 2002*

"A much needed addition to the Omnigraphics *Health Reference Series*. A current reference work to provide people with disabilities, their families, caregivers or those who work with them, a broad range of information in one volume, has not been available until now. . . . It is recommended for all public and academic library reference collections." *— E-Streams, May '01*

"An excellent source book in easy-to-read format covering many current topics; highly recommended for all libraries." *— Choice, Association of College and Research Libraries, Jan '01*

"Recommended reference source."
—Booklist, American Library Association, Jul '00

■

Domestic Violence Sourcebook, 2nd Edition

Basic Consumer Health Information about the Causes and Consequences of Abusive Relationships, Including Physical Violence, Sexual Assault, Battery, Stalking, and Emotional Abuse, and Facts about the Effects of Violence on Women, Men, Young Adults, and the Elderly, with Reports about Domestic Violence in Selected Populations, and Featuring Facts about Medical Care, Victim Assistance and Protection, Prevention Strategies, Mental Health Services, and Legal Issues

Along with a Glossary of Related Terms and Resources for Additional Help and Information

Edited by Dawn D. Matthews. 628 pages. 2004. 0-7808-0669-7. $78.

ALSO AVAILABLE: Domestic Violence & Child Abuse Sourcebook, 1st Edition. Edited by Helene Henderson. 1,064 pages. 2001. 0-7808-0235-7. $78.

"Interested lay persons should find the book extremely beneficial. . . . A copy of *Domestic Violence and Child Abuse Sourcebook* should be in every public library in the United States."
— *Social Science & Medicine, No. 56, 2003*

"This is important information. The Web has many resources but this sourcebook fills an important societal need. I am not aware of any other resources of this type." — *Doody's Review Service, Sep '01*

"Recommended for all libraries, scholars, and practitioners." — *Choice,*
Association of College & Research Libraries, Jul '01

"Recommended reference source."
— *Booklist, American Library Association, Apr '01*

"Important pick for college-level health reference libraries." — *The Bookwatch, Mar '01*

"Because this problem is so widespread and because this book includes a lot of issues within one volume, this work is recommended for all public libraries."
— *American Reference Books Annual, 2001*

■

Drug Abuse Sourcebook, 2nd Edition

Basic Consumer Health Information about Illicit Substances of Abuse and the Misuse of Prescription and Over-the-Counter Medications, Including Depressants, Hallucinogens, Inhalants, Marijuana, Stimulants, and Anabolic Steroids

Along with Facts about Related Health Risks, Treatment Programs, Prevention Programs, a Glossary of Abuse and Addiction Terms, a Glossary of Drug-Related Street Terms, and a Directory Resources for More Information

Edited by Catherine Ginther. 600 pages. 2004. 0-7808-0740-5. $78.

ALSO AVAILABLE: Drug Abuse Sourcebook, 1st Edition. Edited by Karen Bellenir. 629 pages. 2000. 0-7808-0242-X. $78.

"Containing a wealth of information . . . . This resource belongs in libraries that serve a lower-division undergraduate or community college clientele as well as the general public." — *Choice, Association of*
College and Research Libraries, Jun '01

"Recommended reference source."
— *Booklist, American Library Association, Feb '01*

"Highly recommended." — *The Bookwatch, Jan '01*

"Even though there is a plethora of books on drug abuse, this volume is recommended for school, public, and college libraries."
— *American Reference Books Annual, 2001*

SEE ALSO Alcoholism Sourcebook, Substance Abuse Sourcebook

Ear, Nose & Throat Disorders Sourcebook

Basic Information about Disorders of the Ears, Nose, Sinus Cavities, Pharynx, and Larynx, Including Ear Infections, Tinnitus, Vestibular Disorders, Allergic and Non-Allergic Rhinitis, Sore Throats, Tonsillitis, and Cancers That Affect the Ears, Nose, Sinuses, and Throat

Along with Reports on Current Research Initiatives, a Glossary of Related Medical Terms, and a Directory of Sources for Further Help and Information

Edited by Karen Bellenir and Linda M. Shin. 576 pages. 1998. 0-7808-0206-3. $78.

"Overall, this sourcebook is helpful for the consumer seeking information on ENT issues. It is recommended for public libraries."
— *American Reference Books Annual, 1999*

"Recommended reference source."
— *Booklist, American Library Association, Dec '98*

■

Eating Disorders Sourcebook

Basic Consumer Health Information about Eating Disorders, Including Information about Anorexia Nervosa, Bulimia Nervosa, Binge Eating, Body Dysmorphic Disorder, Pica, Laxative Abuse, and Night Eating Syndrome

Along with Information about Causes, Adverse Effects, and Treatment and Prevention Issues, and Featuring a Section on Concerns Specific to Children and Adolescents, a Glossary, and Resources for Further Help and Information

Edited by Dawn D. Matthews. 322 pages. 2001. 0-7808-0335-3. $78.

"Recommended for health science libraries that are open to the public, as well as hospital libraries. This book is a good resource for the consumer who is concerned about eating disorders." — *E-Streams, Mar '02*

"This volume is another convenient collection of excerpted articles. Recommended for school and public library patrons; lower-division undergraduates; and two-year technical program students." — *Choice,*
Association of College & Research Libraries, Jan '02

"Recommended reference source." — *Booklist,*
American Library Association, Oct '01

SEE ALSO Diet & Nutrition Sourcebook, Digestive Diseases & Disorders Sourcebook, Gastrointestinal Diseases & Disorders Sourcebook

■

Emergency Medical Services Sourcebook

Basic Consumer Health Information about Preventing, Preparing for, and Managing Emergency Situations, When and Who to Call for Help, What to Expect in the Emergency Room, the Emergency Medical Team, Patient Issues, and Current Topics in Emergency Medicine

Along with Statistical Data, a Glossary, and Sources of Additional Help and Information

Edited by Jenni Lynn Colson. 494 pages. 2002. 0-7808-0420-1. $78.

"Handy and convenient for home, public, school, and college libraries. Recommended."
— *Choice, Association of College and Research Libraries, Apr '03*

"This reference can provide the consumer with answers to most questions about emergency care in the United States, or it will direct them to a resource where the answer can be found."
— *American Reference Books Annual, 2003*

"Recommended reference source."
— *Booklist, American Library Association, Feb '03*

■

Endocrine & Metabolic Disorders Sourcebook

Basic Information for the Layperson about Pancreatic and Insulin-Related Disorders Such as Pancreatitis, Diabetes, and Hypoglycemia; Adrenal Gland Disorders Such as Cushing's Syndrome, Addison's Disease, and Congenital Adrenal Hyperplasia; Pituitary Gland Disorders Such as Growth Hormone Deficiency, Acromegaly, and Pituitary Tumors; Thyroid Disorders Such as Hypothyroidism, Graves' Disease, Hashimoto's Disease, and Goiter; Hyperparathyroidism; and Other Diseases and Syndromes of Hormone Imbalance or Metabolic Dysfunction

Along with Reports on Current Research Initiatives

Edited by Linda M. Shin. 574 pages. 1998. 0-7808-0207-1. $78.

"Omnigraphics has produced another needed resource for health information consumers."
— *American Reference Books Annual, 2000*

"Recommended reference source."
— *Booklist, American Library Association, Dec '98*

■

Environmental Health Sourcebook, 2nd Edition

Basic Consumer Health Information about the Environment and Its Effect on Human Health, Including the Effects of Air Pollution, Water Pollution, Hazardous Chemicals, Food Hazards, Radiation Hazards, Biological Agents, Household Hazards, Such as Radon, Asbestos, Carbon Monoxide, and Mold, and Information about Associated Diseases and Disorders, Including Cancer, Allergies, Respiratory Problems, and Skin Disorders

Along with Information about Environmental Concerns for Specific Populations, a Glossary of Related Terms, and Resources for Further Help and Information

Edited by Dawn D. Matthews. 673 pages. 2003. 0-7808-0632-8. $78.

ALSO AVAILABLE: Environmentally Induced Disorders Sourcebook, 1st Edition. Edited by Allan R. Cook. 620 pages. 1997. 0-7808-0083-4. $78.

"This recently updated edition continues the level of quality and the reputation of the numerous other volumes in Omnigraphics' *Health Reference Series.*"
— *American Reference Books Annual, 2004*

"Recommended reference source."
— *Booklist, American Library Association, Sep '98*

"This book will be a useful addition to anyone's library." — *Choice Health Sciences Supplement, Association of College and Research Libraries, May '98*

". . . a good survey of numerous environmentally induced physical disorders . . . a useful addition to anyone's library."
— *Doody's Health Sciences Book Reviews, Jan '98*

". . . provide[s] introductory information from the best authorities around. Since this volume covers topics that potentially affect everyone, it will surely be one of the most frequently consulted volumes in the *Health Reference Series.*" — *Rettig on Reference, Nov '97*

■

Environmentally Induced Disorders Sourcebook, 1st Edition

SEE Environmental Health Sourcebook, 2nd Edition

■

Ethnic Diseases Sourcebook

Basic Consumer Health Information for Ethnic and Racial Minority Groups in the United States, Including General Health Indicators and Behaviors, Ethnic Diseases, Genetic Testing, the Impact of Chronic Diseases, Women's Health, Mental Health Issues, and Preventive Health Care Services

Along with a Glossary and a Listing of Additional Resources

Edited by Joyce Brennfleck Shannon. 664 pages. 2001. 0-7808-0336-1. $78.

"Recommended for health sciences libraries where public health programs are a priority."
— *E-Streams, Jan '02*

"Not many books have been written on this topic to date, and the *Ethnic Diseases Sourcebook* is a strong addition to the list. It will be an important introductory resource for health consumers, students, health care personnel, and social scientists. It is recommended for public, academic, and large hospital libraries."
— *American Reference Books Annual 2002*

"Recommended reference source."
— *Booklist, American Library Association, Oct '01*

"Will prove valuable to any library seeking to maintain a current, comprehensive reference collection of health resources. . . . An excellent source of health information about genetic disorders which affect particular ethnic and racial minorities in the U.S."
— *The Bookwatch, Aug '01*

Eye Care Sourcebook, 2nd Edition

Basic Consumer Health Information about Eye Care and Eye Disorders, Including Facts about the Diagnosis, Prevention, and Treatment of Common Refractive Problems Such as Myopia, Hyperopia, Astigmatism, and Presbyopia, and Eye Diseases, Including Glaucoma, Cataract, Age-Related Macular Degeneration, and Diabetic Retinopathy

Along with a Section on Vision Correction and Refractive Surgeries, Including LASIK and LASEK, a Glossary, and Directories of Resources for Additional Help and Information

Edited by Amy L. Sutton. 543 pages. 2003. 0-7808-0635-2. $78.

ALSO AVAILABLE: Ophthalmic Disorders Sourcebook, 1st Edition. Edited by Linda M. Ross. 631 pages. 1996. 0-7808-0081-8. $78.

". . . a solid reference tool for eye care and a valuable addition to a collection."
— *American Reference Books Annual, 2004*

■

Family Planning Sourcebook

Basic Consumer Health Information about Planning for Pregnancy and Contraception, Including Traditional Methods, Barrier Methods, Hormonal Methods, Permanent Methods, Future Methods, Emergency Contraception, and Birth Control Choices for Women at Each Stage of Life

Along with Statistics, a Glossary, and Sources of Additional Information

Edited by Amy Marcaccio Keyzer. 520 pages. 2001. 0-7808-0379-5. $78.

"Recommended for public, health, and undergraduate libraries as part of the circulating collection."
— *E-Streams, Mar '02*

"Information is presented in an unbiased, readable manner, and the sourcebook will certainly be a necessary addition to those public and high school libraries where Internet access is restricted or otherwise problematic." — *American Reference Books Annual 2002*

"Recommended reference source."
— *Booklist, American Library Association, Oct '01*

"Will prove valuable to any library seeking to maintain a current, comprehensive reference collection of health resources. . . . Excellent reference."
— *The Bookwatch, Aug '01*

SEE ALSO Pregnancy & Birth Sourcebook

■

Fitness & Exercise Sourcebook, 2nd Edition

Basic Consumer Health Information about the Fundamentals of Fitness and Exercise, Including How to Begin and Maintain a Fitness Program, Fitness as a Lifestyle, the Link between Fitness and Diet, Advice for Specific Groups of People, Exercise as It Relates to Specific Medical Conditions, and Recent Research in Fitness and Exercise

Along with a Glossary of Important Terms and Resources for Additional Help and Information

Edited by Kristen M. Gledhill. 646 pages. 2001. 0-7808-0334-5. $78.

ALSO AVAILABLE: Fitness & Exercise Sourcebook, 1st Edition. Edited by Dan R. Harris. 663 pages. 1996. 0-7808-0186-5. $78.

"This work is recommended for all general reference collections."
— *American Reference Books Annual 2002*

"Highly recommended for public, consumer, and school grades fourth through college."
— *E-Streams, Nov '01*

"Recommended reference source." — *Booklist, American Library Association, Oct '01*

"The information appears quite comprehensive and is considered reliable. . . . This second edition is a welcomed addition to the series."
— *Doody's Review Service, Sep '01*

"This reference is a valuable choice for those who desire a broad source of information on exercise, fitness, and chronic-disease prevention through a healthy lifestyle." — *American Medical Writers Association Journal, Fall '01*

"Will prove valuable to any library seeking to maintain a current, comprehensive reference collection of health resources. . . . Excellent reference."
— *The Bookwatch, Aug '01*

■

Food & Animal Borne Diseases Sourcebook

Basic Information about Diseases That Can Be Spread to Humans through the Ingestion of Contaminated Food or Water or by Contact with Infected Animals and Insects, Such as Botulism, E. Coli, Hepatitis A, Trichinosis, Lyme Disease, and Rabies

Along with Information Regarding Prevention and Treatment Methods, and Including a Special Section for International Travelers Describing Diseases Such as Cholera, Malaria, Travelers' Diarrhea, and Yellow Fever, and Offering Recommendations for Avoiding Illness

Edited by Karen Bellenir and Peter D. Dresser. 535 pages. 1995. 0-7808-0033-8. $78.

"Targeting general readers and providing them with a single, comprehensive source of information on selected topics, this book continues, with the excellent caliber of its predecessors, to catalog topical information on health matters of general interest. Readable and thorough, this valuable resource is highly recommended for all libraries."
— *Academic Library Book Review, Summer '96*

"A comprehensive collection of authoritative information." — *Emergency Medical Services, Oct '95*

Food Safety Sourcebook

Basic Consumer Health Information about the Safe Handling of Meat, Poultry, Seafood, Eggs, Fruit Juices, and Other Food Items, and Facts about Pesticides, Drinking Water, Food Safety Overseas, and the Onset, Duration, and Symptoms of Foodborne Illnesses, Including Types of Pathogenic Bacteria, Parasitic Protozoa, Worms, Viruses, and Natural Toxins

Along with the Role of the Consumer, the Food Handler, and the Government in Food Safety; a Glossary, and Resources for Additional Help and Information

Edited by Dawn D. Matthews. 339 pages. 1999. 0-7808-0326-4. $78.

"This book is recommended for public libraries and universities with home economic and food science programs." — *E-Streams, Nov '00*

"Recommended reference source."
— *Booklist, American Library Association, May '00*

"This book takes the complex issues of food safety and foodborne pathogens and presents them in an easily understood manner. [It does] an excellent job of covering a large and often confusing topic."
— *American Reference Books Annual, 2000*

■

Forensic Medicine Sourcebook

Basic Consumer Information for the Layperson about Forensic Medicine, Including Crime Scene Investigation, Evidence Collection and Analysis, Expert Testimony, Computer-Aided Criminal Identification, Digital Imaging in the Courtroom, DNA Profiling, Accident Reconstruction, Autopsies, Ballistics, Drugs and Explosives Detection, Latent Fingerprints, Product Tampering, and Questioned Document Examination

Along with Statistical Data, a Glossary of Forensics Terminology, and Listings of Sources for Further Help and Information

Edited by Annemarie S. Muth. 574 pages. 1999. 0-7808-0232-2. $78.

"Given the expected widespread interest in its content and its easy to read style, this book is recommended for most public and all college and university libraries."
— *E-Streams, Feb '01*

"Recommended for public libraries."
— *Reference & User Services Quarterly, American Library Association, Spring 2000*

"Recommended reference source."
— *Booklist, American Library Association, Feb '00*

"A wealth of information, useful statistics, references are up-to-date and extremely complete. This wonderful collection of data will help students who are interested in a career in any type of forensic field. It is a great resource for attorneys who need information about types of expert witnesses needed in a particular case. It also offers useful information for fiction and nonfiction writers whose work involves a crime. A fascinating compilation. All levels." — *Choice, Association of College and Research Libraries, Jan 2000*

"There are several items that make this book attractive to consumers who are seeking certain forensic data.... This is a useful current source for those seeking general forensic medical answers."
— *American Reference Books Annual, 2000*

■

Gastrointestinal Diseases & Disorders Sourcebook

Basic Information about Gastroesophageal Reflux Disease (Heartburn), Ulcers, Diverticulosis, Irritable Bowel Syndrome, Crohn's Disease, Ulcerative Colitis, Diarrhea, Constipation, Lactose Intolerance, Hemorrhoids, Hepatitis, Cirrhosis, and Other Digestive Problems, Featuring Statistics, Descriptions of Symptoms, and Current Treatment Methods of Interest for Persons Living with Upper and Lower Gastrointestinal Maladies

Edited by Linda M. Ross. 413 pages. 1996. 0-7808-0078-8. $78.

". . . very readable form. The successful editorial work that brought this material together into a useful and understandable reference makes accessible to all readers information that can help them more effectively understand and obtain help for digestive tract problems."
— *Choice, Association of College & Research Libraries, Feb '97*

SEE ALSO *Diet & Nutrition Sourcebook, Digestive Diseases & Disorders, Eating Disorders Sourcebook*

■

Genetic Disorders Sourcebook, 3rd Edition

Basic Consumer Health Information about Hereditary Diseases and Disorders, Including Facts about the Human Genome, Genetic Inheritance Patterns, Disorders Associated with Specific Genes, such as Sickle Cell Disease, Hemophilia, and Cystic Fibrosis, Chromosome Disorders, such as Down Syndrome, Fragile X Syndrome, and Turner Syndrome, and Complex Diseases and Disorders Resulting from the Interaction of Environmental and Genetic Factors, such as Allergies, Cancer, and Obesity

Along with Facts about Genetic Testing, Suggestions for Parents of Children with Special Needs, Reports on Current Research Initiatives, a Glossary of Genetic Terminology, and Resources for Additional Help and Information

Edited by Karen Bellenir. 777 pages. 2004. 0-7808-0742-1. $78.

ALSO AVAILABLE: *Genetic Disorders Sourcebook, 1st Edition.* Edited by Karen Bellenir. 642 pages. 1996. 0-7808-0034-6. $78.

Genetic Disorders Sourcebook, 2nd Edition. Edited by Kathy Massimini. 768 pages. 2001. 0-7808-0241-1. $78.

"Recommended for public libraries and medical and hospital libraries with consumer health collections."
— *E-Streams, May '01*

"Recommended reference source."
— *Booklist, American Library Association, Apr '01*

"Important pick for college-level health reference libraries." — *The Bookwatch, Mar '01*

"Provides essential medical information to both the general public and those diagnosed with a serious or fatal genetic disease or disorder." — *Choice, Association of College and Research Libraries, Jan '97*

■

Head Trauma Sourcebook

Basic Information for the Layperson about Open-Head and Closed-Head Injuries, Treatment Advances, Recovery, and Rehabilitation

Along with Reports on Current Research Initiatives

Edited by Karen Bellenir. 414 pages. 1997. 0-7808-0208-X. $78.

■

Headache Sourcebook

Basic Consumer Health Information about Migraine, Tension, Cluster, Rebound and Other Types of Headaches, with Facts about the Cause and Prevention of Headaches, the Effects of Stress and the Environment, Headaches during Pregnancy and Menopause, and Childhood Headaches

Along with a Glossary and Other Resources for Additional Help and Information

Edited by Dawn D. Matthews. 362 pages. 2002. 0-7808-0337-X. $78.

"Highly recommended for academic and medical reference collections." — *Library Bookwatch, Sep '02*

■

Health Insurance Sourcebook

Basic Information about Managed Care Organizations, Traditional Fee-for-Service Insurance, Insurance Portability and Pre-Existing Conditions Clauses, Medicare, Medicaid, Social Security, and Military Health Care

Along with Information about Insurance Fraud

Edited by Wendy Wilcox. 530 pages. 1997. 0-7808-0222-5. $78.

"Particularly useful because it brings much of this information together in one volume. This book will be a handy reference source in the health sciences library, hospital library, college and university library, and medium to large public library." — *Medical Reference Services Quarterly, Fall '98*

Awarded "Books of the Year Award" — *American Journal of Nursing, 1997*

"The layout of the book is particularly helpful as it provides easy access to reference material. A most useful addition to the vast amount of information about health insurance. The use of data from U.S. government agencies is most commendable. Useful in a library or learning center for healthcare professional students." — *Doody's Health Sciences Book Reviews, Nov '97*

Health Reference Series Cumulative Index 1999

A Comprehensive Index to the Individual Volumes of the Health Reference Series, Including a Subject Index, Name Index, Organization Index, and Publication Index

Along with a Master List of Acronyms and Abbreviations

Edited by Edward J. Prucha, Anne Holmes, and Robert Rudnick. 990 pages. 2000. 0-7808-0382-5. $78.

"This volume will be most helpful in libraries that have a relatively complete collection of the Health Reference Series." — *American Reference Books Annual, 2001*

"Essential for collections that hold any of the numerous *Health Reference Series* titles." — *Choice, Association of College and Research Libraries, Nov '00*

■

Healthy Aging Sourcebook

Basic Consumer Health Information about Maintaining Health through the Aging Process, Including Advice on Nutrition, Exercise, and Sleep, Help in Making Decisions about Midlife Issues and Retirement, and Guidance Concerning Practical and Informed Choices in Health Consumerism

Along with Data Concerning the Theories of Aging, Different Experiences in Aging by Minority Groups, and Facts about Aging Now and Aging in the Future; and Featuring a Glossary, a Guide to Consumer Help, Additional Suggested Reading, and Practical Resource Directory

Edited by Jenifer Swanson. 536 pages. 1999. 0-7808-0390-6. $78.

"Recommended reference source." — *Booklist, American Library Association, Feb '00*

SEE ALSO Physical & Mental Issues in Aging Sourcebook

■

Healthy Children Sourcebook

Basic Consumer Health Information about the Physical and Mental Development of Children between the Ages of 3 and 12, Including Routine Health Care, Preventative Health Services, Safety and First Aid, Healthy Sleep, Dental Care, Nutrition, and Fitness, and Featuring Parenting Tips on Such Topics as Bedwetting, Choosing Day Care, Monitoring TV and Other Media, and Establishing a Foundation for Substance Abuse Prevention

Along with a Glossary of Commonly Used Pediatric Terms and Resources for Additional Help and Information.

Edited by Chad T. Kimball. 647 pages. 2003. 0-7808-0247-0. $78.

"It is hard to imagine that any other single resource exists that would provide such a comprehensive guide of timely information on health promotion and disease prevention for children aged 3 to 12."

—*American Reference Books Annual, 2004*

"The strengths of this book are many. It is clearly written, presented and structured."

—*Journal of the National Medical Association, 2004*

■

Healthy Heart Sourcebook for Women

Basic Consumer Health Information about Cardiac Issues Specific to Women, Including Facts about Major Risk Factors and Prevention, Treatment and Control Strategies, and Important Dietary Issues

Along with a Special Section Regarding the Pros and Cons of Hormone Replacement Therapy and Its Impact on Heart Health, and Additional Help, Including Recipes, a Glossary, and a Directory of Resources

Edited by Dawn D. Matthews. 336 pages. 2000. 0-7808-0329-9. $78.

"A good reference source and recommended for all public, academic, medical, and hospital libraries."

—*Medical Reference Services Quarterly, Summer '01*

"Because of the lack of information specific to women on this topic, this book is recommended for public libraries and consumer libraries."

—*American Reference Books Annual, 2001*

"Contains very important information about coronary artery disease that all women should know. The information is current and presented in an easy-to-read format. The book will make a good addition to any library."

—*American Medical Writers Association Journal, Summer '00*

"Important, basic reference."

—*Reviewer's Bookwatch, Jul '00*

SEE ALSO *Heart Diseases & Disorders Sourcebook, Women's Health Concerns Sourcebook*

■

Heart Diseases & Disorders Sourcebook, 2nd Edition

Basic Consumer Health Information about Heart Attacks, Angina, Rhythm Disorders, Heart Failure, Valve Disease, Congenital Heart Disorders, and More, Including Descriptions of Surgical Procedures and Other Interventions, Medications, Cardiac Rehabilitation, Risk Identification, and Prevention Tips

Along with Statistical Data, Reports on Current Research Initiatives, a Glossary of Cardiovascular Terms, and Resource Directory

Edited by Karen Bellenir. 612 pages. 2000. 0-7808-0238-1. $78.

ALSO AVAILABLE: *Cardiovascular Diseases & Disorders Sourcebook, 1st Edition.* Edited by Karen Bellenir and Peter D. Dresser. 683 pages. 1995. 0-7808-0032-X. $78.

"This work stands out as an imminently accessible resource for the general public. It is recommended for the reference and circulating shelves of school, public, and academic libraries."

—*American Reference Books Annual, 2001*

"Recommended reference source."

—*Booklist, American Library Association, Dec '00*

"Provides comprehensive coverage of matters related to the heart. This title is recommended for health sciences and public libraries with consumer health collections."

—*E-Streams, Oct '00*

SEE ALSO *Healthy Heart Sourcebook for Women*

■

Household Safety Sourcebook

Basic Consumer Health Information about Household Safety, Including Information about Poisons, Chemicals, Fire, and Water Hazards in the Home

Along with Advice about the Safe Use of Home Maintenance Equipment, Choosing Toys and Nursery Furniture, Holiday and Recreation Safety, a Glossary, and Resources for Further Help and Information

Edited by Dawn D. Matthews. 606 pages. 2002. 0-7808-0338-8. $78.

"This work will be useful in public libraries with large consumer health and wellness departments."

—*American Reference Books Annual, 2003*

"As a sourcebook on household safety this book meets its mark. It is encyclopedic in scope and covers a wide range of safety issues that are commonly seen in the home."

—*E-Streams, Jul '02*

■

Hypertension Sourcebook

Basic Consumer Health Information about the Causes, Diagnosis, and Treatment of High Blood Pressure, with Facts about Consequences, Complications, and Co-Occurring Disorders, Such as Coronary Heart Disease, Diabetes, Stroke, Kidney Disease, and Hypertensive Retinopathy, and Issues in Blood Pressure Control, Including Dietary Choices, Stress Management, and Medications

Along with Reports on Current Research Initiatives and Clinical Trials, a Glossary, and Resources for Additional Help and Information

Edited by Dawn D. Matthews and Karen Bellenir. 613 pages. 2004. 0-7808-0674-3. $78.

■

Immune System Disorders Sourcebook

Basic Information about Lupus, Multiple Sclerosis, Guillain-Barré Syndrome, Chronic Granulomatous Disease, and More

Along with Statistical and Demographic Data and Reports on Current Research Initiatives

Edited by Allan R. Cook. 608 pages. 1997. 0-7808-0209-8. $78.

Infant & Toddler Health Sourcebook

Basic Consumer Health Information about the Physical and Mental Development of Newborns, Infants, and Toddlers, Including Neonatal Concerns, Nutrition Recommendations, Immunization Schedules, Common Pediatric Disorders, Assessments and Milestones, Safety Tips, and Advice for Parents and Other Caregivers

Along with a Glossary of Terms and Resource Listings for Additional Help

Edited by Jenifer Swanson. 585 pages. 2000. 0-7808-0246-2. $78.

"As a reference for the general public, this would be useful in any library." —E-Streams, May '01

"Recommended reference source."
—Booklist, American Library Association, Feb '01

"This is a good source for general use."
—American Reference Books Annual, 2001

■

Infectious Diseases Sourcebook

Basic Consumer Health Information about Non-Contagious Bacterial, Viral, Prion, Fungal, and Parasitic Diseases Spread by Food and Water, Insects and Animals, or Environmental Contact, Including Botulism, E. Coli, Encephalitis, Legionnaires' Disease, Lyme Disease, Malaria, Plague, Rabies, Salmonella, Tetanus, and Others, and Facts about Newly Emerging Diseases, Such as Hantavirus, Mad Cow Disease, Monkeypox, and West Nile Virus

Along with Information about Preventing Disease Transmission, the Threat of Bioterrorism, and Current Research Initiatives, with a Glossary and Directory of Resources for More Information

Edited by Karen Bellenir. 634 pages. 2004. 0-7808-0675-1. $78.

■

Injury & Trauma Sourcebook

Basic Consumer Health Information about the Impact of Injury, the Diagnosis and Treatment of Common and Traumatic Injuries, Emergency Care, and Specific Injuries Related to Home, Community, Workplace, Transportation, and Recreation

Along with Guidelines for Injury Prevention, a Glossary, and a Directory of Additional Resources

Edited by Joyce Brennfleck Shannon. 696 pages. 2002. 0-7808-0421-X. $78.

"This publication is the most comprehensive work of its kind about injury and trauma."
—American Reference Books Annual, 2003

"This sourcebook provides concise, easily readable, basic health information about injuries. . . . This book is well organized and an easy to use reference resource suitable for hospital, health sciences and public libraries with consumer health collections."
—E-Streams, Nov '02

"Practitioners should be aware of guides such as this in order to facilitate their use by patients and their families." —Doody's Health Sciences Book Review Journal, Sep-Oct '02

"Recommended reference source."
—Booklist, American Library Association, Sep '02

"Highly recommended for academic and medical reference collections." —Library Bookwatch, Sep '02

■

Kidney & Urinary Tract Diseases & Disorders Sourcebook

Basic Information about Kidney Stones, Urinary Incontinence, Bladder Disease, End Stage Renal Disease, Dialysis, and More

Along with Statistical and Demographic Data and Reports on Current Research Initiatives

Edited by Linda M. Ross. 602 pages. 1997. 0-7808-0079-6. $78.

■

Learning Disabilities Sourcebook, 2nd Edition

Basic Consumer Health Information about Learning Disabilities, Including Dyslexia, Developmental Speech and Language Disabilities, Non-Verbal Learning Disorders, Developmental Arithmetic Disorder, Developmental Writing Disorder, and Other Conditions That Impede Learning Such as Attention Deficit/ Hyperactivity Disorder, Brain Injury, Hearing Impairment, Klinefelter Syndrome, Dyspraxia, and Tourette Syndrome

Along with Facts about Educational Issues and Assistive Technology, Coping Strategies, a Glossary of Related Terms, and Resources for Further Help and Information

Edited by Dawn D. Matthews. 621 pages. 2003. 0-7808-0626-3. $78.

ALSO AVAILABLE: Learning Disabilities Sourcebook, 1st Edition. Edited by Linda M. Shin. 579 pages. 1998. 0-7808-0210-1. $78.

"The second edition of Learning Disabilities Sourcebook far surpasses the earlier edition in that it is more focused on information that will be useful as a consumer health resource."
—American Reference Books Annual, 2004

"Teachers as well as consumers will find this an essential guide to understanding various syndromes and their latest treatments. [An] invaluable reference for public and school library collections alike."
—Library Bookwatch, Apr '03

Named "Outstanding Reference Book of 1999."
—New York Public Library, Feb 2000

"An excellent candidate for inclusion in a public library reference section. It's a great source of information. Teachers will also find the book useful. Definitely worth reading."
—Journal of Adolescent & Adult Literacy, Feb 2000

"Readable . . . provides a solid base of information regarding successful techniques used with individuals who have learning disabilities, as well as practical suggestions for educators and family members. Clear language, concise descriptions, and pertinent information for contacting multiple resources add to the strength of this book as a useful tool." —Choice, Association of College and Research Libraries, Feb '99

"Recommended reference source."
—Booklist, American Library Association, Sep '98

"A useful resource for libraries and for those who don't have the time to identify and locate the individual publications." —Disability Resources Monthly, Sep '98

■

Leukemia Sourcebook

Basic Consumer Health Information about Adult and Childhood Leukemias, Including Acute Lymphocytic Leukemia (ALL), Chronic Lymphocytic Leukemia (CLL), Acute Myelogenous Leukemia (AML), Chronic Myelogenous Leukemia (CML), and Hairy Cell Leukemia, and Treatments Such as Chemotherapy, Radiation Therapy, Peripheral Blood Stem Cell and Marrow Transplantation, and Immunotherapy

Along with Tips for Life During and After Treatment, a Glossary, and Directories of Additional Resources

Edited by Joyce Brennfleck Shannon. 587 pages. 2003. 0-7808-0627-1. $78.

"Unlike other medical books for the layperson, . . . the language does not talk down to the reader. . . . This volume is highly recommended for all libraries."
—American Reference Books Annual, 2004

■

Liver Disorders Sourcebook

Basic Consumer Health Information about the Liver and How It Works; Liver Diseases, Including Cancer, Cirrhosis, Hepatitis, and Toxic and Drug Related Diseases; Tips for Maintaining a Healthy Liver; Laboratory Tests, Radiology Tests, and Facts about Liver Transplantation

Along with a Section on Support Groups, a Glossary, and Resource Listings

Edited by Joyce Brennfleck Shannon. 591 pages. 2000. 0-7808-0383-3. $78.

"A valuable resource."
—American Reference Books Annual, 2001

"This title is recommended for health sciences and public libraries with consumer health collections."
—E-Streams, Oct '00

"Recommended reference source."
—Booklist, American Library Association, Jun '00

■

Lung Disorders Sourcebook

Basic Consumer Health Information about Emphysema, Pneumonia, Tuberculosis, Asthma, Cystic Fibrosis, and Other Lung Disorders, Including Facts about

Diagnostic Procedures, Treatment Strategies, Disease Prevention Efforts, and Such Risk Factors as Smoking, Air Pollution, and Exposure to Asbestos, Radon, and Other Agents

Along with a Glossary and Resources for Additional Help and Information

Edited by Dawn D. Matthews. 678 pages. 2002. 0-7808-0339-6. $78.

"This title is a great addition for public and school libraries because it provides concise health information on the lungs."
—American Reference Books Annual, 2003

"Highly recommended for academic and medical reference collections." —Library Bookwatch, Sep '02

■

Medical Tests Sourcebook, 2nd Edition

Basic Consumer Health Information about Medical Tests, Including Age-Specific Health Tests, Important Health Screenings and Exams, Home-Use Tests, Blood and Specimen Tests, Electrical Tests, Scope Tests, Genetic Testing, and Imaging Tests, Such as X-Rays, Ultrasound, Computed Tomography, Magnetic Resonance Imaging, Angiography, and Nuclear Medicine

Along with a Glossary and Directory of Additional Resources

Edited by Joyce Brennfleck Shannon. 654 pages. 2004. 0-7808-0670-0. $78.

ALSO AVAILABLE: Medical Tests, 1st Edition. Edited by Joyce Brennfleck Shannon. 691 pages. 1999. 0-7808-0243-8. $78.

"Recommended for hospital and health sciences libraries with consumer health collections."
—E-Streams, Mar '00

"This is an overall excellent reference with a wealth of general knowledge that may aid those who are reluctant to get vital tests performed."
—Today's Librarian, Jan 2000

"A valuable reference guide."
—American Reference Books Annual, 2000

■

Men's Health Concerns Sourcebook, 2nd Edition

Basic Consumer Health Information about the Medical and Mental Concerns of Men, Including Theories about the Shorter Male Lifespan, the Leading Causes of Death and Disability, Physical Concerns of Special Significance to Men, Reproductive and Sexual Concerns, Sexually Transmitted Diseases, Men's Mental and Emotional Health, and Lifestyle Choices That Affect Wellness, Such as Nutrition, Fitness, and Substance Use

Along with a Glossary of Related Terms and a Directory of Organizational Resources in Men's Health

Edited by Robert Aquinas McNally. 644 pages. 2004. 0-7808-0671-9. $78.

■

Mental Health Disorders Sourcebook, 2nd Edition

Basic Consumer Health Information about Anxiety Disorders, Depression and Other Mood Disorders, Eating Disorders, Personality Disorders, Schizophrenia, and More, Including Disease Descriptions, Treatment Options, and Reports on Current Research Initiatives

Along with Statistical Data, Tips for Maintaining Mental Health, a Glossary, and Directory of Sources for Additional Help and Information

Edited by Karen Bellenir. 605 pages. 2000. 0-7808-0240-3. $78.

■

Mental Retardation Sourcebook

Basic Consumer Health Information about Mental Retardation and Its Causes, Including Down Syndrome, Fetal Alcohol Syndrome, Fragile X Syndrome, Genetic Conditions, Injury, and Environmental Sources

Along with Preventive Strategies, Parenting Issues, Educational Implications, Health Care Needs, Employment and Economic Matters, Legal Issues, a Glossary, and a Resource Listing for Additional Help and Information

Edited by Joyce Brennfleck Shannon. 642 pages. 2000. 0-7808-0377-9. $78.

Movement Disorders Sourcebook

Basic Consumer Health Information about Neurological Movement Disorders, Including Essential Tremor, Parkinson's Disease, Dystonia, Cerebral Palsy, Huntington's Disease, Myasthenia Gravis, Multiple Sclerosis, and Other Early-Onset and Adult-Onset Movement Disorders, Their Symptoms and Causes, Diagnostic Tests, and Treatments

Along with Mobility and Assistive Technology Information, a Glossary, and a Directory of Additional Resources

Edited by Joyce Brennfleck Shannon. 655 pages. 2003. 0-7808-0628-X. $78.

■

Muscular Dystrophy Sourcebook

Basic Consumer Health Information about Congenital, Childhood-Onset, and Adult-Onset Forms of Muscular Dystrophy, Such as Duchenne, Becker, Emery-Dreifuss, Distal, Limb-Girdle, Facioscapulohumeral (FSHD), Myotonic, and Ophthalmoplegic Muscular Dystrophies, Including Facts about Diagnostic Tests, Medical and Physical Therapies, Management of Co-Occurring Conditions, and Parenting Guidelines

Along with Practical Tips for Home Care, a Glossary, and Directories of Additional Resources

Edited by Joyce Brennfleck Shannon. 577 pages. 2004. 0-7808-0676-X. $78.

■

Obesity Sourcebook

Basic Consumer Health Information about Diseases and Other Problems Associated with Obesity, and Including Facts about Risk Factors, Prevention Issues, and Management Approaches

Along with Statistical and Demographic Data, Information about Special Populations, Research Updates, a Glossary, and Source Listings for Further Help and Information

Edited by Wilma Caldwell and Chad T. Kimball. 376 pages. 2001. 0-7808-0333-7. $78.

Ophthalmic Disorders Sourcebook, 1st Edition

SEE Eye Care Sourcebook, 2nd Edition

■

Oral Health Sourcebook

SEE Dental Care & Oral Health Sourcebook, 2nd Ed.

■

Osteoporosis Sourcebook

Basic Consumer Health Information about Primary and Secondary Osteoporosis and Juvenile Osteoporosis and Related Conditions, Including Fibrous Dysplasia, Gaucher Disease, Hyperthyroidism, Hypophosphatasia, Myeloma, Osteopetrosis, Osteogenesis Imperfecta, and Paget's Disease

Along with Information about Risk Factors, Treatments, Traditional and Non-Traditional Pain Management, a Glossary of Related Terms, and a Directory of Resources

Edited by Allan R. Cook. 584 pages. 2001. 0-7808-0239-X. $78.

"This would be a book to be kept in a staff or patient library. The targeted audience is the layperson, but the therapist who needs a quick bit of information on a particular topic will also find the book useful."
— *Physical Therapy, Jan '02*

"This resource is recommended as a great reference source for public, health, and academic libraries, and is another triumph for the editors of Omnigraphics."
— *American Reference Books Annual 2002*

"Recommended for all public libraries and general health collections, especially those supporting patient education or consumer health programs."
— *E-Streams, Nov '01*

"Will prove valuable to any library seeking to maintain a current, comprehensive reference collection of health resources. . . . From prevention to treatment and associated conditions, this provides an excellent survey."
— *The Bookwatch, Aug '01*

"Recommended reference source."
— *Booklist, American Library Association, July '01*

SEE ALSO Women's Health Concerns Sourcebook

■

Pain Sourcebook, 2nd Edition

Basic Consumer Health Information about Specific Forms of Acute and Chronic Pain, Including Muscle and Skeletal Pain, Nerve Pain, Cancer Pain, and Disorders Characterized by Pain, Such as Fibromyalgia, Shingles, Angina, Arthritis, and Headaches

Along with Information about Pain Medications and Management Techniques, Complementary and Alternative Pain Relief Options, Tips for People Living with Chronic Pain, a Glossary, and a Directory of Sources for Further Information

Edited by Karen Bellenir. 670 pages. 2002. 0-7808-0612-3. $78.

ALSO AVAILABLE: Pain Sourcebook, 1st Edition. Edited by Allan R. Cook. 667 pages. 1997. 0-7808-0213-6. $78.

"A source of valuable information. . . . This book offers help to nonmedical people who need information about pain and pain management. It is also an excellent reference for those who participate in patient education."
— *Doody's Review Service, Sep '02*

"The text is readable, easily understood, and well indexed. This excellent volume belongs in all patient education libraries, consumer health sections of public libraries, and many personal collections."
— *American Reference Books Annual, 1999*

"A beneficial reference." — *Booklist Health Sciences Supplement, American Library Association, Oct '98*

"The information is basic in terms of scholarship and is appropriate for general readers. Written in journalistic style . . . intended for non-professionals. Quite thorough in its coverage of different pain conditions and summarizes the latest clinical information regarding pain treatment."
— *Choice, Association of College and Research Libraries, Jun '98*

"Recommended reference source."
— *Booklist, American Library Association, Mar '98*

■

Pediatric Cancer Sourcebook

Basic Consumer Health Information about Leukemias, Brain Tumors, Sarcomas, Lymphomas, and Other Cancers in Infants, Children, and Adolescents, Including Descriptions of Cancers, Treatments, and Coping Strategies

Along with Suggestions for Parents, Caregivers, and Concerned Relatives, a Glossary of Cancer Terms, and Resource Listings

Edited by Edward J. Prucha. 587 pages. 1999. 0-7808-0245-4. $78.

"An excellent source of information. Recommended for public, hospital, and health science libraries with consumer health collections."
— *E-Streams, Jun '00*

"Recommended reference source."
— *Booklist, American Library Association, Feb '00*

"A valuable addition to all libraries specializing in health services and many public libraries."
— *American Reference Books Annual, 2000*

■

Physical & Mental Issues in Aging Sourcebook

Basic Consumer Health Information on Physical and Mental Disorders Associated with the Aging Process, Including Concerns about Cardiovascular Disease, Pulmonary Disease, Oral Health, Digestive Disorders, Musculoskeletal and Skin Disorders, Metabolic Changes, Sexual and Reproductive Issues, and Changes in Vision, Hearing, and Other Senses

Along with Data about Longevity and Causes of Death, Information on Acute and Chronic Pain, Descriptions of Mental Concerns, a Glossary of Terms, and Resource Listings for Additional Help

Edited by Jenifer Swanson. 660 pages. 1999. 0-7808-0233-0. $78.

"This is a treasure of health information for the layperson." — *Choice Health Sciences Supplement, Association of College & Research Libraries, May 2000*

"Recommended for public libraries."
—*American Reference Books Annual, 2000*

"Recommended reference source."
—*Booklist, American Library Association, Oct '99*

SEE ALSO Healthy Aging Sourcebook

Podiatry Sourcebook

Basic Consumer Health Information about Foot Conditions, Diseases, and Injuries, Including Bunions, Corns, Calluses, Athlete's Foot, Plantar Warts, Hammertoes and Clawtoes, Clubfoot, Heel Pain, Gout, and More

Along with Facts about Foot Care, Disease Prevention, Foot Safety, Choosing a Foot Care Specialist, a Glossary of Terms, and Resource Listings for Additional Information

Edited by M. Lisa Weatherford. 380 pages. 2001. 0-7808-0215-2. $78.

"Recommended reference source."
—*Booklist, American Library Association, Feb '02*

"There is a lot of information presented here on a topic that is usually only covered sparingly in most larger comprehensive medical encyclopedias."
—*American Reference Books Annual 2002*

Pregnancy & Birth Sourcebook, 2nd Edition

Basic Consumer Health Information about Conception and Pregnancy, Including Facts about Fertility, Infertility, Pregnancy Symptoms and Complications, Fetal Growth and Development, Labor, Delivery, and the Postpartum Period, as Well as Information about Maintaining Health and Wellness during Pregnancy and Caring for a Newborn

Along with Information about Public Health Assistance for Low-Income Pregnant Women, a Glossary, and Directories of Agencies and Organizations Providing Help and Support

Edited by Amy L. Sutton. 626 pages. 2004. 0-7808-0672-7. $78.

ALSO AVAILABLE: *Pregnancy & Birth Sourcebook, 1st Edition.* Edited by Heather E. Aldred. 737 pages. 1997. 0-7808-0216-0. $78.

"A well-organized handbook. Recommended."
— *Choice, Association of College and Research Libraries, Apr '98*

"Recommended reference source."
—*Booklist, American Library Association, Mar '98*

"Recommended for public libraries."
—*American Reference Books Annual, 1998*

SEE ALSO Congenital Disorders Sourcebook, Family Planning Sourcebook

---

Prostate Cancer Sourcebook

Basic Consumer Health Information about Prostate Cancer, Including Information about the Associated Risk Factors, Detection, Diagnosis, and Treatment of Prostate Cancer

Along with Information on Non-Malignant Prostate Conditions, and Featuring a Section Listing Support and Treatment Centers and a Glossary of Related Terms

Edited by Dawn D. Matthews. 358 pages. 2001. 0-7808-0324-8. $78.

"Recommended reference source."
—*Booklist, American Library Association, Jan '02*

"A valuable resource for health care consumers seeking information on the subject. . . . All text is written in a clear, easy-to-understand language that avoids technical jargon. Any library that collects consumer health resources would strengthen their collection with the addition of the *Prostate Cancer Sourcebook*."
—*American Reference Books Annual 2002*

Public Health Sourcebook

Basic Information about Government Health Agencies, Including National Health Statistics and Trends, Healthy People 2000 Program Goals and Objectives, the Centers for Disease Control and Prevention, the Food and Drug Administration, and the National Institutes of Health

Along with Full Contact Information for Each Agency

Edited by Wendy Wilcox. 698 pages. 1998. 0-7808-0220-9. $78.

"Recommended reference source."
—*Booklist, American Library Association, Sep '98*

"This consumer guide provides welcome assistance in navigating the maze of federal health agencies and their data on public health concerns."
—*SciTech Book News, Sep '98*

Reconstructive & Cosmetic Surgery Sourcebook

Basic Consumer Health Information on Cosmetic and Reconstructive Plastic Surgery, Including Statistical Information about Different Surgical Procedures, Things to Consider Prior to Surgery, Plastic Surgery Techniques and Tools, Emotional and Psychological Considerations, and Procedure-Specific Information

Along with a Glossary of Terms and a Listing of Resources for Additional Help and Information

Edited by M. Lisa Weatherford. 374 pages. 2001. 0-7808-0214-4. $78.

"An excellent reference that addresses cosmetic and medically necessary reconstructive surgeries. . . . The

style of the prose is calm and reassuring, discussing the many positive outcomes now available due to advances in surgical techniques."
— *American Reference Books Annual 2002*

"Recommended for health science libraries that are open to the public, as well as hospital libraries that are open to the patients. This book is a good resource for the consumer interested in plastic surgery."
— *E-Streams, Dec '01*

"Recommended reference source."
— *Booklist, American Library Association, July '01*

◼

Rehabilitation Sourcebook

Basic Consumer Health Information about Rehabilitation for People Recovering from Heart Surgery, Spinal Cord Injury, Stroke, Orthopedic Impairments, Amputation, Pulmonary Impairments, Traumatic Injury, and More, Including Physical Therapy, Occupational Therapy, Speech/ Language Therapy, Massage Therapy, Dance Therapy, Art Therapy, and Recreational Therapy

Along with Information on Assistive and Adaptive Devices, a Glossary, and Resources for Additional Help and Information

Edited by Dawn D. Matthews. 531 pages. 1999. 0-7808-0236-5. $78.

"This is an excellent resource for public library reference and health collections."
— *American Reference Books Annual, 2001*

"Recommended reference source."
— *Booklist, American Library Association, May '00*

◼

Respiratory Diseases & Disorders Sourcebook

Basic Information about Respiratory Diseases and Disorders, Including Asthma, Cystic Fibrosis, Pneumonia, the Common Cold, Influenza, and Others, Featuring Facts about the Respiratory System, Statistical and Demographic Data, Treatments, Self-Help Management Suggestions, and Current Research Initiatives

Edited by Allan R. Cook and Peter D. Dresser. 771 pages. 1995. 0-7808-0037-0. $78.

"Designed for the layperson and for patients and their families coping with respiratory illness. . . . an extensive array of information on diagnosis, treatment, management, and prevention of respiratory illnesses for the general reader." — *Choice, Association of College and Research Libraries, Jun '96*

"A highly recommended text for all collections. It is a comforting reminder of the power of knowledge that good books carry between their covers."
— *Academic Library Book Review, Spring '96*

"A comprehensive collection of authoritative information presented in a nontechnical, humanitarian style for patients, families, and caregivers." — *Association of Operating Room Nurses, Sep/Oct '95*

SEE ALSO Lung Disorders Sourcebook

Sexually Transmitted Diseases Sourcebook, 2nd Edition

Basic Consumer Health Information about Sexually Transmitted Diseases, Including Information on the Diagnosis and Treatment of Chlamydia, Gonorrhea, Hepatitis, Herpes, HIV, Mononucleosis, Syphilis, and Others

Along with Information on Prevention, Such as Condom Use, Vaccines, and STD Education; And Featuring a Section on Issues Related to Youth and Adolescents, a Glossary, and Resources for Additional Help and Information

Edited by Dawn D. Matthews. 538 pages. 2001. 0-7808-0249-7. $78.

ALSO AVAILABLE: Sexually Transmitted Diseases Sourcebook, 1st Edition. Edited by Linda M. Ross. 550 pages. 1997. 0-7808-0217-9. $78.

"Recommended for consumer health collections in public libraries, and secondary school and community college libraries."
— *American Reference Books Annual 2002*

"Every school and public library should have a copy of this comprehensive and user-friendly reference book."
— *Choice, Association of College & Research Libraries, Sep '01*

"This is a highly recommended book. This is an especially important book for all school and public libraries." — *AIDS Book Review Journal, Jul-Aug '01*

"Recommended reference source."
— *Booklist, American Library Association, Apr '01*

"Recommended pick both for specialty health library collections and any general consumer health reference collection." — *The Bookwatch, Apr '01*

◼

Skin Disorders Sourcebook

Basic Information about Common Skin and Scalp Conditions Caused by Aging, Allergies, Immune Reactions, Sun Exposure, Infectious Organisms, Parasites, Cosmetics, and Skin Traumas, Including Abrasions, Cuts, and Pressure Sores

Along with Information on Prevention and Treatment

Edited by Allan R. Cook. 647 pages. 1997. 0-7808-0080-X. $78.

". . . comprehensive, easily read reference book."
— *Doody's Health Sciences Book Reviews, Oct '97*

SEE ALSO Burns Sourcebook

◼

Sleep Disorders Sourcebook

Basic Consumer Health Information about Sleep and Its Disorders, Including Insomnia, Sleepwalking, Sleep Apnea, Restless Leg Syndrome, and Narcolepsy

Along with Data about Shiftwork and Its Effects, Information on the Societal Costs of Sleep Deprivation, Descriptions of Treatment Options, a Glossary of Terms, and Resource Listings for Additional Help

Edited by Jenifer Swanson. 439 pages. 1998. 0-7808-0234-9. $78.

"This text will complement any home or medical library. It is user-friendly and ideal for the adult reader."
— *American Reference Books Annual, 2000*

"A useful resource that provides accurate, relevant, and accessible information on sleep to the general public. Health care providers who deal with sleep disorders patients may also find it helpful in being prepared to answer some of the questions patients ask."
— *Respiratory Care, Jul '99*

"Recommended reference source."
— *Booklist, American Library Association, Feb '99*

■

Smoking Concerns Sourcebook

Basic Consumer Health Information about Nicotine Addiction and Smoking Cessation, Featuring Facts about the Health Effects of Tobacco Use, Including Lung and Other Cancers, Heart Disease, Stroke, and Respiratory Disorders, Such as Emphysema and Chronic Bronchitis

Along with Information about Smoking Prevention Programs, Suggestions for Achieving and Maintaining a Smoke-Free Lifestyle, Statistics about Tobacco Use, Reports on Current Research Initiatives, a Glossary of Related Terms, and Directories of Resources for Additional Help and Information

Edited by Karen Bellenir. 621 pages. 2004. 0-7808-0323-X. $78.

■

Sports Injuries Sourcebook, 2nd Edition

Basic Consumer Health Information about the Diagnosis, Treatment, and Rehabilitation of Common Sports-Related Injuries in Children and Adults

Along with Suggestions for Conditioning and Training, Information and Prevention Tips for Injuries Frequently Associated with Specific Sports and Special Populations, a Glossary, and a Directory of Additional Resources

Edited by Joyce Brennfleck Shannon. 614 pages. 2002. 0-7808-0604-2. $78.

ALSO AVAILABLE: *Sports Injuries Sourcebook, 1st Edition.* Edited by Heather E. Aldred. 624 pages. 1999. 0-7808-0218-7. $78.

"This is an excellent reference for consumers and it is recommended for public, community college, and undergraduate libraries."
— *American Reference Books Annual, 2003*

"Recommended reference source."
— *Booklist, American Library Association, Feb '03*

Stress-Related Disorders Sourcebook

Basic Consumer Health Information about Stress and Stress-Related Disorders, Including Stress Origins and Signals, Environmental Stress at Work and Home, Mental and Emotional Stress Associated with Depression, Post-Traumatic Stress Disorder, Panic Disorder, Suicide, and the Physical Effects of Stress on the Cardiovascular, Immune, and Nervous Systems

Along with Stress Management Techniques, a Glossary, and a Listing of Additional Resources

Edited by Joyce Brennfleck Shannon. 610 pages. 2002. 0-7808-0560-7. $78.

"Well written for a general readership, the *Stress-Related Disorders Sourcebook* is a useful addition to the health reference literature."
— *American Reference Books Annual, 2003*

"I am impressed by the amount of information. It offers a thorough overview of the causes and consequences of stress for the layperson. . . . A well-done and thorough reference guide for professionals and nonprofessionals alike."
— *Doody's Review Service, Dec '02*

■

Stroke Sourcebook

Basic Consumer Health Information about Stroke, Including Ischemic, Hemorrhagic, Transient Ischemic Attack (TIA), and Pediatric Stroke, Stroke Triggers and Risks, Diagnostic Tests, Treatments, and Rehabilitation Information

Along with Stroke Prevention Guidelines, Legal and Financial Information, a Glossary, and a Directory of Additional Resources

Edited by Joyce Brennfleck Shannon. 606 pages. 2003. 0-7808-0630-1. $78.

"This volume is highly recommended and should be in every medical, hospital, and public library."
— *American Reference Books Annual, 2004*

■

Substance Abuse Sourcebook

Basic Health-Related Information about the Abuse of Legal and Illegal Substances Such as Alcohol, Tobacco, Prescription Drugs, Marijuana, Cocaine, and Heroin; and Including Facts about Substance Abuse Prevention Strategies, Intervention Methods, Treatment and Recovery Programs, and a Section Addressing the Special Problems Related to Substance Abuse during Pregnancy

Edited by Karen Bellenir. 573 pages. 1996. 0-7808-0038-9. $78.

"A valuable addition to any health reference section. Highly recommended."
— *The Book Report, Mar/Apr '97*

". . . a comprehensive collection of substance abuse information that's both highly readable and compact. Families and caregivers of substance abusers will find

the information enlightening and helpful, while teachers, social workers and journalists should benefit from the concise format. Recommended."
— *Drug Abuse Update, Winter '96/'97*

SEE ALSO *Alcoholism Sourcebook, Drug Abuse Sourcebook*

■

Surgery Sourcebook

Basic Consumer Health Information about Inpatient and Outpatient Surgeries, Including Cardiac, Vascular, Orthopedic, Ocular, Reconstructive, Cosmetic, Gynecologic, and Ear, Nose, and Throat Procedures and More

Along with Information about Operating Room Policies and Instruments, Laser Surgery Techniques, Hospital Errors, Statistical Data, a Glossary, and Listings of Sources for Further Help and Information

Edited by Annemarie S. Muth and Karen Bellenir. 596 pages. 2002. 0-7808-0380-9. $78.

"Large public libraries and medical libraries would benefit from this material in their reference collections."
— *American Reference Books Annual, 2004*

"Invaluable reference for public and school library collections alike." — *Library Bookwatch, Apr '03*

■

Transplantation Sourcebook

Basic Consumer Health Information about Organ and Tissue Transplantation, Including Physical and Financial Preparations, Procedures and Issues Relating to Specific Solid Organ and Tissue Transplants, Rehabilitation, Pediatric Transplant Information, the Future of Transplantation, and Organ and Tissue Donation

Along with a Glossary and Listings of Additional Resources

Edited by Joyce Brennfleck Shannon. 628 pages. 2002. 0-7808-0322-1. $78.

"Along with these advances [in transplantation technology] have come a number of daunting questions for potential transplant patients, their families, and their health care providers. This reference text is the best single tool to address many of these questions. . . . It will be a much-needed addition to the reference collections in health care, academic, and large public libraries."
— *American Reference Books Annual, 2003*

"Recommended for libraries with an interest in offering consumer health information." — *E-Streams, Jul '02*

"This is a unique and valuable resource for patients facing transplantation and their families."
— *Doody's Review Service, Jun '02*

■

Traveler's Health Sourcebook

Basic Consumer Health Information for Travelers, Including Physical and Medical Preparations, Transportation Health and Safety, Essential Information about Food and Water, Sun Exposure, Insect and Snake Bites, Camping and Wilderness Medicine, and Travel with Physical or Medical Disabilities

Along with International Travel Tips, Vaccination Recommendations, Geographical Health Issues, Disease Risks, a Glossary, and a Listing of Additional Resources

Edited by Joyce Brennfleck Shannon. 613 pages. 2000. 0-7808-0384-1. $78.

"Recommended reference source."
— *Booklist, American Library Association, Feb '01*

"This book is recommended for any public library, any travel collection, and especially any collection for the physically disabled."
— *American Reference Books Annual, 2001*

■

Vegetarian Sourcebook

Basic Consumer Health Information about Vegetarian Diets, Lifestyle, and Philosophy, Including Definitions of Vegetarianism and Veganism, Tips about Adopting Vegetarianism, Creating a Vegetarian Pantry, and Meeting Nutritional Needs of Vegetarians, with Facts Regarding Vegetarianism's Effect on Pregnant and Lactating Women, Children, Athletes, and Senior Citizens

Along with a Glossary of Commonly Used Vegetarian Terms and Resources for Additional Help and Information

Edited by Chad T. Kimball. 360 pages. 2002. 0-7808-0439-2. $78.

"Organizes into one concise volume the answers to the most common questions concerning vegetarian diets and lifestyles. This title is recommended for public and secondary school libraries." — *E-Streams, Apr '03*

"Invaluable reference for public and school library collections alike." — *Library Bookwatch, Apr '03*

"The articles in this volume are easy to read and come from authoritative sources. The book does not necessarily support the vegetarian diet but instead provides the pros and cons of this important decision. The *Vegetarian Sourcebook* is recommended for public libraries and consumer health libraries."
— *American Reference Books Annual, 2003*

■

Women's Health Concerns Sourcebook, 2nd Edition

Basic Consumer Health Information about the Medical and Mental Concerns of Women, Including Maintaining Health and Wellness, Gynecological Concerns, Breast Health, Sexuality and Reproductive Issues, Menopause, Cancer in Women, the Leading Causes of Death and Disability among Women, Physical Concerns of Special Significance to Women, and Women's Mental and Emotional Health

Along with a Glossary of Related Terms and Directories of Resources for Additional Help and Information

Edited by Amy L. Sutton. 748 pages. 2004. 0-7808-0673-5. $78.

ALSO AVAILABLE: *Women's Health Concerns Sourcebook, 1st Edition.* Edited by Heather E. Aldred. 567 pages. 1997. 0-7808-0219-5. $78.

"Handy compilation. There is an impressive range of diseases, devices, disorders, procedures, and other physical and emotional issues covered . . . well organized, illustrated, and indexed." — *Choice*, *Association of College and Research Libraries, Jan '98*

SEE ALSO *Breast Cancer Sourcebook, Cancer Sourcebook for Women, Healthy Heart Sourcebook for Women, Osteoporosis Sourcebook*

Workplace Health & Safety Sourcebook

Basic Consumer Health Information about Workplace Health and Safety, Including the Effect of Workplace Hazards on the Lungs, Skin, Heart, Ears, Eyes, Brain, Reproductive Organs, Musculoskeletal System, and Other Organs and Body Parts

Along with Information about Occupational Cancer, Personal Protective Equipment, Toxic and Hazardous Chemicals, Child Labor, Stress, and Workplace Violence

Edited by Chad T. Kimball. 626 pages. 2000. 0-7808-0231-4. $78.

"As a reference for the general public, this would be useful in any library." —*E-Streams, Jun '01*

"Provides helpful information for primary care physicians and other caregivers interested in occupational medicine. . . . General readers; professionals." — *Choice, Association of College & Research Libraries, May '01*

"Recommended reference source." — *Booklist, American Library Association, Feb '01*

"Highly recommended." — *The Bookwatch, Jan '01*

Worldwide Health Sourcebook

Basic Information about Global Health Issues, Including Malnutrition, Reproductive Health, Disease Dispersion and Prevention, Emerging Diseases, Risky Health Behaviors, and the Leading Causes of Death

Along with Global Health Concerns for Children, Women, and the Elderly, Mental Health Issues, Research and Technology Advancements, and Economic, Environmental, and Political Health Implications, a Glossary, and a Resource Listing for Additional Help and Information

Edited by Joyce Brennfleck Shannon. 614 pages. 2001. 0-7808-0330-2. $78.

"Named an Outstanding Academic Title." —*Choice, Association of College & Research Libraries, Jan '02*

"Yet another handy but also unique compilation in the extensive Health Reference Series, this is a useful work because many of the international publications reprinted or excerpted are not readily available. Highly recommended." —*Choice, Association of College & Research Libraries, Nov '01*

"Recommended reference source." —*Booklist, American Library Association, Oct '01*

Teen Health Series

Helping Young Adults Understand, Manage, and Avoid Serious Illness

Alcohol Information For Teens

Health Tips About Alcohol And Alcoholism

Including Facts about Underage Drinking, Preventing Teen Alcohol Use, Alcohol's Effects on the Brain and the Body, Alcohol Abuse Treatment, Help for Children of Alcoholics, and More

Edited by Joyce Brennfleck Shannon. 400 pages. 2005. 0-7808-0741-3. $58.

■

Cancer Information for Teens

Health Tips about Cancer Awareness, Prevention, Diagnosis, and Treatment

Including Facts about Frequently Occurring Cancers, Cancer Risk Factors, and Coping Strategies for Teens Fighting Cancer or Dealing with Cancer in Friends or Family Members

Edited by Wilma R. Caldwell. 428 pages. 2004. 0-7808-0678-6. $58.

■

Diet Information for Teens

Health Tips about Diet and Nutrition

Including Facts about Nutrients, Dietary Guidelines, Breakfasts, School Lunches, Snacks, Party Food, Weight Control, Eating Disorders, and More

Edited by Karen Bellenir. 399 pages. 2001. 0-7808-0441-4. $58.

"Full of helpful insights and facts throughout the book. . . . An excellent resource to be placed in public libraries or even in personal collections."
—*American Reference Books Annual 2002*

"Recommended for middle and high school libraries and media centers as well as academic libraries that educate future teachers of teenagers. It is also a suitable addition to health science libraries that serve patrons who are interested in teen health promotion and education."
—*E-Streams, Oct '01*

"This comprehensive book would be beneficial to collections that need information about nutrition, dietary guidelines, meal planning, and weight control. . . . This reference is so easy to use that its purchase is recommended."
—*The Book Report, Sep-Oct '01*

"This book is written in an easy to understand format describing issues that many teens face every day, and then provides thoughtful explanations so that teens can make informed decisions. This is an interesting book that provides important facts and information for today's teens."
—*Doody's Health Sciences Book Review Journal, Jul-Aug '01*

"A comprehensive compendium of diet and nutrition. The information is presented in a straightforward, plain-spoken manner. This title will be useful to those working on reports on a variety of topics, as well as to general readers concerned about their dietary health."
—*School Library Journal, Jun '01*

■

Drug Information for Teens

Health Tips about the Physical and Mental Effects of Substance Abuse

Including Facts about Alcohol, Anabolic Steroids, Club Drugs, Cocaine, Depressants, Hallucinogens, Herbal Products, Inhalants, Marijuana, Narcotics, Stimulants, Tobacco, and More

Edited by Karen Bellenir. 452 pages. 2002. 0-7808-0444-9. $58.

"A clearly written resource for general readers and researchers alike."
—*School Library Journal*

"The chapters are quick to make a connection to their teenage reading audience. The prose is straightforward and the book lends itself to spot reading. It should be useful both for practical information and for research, and it is suitable for public and school libraries."
—*American Reference Books Annual, 2003*

"Recommended reference source."
—*Booklist, American Library Association, Feb '03*

"This is an excellent resource for teens and their parents. Education about drugs and substances is key to discouraging teen drug abuse and this book provides this much needed information in a way that is interesting and factual."
—*Doody's Review Service, Dec '02*

■

Fitness Information for Teens

Health Tips about Exercise, Physical Well-Being, and Health Maintenance

Including Facts about Aerobic and Anaerobic Conditioning, Stretching, Body Shape and Body Image, Sports Training, Nutrition, and Activities for Non-Athletes

Edited by Karen Bellenir. 425 pages. 2004. 0-7808-0679-4. $58.

Mental Health Information for Teens

Health Tips about Mental Health and Mental Illness

Including Facts about Anxiety, Depression, Suicide, Eating Disorders, Obsessive-Compulsive Disorders, Panic Attacks, Phobias, Schizophrenia, and More

Edited by Karen Bellenir. 406 pages. 2001. 0-7808-0442-2. $58.

"In both language and approach, this user-friendly entry in the *Teen Health Series* is on target for teens needing information on mental health concerns." —*Booklist, American Library Association, Jan '02*

"Readers will find the material accessible and informative, with the shaded notes, facts, and embedded glossary insets adding appropriately to the already interesting and succinct presentation." —*School Library Journal, Jan '02*

"This title is highly recommended for any library that serves adolescents and parents/caregivers of adolescents." —*E-Streams, Jan '02*

"Recommended for high school libraries and young adult collections in public libraries. Both health professionals and teenagers will find this book useful." —*American Reference Books Annual 2002*

"This is a nice book written to enlighten the society, primarily teenagers, about common teen mental health issues. It is highly recommended to teachers and parents as well as adolescents." —*Doody's Review Service, Dec '01*

Sexual Health Information for Teens

Health Tips about Sexual Development, Human Reproduction, and Sexually Transmitted Diseases

Including Facts about Puberty, Reproductive Health, Chlamydia, Human Papillomavirus, Pelvic Inflammatory Disease, Herpes, AIDS, Contraception, Pregnancy, and More

Edited by Deborah A. Stanley. 391 pages. 2003. 0-7808-0445-7. $58.

"This work should be included in all high school libraries and many larger public libraries. . . . highly recommended." —*American Reference Books Annual 2004*

"Sexual Health approaches its subject with appropriate seriousness and offers easily accessible advice and information." —*School Library Journal, Feb. 2004*

Skin Health Information For Teens

Health Tips about Dermatological Concerns and Skin Cancer Risks

Including Facts about Acne, Warts, Hives, and Other Conditions and Lifestyle Choices, Such as Tanning, Tattooing, and Piercing, That Affect the Skin, Nails, Scalp, and Hair

Edited by Robert Aquinas McNally. 430 pages. 2003. 0-7808-0446-5. $58.

"This volume, as with others in the series, will be a useful addition to school and public library collections." —*American Reference Books Annual 2004*

"This volume serves as a one-stop source and should be a necessity for any health collection." —*Library Media Connection*

Sports Injuries Information For Teens

Health Tips about Sports Injuries and Injury Protection

Including Facts about Specific Injuries, Emergency Treatment, Rehabilitation, Sports Safety, Competition Stress, Fitness, Sports Nutrition, Steroid Risks, and More

Edited by Joyce Brennfleck Shannon. 425 pages. 2003. 0-7808-0447-3. $58.

"This work will be useful in the young adult collections of public libraries as well as high school libraries." —*American Reference Books Annual 2004*

Suicide Information for Teens

Health Tips about Suicide Causes and Prevention

Including Facts about Depression, Risk Factors, Getting Help, Survivor Support, and More

Edited by Joyce Brennfleck Shannon. 400 pages. 2004. 0-7808-0737-5. $58.

Health Reference Series

Adolescent Health Sourcebook

AIDS Sourcebook, 3rd Edition

Alcoholism Sourcebook

Allergies Sourcebook, 2nd Edition

Alternative Medicine Sourcebook, 2nd Edition

Alzheimer's Disease Sourcebook, 3rd Edition

Arthritis Sourcebook

Asthma Sourcebook

Attention Deficit Disorder Sourcebook

Back & Neck Disorders Sourcebook

Blood & Circulatory Disorders Sourcebook

Brain Disorders Sourcebook

Breast Cancer Sourcebook

Breastfeeding Sourcebook

Burns Sourcebook

Cancer Sourcebook, 4th Edition

Cancer Sourcebook for Women, 2nd Edition

Caregiving Sourcebook

Child Abuse Sourcebook

Childhood Diseases & Disorders Sourcebook

Colds, Flu & Other Common Ailments Sourcebook

Communication Disorders Sourcebook

Congenital Disorders Sourcebook

Consumer Issues in Health Care Sourcebook

Contagious & Non-Contagious Infectious Diseases Sourcebook

Death & Dying Sourcebook

Dental Care & Oral Health Sourcebook, 2nd Edition

Depression Sourcebook

Diabetes Sourcebook, 3rd Edition

Diet & Nutrition Sourcebook, 2nd Edition

Digestive Diseases & Disorder Sourcebook

Disabilities Sourcebook

Domestic Violence Sourcebook, 2nd Edition

Drug Abuse Sourcebook

Ear, Nose & Throat Disorders Sourcebook

Eating Disorders Sourcebook

Emergency Medical Services Sourcebook

Endocrine & Metabolic Disorders Sourcebook

Environmentally Health Sourcebook, 2nd Edition

Ethnic Diseases Sourcebook

Eye Care Sourcebook, 2nd Edition

Family Planning Sourcebook

Fitness & Exercise Sourcebook, 2nd Edition

Food & Animal Borne Diseases Sourcebook

Food Safety Sourcebook

Forensic Medicine Sourcebook

Gastrointestinal Diseases & Disorders Sourcebook

Genetic Disorders Sourcebook, 2nd Edition

Head Trauma Sourcebook

Headache Sourcebook

Health Insurance Sourcebook

Health Reference Series Cumulative Index 1999

Healthy Aging Sourcebook

Healthy Children Sourcebook